**Sample Size Tables
for Clinical Studies**

To
Oliver, Joshua and Sophie
David, John and Joseph
Lisa and Sophie
Kim San, Geok Yan and Janet

Companion CD-ROM

A companion CD-ROM is included with this book.

The CD contains software that will enable you to implement the sample size calculation methods discussed in the book.

The CD content is referenced throughout the text where you see this symbol $^{S}S_{S}$

See Chapter 17 for full details of the software on the CD and how to install and use it.

Technical requirements:
Operating System: Windows XP, 2000;
CPU: 500 MHz;
RAM: 128 MB;
Disc drive: 16 × CD drive;
Hard drive: 10 MB of free space

Sample Size Tables for Clinical Studies

David Machin
Children's Cancer and Leukaemia Group
University of Leicester, UK;
Division of Clinical Trials and Epidemiological Sciences
National Cancer Centre, Singapore;
Medical Statistics Unit
School of Health and Related Sciences
University of Sheffield, UK

Michael J. Campbell
Medical Statistics Unit
School of Health and Related Research
University of Sheffield, UK

Say Beng Tan
Singapore Clinical Research Institute, Singapore
Duke–NUS Graduate Medical School, Singapore

Sze Huey Tan
Division of Clinical Trials and Epidemiological Sciences
National Cancer Centre, Singapore

THIRD EDITION

WILEY-BLACKWELL
A John Wiley & Sons, Ltd., Publication

Contents

A companion CD-ROM of the sample size software $^{S}S_{S}$ is included in the inside back cover of this book

Preface

It is now more than 20 years since the first edition of this book and 10 years from the second. The need for evidence-based estimates of the required size of a study is now universally recognized. Since the second edition the methodology for sample-size calculation has been widely extended, which is the main reason for a third edition. A second reason is the vastly improved computing power available. For the first edition, the tabulations were extensive to obviate separate calculations. A computer program to extend the range of the tables was available for the second edition.

This edition comes with sample size software SS_S, which we hope will give the user even greater flexibility and easy access to a wide range of designs, and allow design parameters to be tailored more readily to specific problems. Further, as some early phase designs are adaptive in nature and require knowledge of earlier patients' response to determine the relevant options for the next patient, a (secure) database is provided for these.

Designing modern clinical research studies requires the involvement of multidisciplinary teams, with the process of sample size determination not being something that can be done by the statistician alone. So while software is available that can compute sample sizes (even from the internet), we feel that it is necessary that such software be complemented with a book that clearly explains and illustrates the methodology, along with tables. Feedback from users of earlier editions suggests that this can facilitate planning discussions within the research team.

Thus a major consideration has been to present the details, which are often complex, as clearly as possible and to illustrate these with appropriate examples. One objective of this approach is to encourage the wider use of sample size issues at the design stage in areas such as laboratory studies, which have been relatively neglected compared to epidemiological studies and clinical trials.

David Machin
Michael J. Campbell
Say Beng Tan
Sze Huey Tan
Singapore; Leicester and Sheffield, UK

1 Basic design considerations

SUMMARY

This chapter reviews the reasons why sample-size considerations are important when planning a clinical study of any type. The basic elements underlying this process including the null and alternative study hypotheses, effect size, statistical significance level and power are described. We introduce the notation to distinguish the population parameters we are trying to estimate from the study, from their anticipated value at the design stage, and finally their estimated value once the study has been completed. In the context of clinical trials, we emphasise the need for randomised allocation of subjects to treatment.

1.1 Why sample size calculations?

To motivate the statistical issues relevant to sample-size calculations, we will assume that we are planning a two-group clinical trial in which subjects are allocated at random to one of two alternative treatments for a particular medical condition and that a single binary endpoint (success or failure) has been specified in advance. However, it should be emphasised that the basic principles described, the formulae, sample-size tables and associated software included in this book are equally relevant to a wide range of design types covering all areas of medical research: ranging from the epidemiological, to clinical and laboratory-based studies.

Whatever the field of enquiry a well-designed study will have considered the questions posed carefully and, what is the particular focus for us, formally estimated the required sample size and will have recorded the supporting justification for the choice. Awareness of the importance of these has led to the major medical and related journals demanding that a detailed justification of the study size be included in any submitted article as it is a key component for peer reviewers to consider when assessing the scientific credibility of the work undertaken. For example, the *General Statistical Checklist* of the *British Medical Journal*, asks: 'Was a pre-study calculation of study size reported?'

In any event, at a more mundane level, investigators, grant-awarding bodies and medical product development companies will all wish to know how much a study is likely to 'cost' both in terms of time and resource consumed as well as monetary terms. The projected study size will be a key component in this 'cost'. They would also like to be reassured that the allocated resource will be well spent by assessing the likelihood that the study will give unequivocal results. In addition, the regulatory authorities, including the Food and Drug Administration (FDA 1988) in the USA and the Committee for Proprietary Medicinal Products (CPMP 1995) in the European Union, require information on planned study size. These are encapsulated in

Sample Size Tables for Clinical Studies, 3rd edition. By David Machin, Michael J. Campbell, Say Beng Tan, and Sze Huey Tan. Published 2009 by Blackwell Publishing, ISBN: 978-1-4051-4650-0

the guidelines of the International Conference on Harmonisation of Technical Requirements for Registration of Pharmaceuticals for Human Use (1998) ICH Topic E9.

If too few subjects are involved, the study is potentially a misuse of time because realistic medical differences are unlikely to be distinguished from chance variation. Too large a study can be a waste of important resources. Further, it may be argued that ethical considerations also enter into sample size calculations. Thus a small clinical trial with no chance of detecting a clinically useful difference between treatments is unfair to all the patients put to the (possible) risk and discomfort of the trial processes. A trial that is too large may be unfair if one treatment could have been 'proven' to be more effective with fewer patients as, a larger than necessary number of them has received the (now known) inferior treatment.

Providing a sample size for a study is not simply a matter of giving a single number from a set of tables. It is, and should be, a several-stage process. At the preliminary stages, what is required are 'ball-park' figures that enable the investigators to judge whether or not to start the detailed planning of the study. If a decision is made to proceed, then the later stages are to refine the supporting evidence for the early calculations until they make a persuasive case for the final patient numbers chosen which is then included (and justified) in the final study protocol.

Once the final sample size is determined, the protocol prepared and approved by the relevant bodies, it is incumbent on the research team to expedite the recruitment processes as much as possible, ensure the study is conducted to the highest of standards possible and eventually reported comprehensively.

Cautionary note

This book contains formulae for sample-size determination for many different situations. If these formulae are evaluated with the necessary input values provided they will give sample sizes to a mathematical accuracy of a single subject. However, the user should be aware that when planning a study of whatever type, one is planning in the presence of considerable uncertainty with respect to the eventual outcome. This suggests that, in the majority of applications, the number obtained should be rounded upwards to the nearest five, 10 or even more to establish the required sample size. We round upwards as that would give rise to narrower confidence intervals, and hence more 'convincing' evidence.

In some cases statistical research may improve the numerical accuracy of the formulae which depend on approximations (particularly in situations with small sample sizes resulting), but these improvements are likely to have less effect on the subsequent subject numbers obtained than changes in the planning values substituted into the formulae. As a consequence, we have specifically avoided using these refinements if they are computationally intensive. In contrast, and as appropriate, we do provide alternative methods which can easily be evaluated to give the design team a quick check on the accuracy of their computations and some reassurance on the output from ^SS_S and the tables we provide.

1.2 Design and analysis

Notation

In very brief terms the (statistical) objective of any study is to estimate from a sample the value of a population parameter. For example, if we were interested in the mean birth weight of babies born in a certain locality, then we may record the weight of a selected sample of n babies and their mean weight $\overline{w}$ is taken as our estimate of the population mean birth weight denoted ω_{Pop}. The Greek ω distinguished the population value from its estimate Roman $\overline{w}$. When planning a study, we are clearly ignorant of ω_{Pop} and neither do we have the data $\overline{w}$. As we shall see later, when planning a study the investigators will usually need to provide some value for what ω_{Pop} may turn out to be. We term this anticipated value ω_{Plan}. This value then forms (part of) the basis for subsequent sample size calculations. However, because adding 'Plan' as a subscript to the, often several, parameters concerned in the formulae for sample sizes included in this book, makes them even more cumbersome it is usually omitted, so ω_{Plan} becomes simply ω. However to help with maintaining the distinction between 'Plan' and 'Population' values of parameters we have added the subscript 'Pop' to the latter. Unfortunately, although making subsequent chapters easier, this rather complicates the sections immediately below.

The randomised controlled trial

Consider, as an example, a proposed randomised trial of a placebo (control) against acupuncture in the relief of pain in a particular diagnosis. The patients are randomised to receive either placebo or acupuncture (how placebo acupuncture can be administered is clearly an important consideration). In addition, we assume that pain relief is assessed at a fixed time after randomisation and is defined in such a way as to be unambiguously evaluable for each patient as either 'success' or 'failure'. We assume the aim of the trial is to estimate the true difference δ_{Pop} between the true success rate π_{PopA} of Acupuncture and the true success rate π_{PopC} of Control. Thus the key (population) parameter of interest is δ_{Pop} which is a composite of the two (population) parameters π_{PopA} and π_{PopC}.

At the completion of the trial the Acupuncture group of patients yield a treatment success rate p_A which is an estimate of π_{PopA} and the Control group give success rate p_C which is an estimate of π_{PopC}. Thus, the observed difference, $d = p_A - p_C$, provides an estimate of the true difference $\delta_{Pop} = \pi_{PopA} - \pi_{PopC}$.

In contrast, at the design stage of the trial one can only postulate what the size of difference (strictly the minimum size of interest) might be and we denote this by δ_{Plan}.

The number of patients necessary to recruit to a particular study depends on:
- The *anticipated* clinical difference between the alternative treatments;
- The *level* of statistical significance, α;
- The *chance* of detecting the *anticipated* clinical difference, $1 - \beta$.

The null and alternative hypotheses, and effect size

Null hypothesis

In our example, the null hypothesis, termed H_{Null}, implies that acupuncture and placebo are equally effective or that $\pi_{PopA} = \pi_{PopC}$. Even when that null hypothesis is true, observed differences, $d = p_A - p_C$ other than zero, will occur. The probability of obtaining the observed difference d or a more extreme one given that $\pi_{PopA} = \pi_{PopC}$ can be calculated. If, under this null hypothesis, the resulting probability or p-value was very small, then we would reject the null hypothesis. We then conclude the two treatments do indeed differ in efficacy.

Alternative hypothesis

Usually in statistical significance testing, by rejecting the null hypothesis, we do not specifically accept any alternative hypothesis and it is usual to report the range of plausible population values with a confidence interval (CI). However, sample-size calculations are usually posed in a hypothesis test framework, and this requires us to specify an alternative hypothesis, termed H_{Alt}, that is, $\pi_{PopA} - \pi_{PopC} = \delta_{Pop}$ with $\delta_{Pop} \neq 0$. The value δ_{Pop} is known as the true *effect size*.

Establishing the effect size

Of the parameters that have to be pre-specified before the sample size can be determined, the true effect size is the most critical and, in order to estimate sample size, one must first identify the magnitude of the difference one wishes to detect by means of δ_{Plan}.

Sometimes there is prior knowledge that enables an investigator to anticipate what treatment benefit is likely to be observed, and the role of the trial is to confirm that expectation. At other times it may be possible to say that, for example, only the prospect of doubling of their median survival would be worthwhile for patients with this type of rapidly fatal disease because the new treatment is so toxic.

One additional problem is that investigators are often optimistic about the effect of new treatments; it can take considerable effort to initiate a trial and so, in many cases, the trial would only be launched if the investigator is enthusiastic about the new treatment and is sufficiently convinced about its potential efficacy. Experience suggests that as trials progress there is often a growing realism that, even at best, the initial expectations were optimistic and there is ample historical evidence to suggest that trials which set out to detect large treatment differences nearly always result in 'no significant difference was detected'. In such cases there may have been a true and worthwhile treatment benefit that has been missed, since the level of detectable differences set by the design was unrealistically high, and hence the sample size too small.

In practice a form of iteration is often used. The clinician team might offer a variety of opinions as to what clinically useful difference will transpire—ranging perhaps from the unduly pessimistic small effect to the optimistic (and unlikely in many situations) large effect. Sample sizes may then be calculated under this range of scenarios with corresponding patient numbers ranging perhaps from extremely large to the relatively small. The importance of the clinical question, and/or the impossibility of recruiting large patient numbers may rule out a very large trial but to conduct a small trial may leave important clinical effects not firmly established. As a consequence, the team may next define a revised aim maybe using a summary derived from the original opinions, and the calculations are repeated. Perhaps the sample size now becomes attainable and forms the basis for the definitive protocol.

There are a number of ways of eliciting useful effect sizes: a Bayesian perspective has been advocated by Spiegelhalter, Freedman and Parmar (1994), an economic approach by Drummond and O'Brien (1993) and one based on patients' perceptions rather than clinicians' perceptions of benefit by Naylor and Llewellyn-Thomas (1994).

Test size, significance level or Type I error

The critical value we take for the p-value is arbitrary, and we denote it by α. If p-value $\leq \alpha$ one rejects the null hypothesis, conversely if p-value $> \alpha$ one does not reject the null hypothesis.

Even when the null hypothesis is in fact true there is a risk of rejecting it and to reject the null hypothesis when it is true is to make a Type I error. The probability of rejecting the null hypothesis when it is true is α. The quantity α can be referred to either as the test size, significance level, probability of a Type I error or the false-positive error. Conventionally $\alpha = 0.05$ is often used.

Type II error and power

The clinical trial could yield an observed difference d that would lead to a p-value $> \alpha$ even though the null hypothesis is really not true, that is, π_{PopA} truly differs from π_{PopC}. In such a situation, we then *fail* to reject the null hypothesis when it is in fact false. This is called a Type II or false-negative error and the probability of this is denoted by β.

The probability of a Type II error is based on the assumption that the null hypothesis is *not* true, that is, $\delta_{\text{Pop}} = \pi_{\text{PopA}} - \pi_{\text{PopC}} \neq 0$. There are clearly many possible values of δ_{Pop} in this instance since many values other than zero satisfy this condition, and each would give a different value for β.

The *power* is defined as one minus the probability of a Type II error, $1 - \beta$. That is, 'power' is the probability of obtaining a 'significant' p-value if the null hypothesis is really false. Conventionally a minimum power of 80% is required in a clinical trial.

One and two-sided significance tests

It is usual for most clinical trials that there is considerable uncertainty about the relative merits of the alternative treatments so that even when the new treatment or intervention under test is thought for scientific reasons to be an improvement over the current standard, the possibility that this is not the case is allowed for. For example, in the clinical trial conducted by Chow, Tai, Tan *et al.* (2002) it was thought at the planning stage that high dose tamoxifen would improve survival over placebo in patients with inoperable hepatocellular carcinoma. This turned out not to be the case and, if anything, tamoxifen was detrimental to the ultimate survival. This is not an isolated example.

Since it is plausible to assume in the acupuncture trial referred to earlier that the placebo is in some sense 'inactive' and that any 'active' treatment will have to perform better than the 'inactive' treatment if it is to be adopted into clinical practice, then the alternative hypothesis may be that the acupuncture has an improved success rate, that is, $\pi_{\text{PopA}} > \pi_{\text{PopC}}$. This leads to a one-sided or one-tailed statistical significance test.

On the other hand, if we cannot make this type of assumption about the new treatment at the design stage, then the alternative hypothesis is that π_{PopA} and π_{PopC} differ, that is, $\pi_{\text{PopA}} \neq \pi_{\text{PopC}}$.

In general, for a given sample size, a one-sided test is more powerful than the corresponding two-sided test. However, a decision to use a one-sided test should never be made after looking at the data and observing the direction of the departure. Such decisions should be made at the design stage and one should use a one-sided test *only* if it is *certain* that departures in the particular direction *not anticipated* will always be ascribed to chance, and therefore regarded as non-significant, however large they are. It will almost always be preferable to carry out two-sided hypothesis tests *but*, if a one-sided test is to be used, this should be indicated and justified for the problem in hand.

Confidence intervals

Medical statisticians often point out that there is an over-emphasis on tests of significance in the reporting of results and they argue that, wherever possible, confidence intervals (CI) should be quoted (see **Chapter** 2). The reason for this is that a p-value alone gives the reader, who wishes to make use of the published results of a particular trial, little practical information. In contrast, quoting an estimate of the effect with the corresponding (usually 95%) confidence interval, enables him or her to better judge the relative efficacy of the alternative treatments. For the purposes of this book, the associated software ^SS_S and in the planning stages of the trial, discussion is easier in terms of statistical significance but nevertheless it should be emphasised that key confidence intervals should always be quoted in the final report of any study of whatever design.

Randomisation

As Machin and Campbell (2005) and many others point out, of fundamental importance to the design of any clinical trial (and to all types of other studies when feasible) is the random allocation of subjects to the options under study. Such allocation safeguards in particular against bias in the estimate of group differences and is the necessary basis for the subsequent statistical tests.

1.3 Practicalities

Power and significance tests

In a clinical trial, two or more forms of therapy or intervention may be compared. However, patients themselves vary both in their baseline characteristics at diagnosis and in their response to subsequent therapy. Hence in a clinical trial, an apparent difference in treatments may be observed due to chance alone, that is, we may observe a difference but it may be explained by the intrinsic characteristics of the patients themselves rather than 'caused' by the different treatments given. As a consequence, it is customary to use a 'significance test' to assess the weight of evidence and to estimate the probability that the observed data could in fact have arisen purely by chance. The results of the significance test, calculated on the assumption that the null hypothesis is true, will be expressed as a 'p-value'. For example, at the end of the trial if the difference between treatments is tested, then a $p < 0.05$ would indicate that so extreme an observed difference could be expected to have arisen by chance alone less than 5% of the time, and so it is quite likely that a treatment difference really is present.

However, if only a few patients were entered into the trial then, even if there really were a true treatment difference, the results are less convincing than if a much larger number of patients had been assessed. Thus, the weight of evidence in favour of concluding that there is a treatment effect will be much less in a small trial than in a large one. In statistical terms, we would say that the 'sample size' is too small, and that the 'power of the test' is very low.

The 'power' of a significance test is a measure of how likely a test is to produce a statistically significant result, given a true difference between the treatments of a certain magnitude.

Sample size and interpretation of significance

Suppose the results of an *observed* treatment difference in a clinical trial are declared 'not statistically significant'. Such a statement only indicates that there was insufficient weight of evidence to be able to declare: 'that the observed difference is *unlikely* to have arisen by chance'. It does *not* imply that there is 'no clinically important difference between the treatments' as, for example, if the sample size was too small the trial might be very unlikely to obtain a significant p-value even when a clinically relevant difference is truly present. Hence it is of crucial importance to consider sample size and power when interpreting statements about 'non-significant' results. In particular, if the power of the test was very low, all one can conclude from a non-significant result is that the question of treatment differences remains unresolved.

Estimation of sample size and power

In estimating the number of patients required for a trial (sample size), it is usual to identify a single major outcome which is regarded as the primary endpoint for comparing treatment differences. In many clinical trials this will be a measure such as response rate, time to wound healing, degree of palliation, or a quality of life index.

It is customary to start by specifying the size of the difference required to be detected, and then to estimate the number of patients necessary to enable the trial to detect this difference if it truly exists. Thus, for example, it might be anticipated that acupuncture could improve the response rate from 20 to 30%, and that since this is a plausible and medically important improvement, it is desired to be reasonably certain of detecting such a difference if it really exists. 'Detecting a difference' is usually taken to mean 'obtain a statistically significant difference with p-value < 0.05'; and similarly the phrase 'to be reasonably certain' is usually interpreted to mean something like 'have a chance of at least 90% of obtaining such a p-value' if there really is an improvement from 20 to 30%. This latter statement corresponds, in statistical terms, to saying that the power of the trial should be 0.9 or 90%.

More than one primary outcome

We have based the above discussion on the assumption that there is a single identifiable end point or outcome, upon which treatment comparisons are based. However, often there is more than one endpoint of interest within the same trial, such as wound healing time, pain levels and methicillin-resistant *Staphylococcus aureus* (MRSA) infection rates. If one of these endpoints is regarded as more important than the others, it can be named as the primary endpoint and sample-size estimates calculated accordingly. A problem arises when there are several outcome measures which are all regarded as *equally* important. A commonly adopted approach is to repeat the sample-size estimates for each outcome measure in turn, and then select the largest number as the sample size required to answer *all* the questions of interest.

Here, it is essential to note the relationship between significance tests and power as it is well recognised that p-values become distorted if many endpoints (from the same patients) are each tested for significance. Often a smaller p-value will be considered necessary for statistical significance to compensate for this. In such cases, the sample-size calculations will use the reduced test size and hence increase the corresponding study size.

Internal pilot studies

In order to calculate the sample size for a trial one must first have available some background information. For example, for a trial using a survival endpoint one must provide the anticipated survival of the control group. Also, one must have some idea as to what is a realistic difference to seek. Sometimes such information is available as rather firm prior knowledge from the work of others, at other times, a pilot study may be conducted to obtain the relevant information.

Traditionally, a pilot study is a distinct preliminary investigation, conducted before embarking on the main trial but several authors, including Browne (1995), have advocated the use of an *internal* pilot study. The idea here is to plan the clinical trial on the basis of the best (current) available information, but to regard the first patients entered as the internal pilot. When data from these patients have been collected, the sample size can be re-estimated with the revised knowledge that the data from these first patients have provided. Two vital features accompany this approach: firstly, the final sample size should only ever be adjusted upwards, never down; and secondly, one should only use the internal pilot information in order to improve the design features which are independent of the treatment variable. This second point is crucial. It means that, for example, if treatments are to be compared using a *t*-test, then a basic ingredient of the sample-size calculation will be the standard deviation (σ_{Plan}) whose value may be amended following the pilot phase and then potentially used to revise upwards the ultimate sample size. No note of the observed difference (the effect) between treatments is made so that δ_{Plan} remains unchanged in the revised calculations.

The advantage of an internal pilot is that it can be relatively large—perhaps half of the anticipated patients. It provides an insurance against misjudgement regarding the baseline planning assumptions. It is, nevertheless, important that the intention to conduct an internal pilot study is recorded at the outset and that full details are given in the study protocol.

More than two groups

The majority of clinical trials involve a simple comparison between two interventions or treatments. When there are more than two treatments the situation is much more complicated. This is because there is no longer one clear alternative hypothesis. Thus, for example, with three groups, although the null hypothesis is that the population means are all equal, there are several potential alternative hypotheses. These include one which postulates that two of the group means are equal but which differ from the third, or one that the means are ordered in some way. Alternatively the investigators may simply wish to compare all three groups, leading to three pairwise comparisons which may not all be equally important.

One problem arising at the time of analysis is that such situations may lead to multiple significance tests, resulting in misleading *p*-values. Various solutions have been proposed, each resulting in different analysis strategies and therefore different design and sample size considerations. One approach that is commonly advocated is to conduct an analysis of variance (ANOVA) or a similar global statistical test, with pairwise or other comparisons of means only being made if the global test is significant. Another approach is to use conventional significance tests but with an adjusted significance level obtained from the Bonferroni correction—essentially reducing the conventional test size (say, 0.05) by dividing by the number of comparisons to be made. However, the simplest strategy is to adopt the approach which regards, for example, a three-treatment groups comparison as little different from carrying out a series of three independent trials, and to use conventional significance tests without adjustment as argued by Saville (1990). As a consequence, and assuming equal numbers of subjects per treatment arm, the sample size is first estimated for the three distinct trial comparisons. Then for each treatment group simply take the maximum of these as the sample size required.

Studies with g (> 2) groups may compare different doses of the same therapy or some other type of ordered treatment groups. Thus, although the null hypothesis would still be that all population means are equal, the alternative will now be H_{Ordered} which is either $\mu_{\text{Pop1}} < \mu_{\text{Pop1}} < \ldots < \mu_{\text{Popg}}$ or $\mu_{\text{Pop1}} > \mu_{\text{Pop1}} > \ldots > \mu_{\text{Popg}}$. In the simplest case, the doses may be equally spaced either on the original or possibly a logarithmic scale, and these may allow H_{Ordered} to be expressed as $\mu_{\text{Pop}} = \alpha_{\text{Pop}} + \beta_{\text{Pop}}(\text{dose})$. The study is then designed to estimate the regression coefficient, β_{Pop}, and the sample size is calculated on the basis of an anticipated value, β_{Plan}.

A rather different situation arises with factorial designs. Suppose that a 2×2 factorial trial is planned to compare two factors, A and B each of two levels, then there will be four groups to be compared with m subjects per group. The design may be particularly useful in circumstances where (say) factor A addresses a major therapeutic question, while factor B poses a more secondary one. For example, A might be the addition of a further drug to an established combination chemotherapy for a cancer while B may the choice of anti-emetic delivered with the drugs. For efficient use of such a design the two main effects, that is the different options within A and those within B, are compared using two means with $2m$ subjects in each group. However, this assumes an absence of interaction between the factors which means that the effect of A remains the same irrespective of which of the options within B the patient receives and vice-versa. If this is not the case, we might then wish to estimate the size of this interaction effect and so have a sufficiently large sample size for this purpose.

In planning a 2×2 factorial trial, the first step would be to assume no interaction was present and consider the sample size for factor A. The second step would be to consider the sample size for factor B which may have a different effect size, test size and power, from the factor A comparison. Clearly, if the resulting sample sizes are similar then there is no difficulty in choosing, perhaps the larger, as the required sample size. If the sample sizes are very disparate then a discussion would ensue as to the most important comparison and perhaps a reasonable compromise reached. This compromise figure could then be used to check what magnitude of interaction (if present) could be detected with such numbers and may have to be increased if there is a strong possibility of an interaction being present.

Rules of thumb

Although we provide in later chapters methods of determining sample sizes in a variety of contexts, it is often very useful (especially at initial planning meetings) to have a 'feel' of the order of magnitude of the sample size that may ultimately be required. Thus some 'rules of thumb' are given in the appropriate chapters for this purpose while Van Belle (2002) provides a more comprehensive review.

1.4 Use of tables and software

It is hoped that the tables and the associated software $^S\!S_S$ will prove useful in a number of ways.

Number of subjects

Before conducting a clinical trial to test the value of acupuncture a researcher believes that the placebo group will yield a response rate of 30%. How many subjects are required to demonstrate an anticipated response rate for acupuncture of 70% at a given significance level and power?

Power of a study

A common situation is one where the number of patients is governed by forces such as time, money, human resources and disease incidence rather than by purely scientific criteria. The researcher may then wish to know what probability he or she has of detecting a certain difference in treatment efficacy with a trial of the intended size.

Size of effect

In this case, the sample size is constrained, and the researcher is interested in exploring the size of effects which could be established for a reasonable power, say, 80%.

1.5 The protocol

As we have indicated the justification of sample size in any study is important. This not only gives an indication of the resources required but also forces the research team to think about issues of design carefully. We give below examples of how the resulting calculations were justified.

Example 1.1—surgical resection for patients with gastric cancer
Cuschieri, Weeden, Fielding *et al.* (1999) compared two forms of surgical resection for patients with gastric cancer. The primary outcome (event of interest) was time to death. The authors state:

> 'Sample size calculations were based on a pre-study survey of 26 gastric surgeons, which indicated that the baseline 5-year survival rate of D_1 surgery was expected to be 20%, and an improvement in survival to 34% (14% change) with D_2 resection would be a realistic expectation. Thus 400 patients (200 in each arm) were to be randomised, providing 90% power to detect such a difference with *p*-value < 0.05'.

Example 1.2—steroid or cyclopsporine for oral lichen planus
The protocol of March 1998 of the subsequently published trial conducted by Poon, Goh, Kim *et al.* (2006) to compare steroid with cyclosporine for the topical treatment of oral lichen planus stated:

'It is anticipated that in patients taking topical steroids, the response rate at 1 month will be approximately 60%. It is anticipated that this may be raised to as much as 80% in those receiving cyclosporine. With two-sided test size 5%, power 80%, then the corresponding number of patients required is approximately 200 (Machin, Campbell, Fayers and Pinol 1997, Table 3.1).'

Example 1.3—sequential hormonal therapy in advanced and metastatic breast cancer
Iaffaioli, Formato, Tortoriello *et al.* (2005) conducted two Phase II trials of sequential hormonal therapy with first-line anastrozole and with second-line exemestane, in advanced and metastatic breast cancer. This example is discussed further in **Chapter 17**.

The authors provide their justification for sample size as follows (we just show the justification for the anastrozole study, a similar justification was provided for the exemestane study):

'The sample size calculation for both single-stage studies was performed as proposed by A'Hern (2001), this method being an exact version of the algorithm first presented by Fleming (1982). The anastrizole evaluation required 93 subjects to decide whether the proportion of patients with a clinical benefit (P) was ≤ 50% or ≥ 65%. If the number of patients with clinical benefit was ≥ 55, the hypothesis that P ≤ 50% was rejected with a target error rate of 0.050 and an actual error rate of 0.048. If the number of patients with clinical benefit was ≤ 54, the hypothesis that P ≥ 65% was rejected with a target error rate of 0.100 and an actual error rate of 0.099.'

1.6 Books on sample-size calculations

Chow SC, Shao J and Wang H (2008). *Sample Size Calculations in Clinical Research*, 2nd edn. Marcel Dekker, New York.

Cohen J (1988). *Statistical Power Analysis for the Behavioral Sciences*, 2nd edn. Lawrence Earlbaum, New Jersey.

Lemeshow S, Hosmar DW, Klar J and Lwanga SK (1990). *Adequacy of Sample Size in Health Studies*. John Wiley & Sons, Chichester.

Lipsey MW (1990). *Design Sensitivity: Statistical Power for Experimental Research*. Sage Publications, London.

Machin D and Campbell MJ (2005). *Design of Studies for Medical Research*, John Wiley & Sons, Chichester.

Schuster JJ (1993). *Practical Handbook of Sample Size Guidelines for Clinical Trials*. CRC Press, FL.

1.7 Software for sample-size calculations

Since sample-size determination is such a critical part of the design process we recommend that all calculations are carefully checked before the final decisions are made. This is particularly important for large and/or resource intensive studies. In-house checking by colleagues is also important.

Biostat (2001). *Power & Precision: Release 2.1.* Englewood, NJ.

Lenth RV (2006). *Java Applets for Power and Sample Size.* URL: http://www.stat.uiowa.edu/ ~rlenth/Power.

National Council for Social Studies (2005). *Power Analysis and Sample Size Software (PASS): Version 2005.* NCSS Statistical Software, Kaysville, UT.

SAS Institute (2004). *Getting Started with the SAS Power and Sample Size Application: Version 9.1.* SAS Institute, Cary, NC.

StataCorp (2007). *Stata Statistical Software: Release 10.* College Station, TX.

Statistical Solutions (2006). *nQuery Adviser: Version 6.0.* Saugus, MA.

1.8 References

A'Hern RP (2001). Sample size tables for exact single stage phase II designs. *Statistics in Medicine,* **20**, 859–866.

Browne RH (1995). On the use of a pilot study for sample size determination. *Statistics in Medicine,* **14**, 1933–1940.

Chow PK-H, Tai B-C, Tan C-K, Machin D, Johnson PJ, Khin M-W and Soo K-C (2002). No role for high-dose tamoxifen in the treatment of inoperable hepatocellular carcinoma: An Asia-Pacific double-blind randomised controlled trial. *Hepatology,* **36**, 1221–1226.

CPMP Working Party on Efficacy of Medicinal Products (1995). Biostatistical methodology in clinical trials in applications for marketing authorizations for medical products. *Statistics in Medicine,* **14**, 1659–1682.

Cuschieri A, Weeden S, Fielding J, Bancewicz J, Craven J, Joypaul V, Sydes M and Fayers P (1999). Patient survival after D_1 and D_2 resections for gastric cancer: long-term results of the MRC randomized surgical trial. *British Journal of Cancer,* **79**, 1522–1530.

Drummond M and O'Brien B (1993). Clinical importance, statistical significance and the assessment of economic and quality-of-life outcomes. *Health Economics,* **2**, 205–212.

FDA (1988). *Guidelines for the Format and Content of the Clinical and Statistics Section of New Drug Applications.* US Department of Health and Human Services, Public Health Service, Food and Drug Administration, Washington D.C.

Fleming TR (1982). One-sample multiple testing procedure for Phase II clinical trial. *Biometrics,* **38**, 143–151.

Iaffaioli RV, Formato R, Tortoriello A, Del Prete S, Caraglia M, Pappagallo G, Pisano A, Fanelli F, Ianniello G, Cigolari S, Pizza C, Marano O, Pezzella G, Pedicini T, Febbraro A, Incoronato P, Manzione L, Ferrari E, Marzano N, Quattrin S, Pisconti S, Nasti G, Giotta G, Colucci G and other Goim authors (2005) Phase II study of sequential hormonal therapy with anastrozole/exemestane in advanced and metastatic breast cancer. *British Journal of Cancer,* **92**, 1621–1625.

International Conference on Harmonisation of Technical Requirements for Registration of Pharmaceuticals for Human Use (1998). *Statistical Principles for Clinical Trials E9.* Available at www.ich.org.

Machin D and Campbell MJ (2005). *Design of Studies for Medical Research.* John Wiley & Sons, Chichester.

Machin D, Campbell MJ, Fayers PM and Pinol A (1997). *Statistical Tables for the Design of Clinical Studies*, 2nd edn. Blackwell Scientific Publications, Oxford.

Naylor CD and Llewellyn-Thomas HA (1994). Can there be a more patients-centred approach to determining clinically important effect size for randomized treatments? *Journal of Clinical Epidemiology*, **47**, 787–795.

Poon CY, Goh BT, Kim M-J, Rajaseharan A, Ahmed S, Thongsprasom K, Chaimusik M, Suresh S, Machin D, Wong-HB and Seldrup J (2006). A randomised controlled trial to compare steroid with cyclosporine for the topical treatment of oral lichen planus. *Oral Surgery, Oral Medicine, Oral Pathology, Oral Radiolology and Endodontics*, **102**, 47–55.

Saville DJ (1990). Multiple comparison procedures: The practical solution. *The American Statistician*, **44**, 174–180.

Speigelhalter DJ, Freedman LS and Parmar MKB (1994). Bayesian approaches to randomized trials (with discussion). *Journal of the Royal Statistical Society (A)*, **157**, 357–416.

Van Belle G (2002). *Statistical Rules of Thumb*. John Wiley & Sons, Chichester.

Distributions and confidence intervals

2

SUMMARY

Five theoretical statistical distributions, the Normal, Binomial, Poisson, Beta and Exponential are described. In particular, the properties of the Normal distribution are stressed and the circumstances (essentially large study size) in which the Binomial and Poisson distributions have an approximately Normal shape are described. Methods for calculating confidence intervals for a population mean are indicated together with (suitably modified) how they can be used for a proportion or rates in larger studies. For the Binomial situation, formulae are also provided where the sample size is not large.

2.1 Normal Distribution

The Normal distribution plays a central role in statistical theory and frequency distributions resembling the Normal distribution form are often observed in practice. Of particular importance is the standardised Normal distribution, which is the Normal distribution that has a mean equal to 0 and a standard deviation equal to 1. The probability density function of such a Normally distributed random variable z is given by

$$\phi(z) = \frac{1}{\sqrt{2\pi}} \exp\left(-\frac{1}{2}z^2\right), \tag{2.1}$$

where π represents the irrational number $3.14159.\ldots$ The curve described by Equation 2.1 is shown in **Figure 2.1**.

For sample size purposes, we shall need to calculate the area under some part of this Normal curve. To do this, use is made of the symmetrical nature of the distribution about the mean of 0, and the fact that the total area under a probability density function is unity.

Any area, like that in **Figure 2.1**, which has area γ (here $\gamma \geq 0.5$) has a corresponding value of z_γ along the horizontal axis that can be calculated. This may be described in mathematical terms by the following integral

$$\gamma = \int_{-\infty}^{z_\gamma} \phi(z)dz = \Phi(z_\gamma). \tag{2.2}$$

For areas with $\gamma < 0.5$ we can use the symmetry of the distribution to calculate the corresponding area. For example if $\gamma = 0.5$, then one can see from **Figure 2.1** that $z_\gamma = z_{0.5} = 0$. It is also useful to be able to find the value of γ for a given value of z_γ and this is tabulated in

Sample Size Tables for Clinical Studies, 3rd edition. By David Machin, Michael J. Campbell, Say Beng Tan, and Sze Huey Tan. Published 2009 by Blackwell Publishing, ISBN: 978-1-4051-4650-0

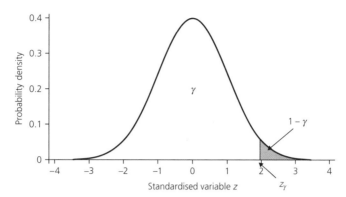

Figure 2.1 The probability density function of a standardised Normal distribution.

Table 2.1. For example if $z_\gamma = 1.9600$ then **Table 2.1** gives $\gamma = 0.97500$. In this case, the unshaded area of **Figure 2.1** is then 0.975 and the shaded area is $1 - 0.975 = 0.025$.

For purposes of sample size estimation, it is the area in the tail, $1 - \gamma$, that is often needed and so we most often need the value of z for a specified area. In relation to test size, we denote the area by α and **Table 2.2** gives the value of z for differing values of α. Thus for *one-sided* $\alpha = 0.025$ we have $z = 1.9600$. As a consequence of the symmetry of **Figure 2.1**, if $z = -1.9600$ then $\alpha = 0.025$ is also in the lower tail of the distribution. Hence the tabular value of $z = 1.9600$ also corresponds to *two-sided* $\alpha = 0.05$. Similarly **Table 2.2** gives the value of z corresponding to the appropriate area under the curve for one-tailed power (see below) $1 - \beta$.

The 'Fundamental Equation'

When the outcome variable of a study is continuous and Normally distributed, the mean, $\bar{x}$, and standard deviation, s, calculated from the data obtained on m subjects provide estimates of the population mean μ_{Pop} and standard deviation σ_{Pop} respectively. The corresponding standard error of the mean is then estimated by $SE(\bar{x}) = \dfrac{s}{\sqrt{m}}$.

In a parallel group trial to compare two treatments, with m patients in each group, the true relative efficacy of the two treatments is $\delta_{\mathrm{Pop}} = \mu_{\mathrm{Pop}1} - \mu_{\mathrm{Pop}2}$, and this is estimated by $d = \bar{x}_1 - \bar{x}_2$, with standard error $SE(d) = \sqrt{\dfrac{s_1^2}{m} + \dfrac{s_2^2}{m}}$. It is usual to assume that the standard deviations are the same in both groups, so $\sigma_{1\mathrm{Pop}} = \sigma_{2\mathrm{Pop}} = \sigma$ (say). In which case a pooled estimate obtained from the data of both groups is $s = \sqrt{(s_1^2 + s_2^2)/2}$, so that $SE(d) = \sqrt{\dfrac{s^2}{m} + \dfrac{s^2}{m}} = s\sqrt{\dfrac{2}{m}}$.

The null hypothesis of no difference between groups is expressed as $H_{\mathrm{Null}} : \mu_{1\mathrm{Pop}} = \mu_{2\mathrm{Pop}}$ or as $\delta = \mu_{1\mathrm{Pop}} - \mu_{2\mathrm{Pop}} = 0$. This corresponds to the left-hand Normal distribution of **Figure 2.2** centred on 0. Provided the groups are sufficiently large then a test of the null hypothesis, $H_0 : \delta = 0$, of equal means calculates $z = \dfrac{d - 0}{SE(d)} = \dfrac{d}{s\sqrt{\dfrac{2}{m}}}$ and, for example, if this is sufficiently large it indicates evidence against the null hypothesis.

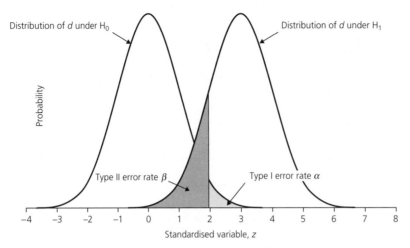

Figure 2.2 Distribution of d under the null ($\delta = 0$) and alternative hypotheses ($\delta > 0$).

Now if this significance test, utilising the data we have collected, is to be *just* significant at some level α, then the corresponding value of z is $z_{1-\alpha}$ and that of d is d_α say. That is if the observed value d equals or exceeds the critical value d_α, then the result is declared significant at significance level α.

At the planning stage of the study, when we have no data, we would express this conceptual result by

$$z_{1-\alpha} = \frac{d_\alpha}{\sigma\sqrt{\dfrac{2}{m}}} \text{ or}$$

$$d_\alpha = z_{1-\alpha}\sigma\sqrt{\frac{2}{m}}. \tag{2.3}$$

The alternative hypothesis, $H_{\text{Alt}} : \delta \neq 0$, we assume $\delta > 0$ for convenience here, corresponds to the right-hand Normal distribution of **Figure 2.2**. If this were the case then we would expect d to be close to δ, so that $d - \delta$ will be close to zero. To just *reject* the hypothesis that $\mu_1 - \mu_2 = \delta$, we require our observed data to provide

$$z = \frac{d - \delta}{SE(d)} = \frac{d - \delta}{s\sqrt{\dfrac{2}{m}}} = -z_{1-\beta}. \tag{2.4}$$

At the planning stage of the study, when we have no data, we would express this conceptual result by

$$d_\alpha = \delta - z_{1-\beta}\sigma\sqrt{\frac{2}{m}}. \tag{2.5}$$

Equating Equations 2.3 and 2.5 for d_α, and rearranging, we obtain the sample size for each group in the trial as

$$m = \frac{2(z_{1-\alpha} + z_{1-\beta})^2}{(\delta/\sigma)^2} = \frac{2(z_{1-\alpha} + z_{1-\beta})^2}{\Delta^2}, \tag{2.6}$$

where $\Delta = \delta/\sigma$ is the (standardised) effect size. As a consequence, the tabulation of the numerator of Equation 2.6, but omitting the multiplier 2, is of particular value for many calculations of sample sizes. This is why it is termed the 'Fundamental Equation'.

The use of Equation 2.6 for the case of a *two-tailed* test, rather than the *one-tailed* test discussed above, involves a slight approximation since d is also statistically significant if it is less than $-d_\alpha$. However, with d positive the associated probability is negligible. Thus, for the case of a two-sided test, we simply replace $z_{1-\alpha}$ in Equation 2.6 by $z_{1-\alpha/2}$.

We denote the *two-tailed* test version of the term in the numerator of Equation 2.6 as $\theta(\alpha, \beta)$, which is tabulated in **Table 2.3**, where

$$\theta(\alpha, \beta) = (z_{1-\alpha/2} + z_{1-\beta})^2. \tag{2.7}$$

In applications discussed in this book, *two-sided* α and *one-sided* β, correspond to the most frequent situation. One-sided α and/or two-sided β are used less often (however, see **Chapter 9**).

In order to design a study comparing two groups the design team supplies:
- The *anticipated effect size*, Δ, which is the size of the anticipated standardised difference between the two groups.
- The significance level, α, of the statistical test to be used in analysis.
- The probability of a Type II error, β, equivalently expressed as the power $1 - \beta$.

Notation

Throughout this book, we denote a *two-sided* (or two-tailed) value for z corresponding to a two-sided significance level, α, by $z_{1-\alpha/2}$ and for a *one-sided* significance level by $z_{1-\alpha}$. The same notation is used in respect to the Type II error β.

Use of tables
Table 2.1
Example 2.1

In retrospectively calculating the power of a completed trial comparing two treatments, an investigator has obtained $z_{1-\beta} = 1.05$, and would like to know the corresponding power, $1 - \beta$.

In the terminology of **Table 2.1**, the investigator needs to find γ for $z_\gamma = 1.05$. Direct reading from the table with $z_\gamma = 1.05$ gives the corresponding $\gamma = 0.85314$. Thus, the power of the test would be approximately $1 - \beta = 0.85$ or 85%.

Table 2.2
Example 2.2

At the planning stage of a randomised trial an investigator is considering using a one-sided or one-tailed test size α of 0.05 and a power 0.8. What are the values of $z_{1-\alpha}$ and $z_{1-\beta}$ that are needed for the calculations?

For a one-tailed test one requires a probability of α in one tail of the corresponding standardized Normal distribution. The investigator thus requires to find $z_\gamma = z_{1-\alpha}$ or $z_{0.95}$. A value of $\gamma = 0.95$ could be found by searching in the body of **Table 2.1**. Such a search gives z as between 1.64 and 1.65. However, direct entry into the first column of **Table 2.2** with $\alpha = 0.05$ gives the corresponding $z = 1.6449$. To find $z_{1-\beta}$ for $1 - \beta = 0.80$, enter the table directly to obtain $z_{0.80} = 0.8416$.

At a later stage in the planning they are led to believe that a two-sided test would be more appropriate; how does this affect the calculations?

For a two-tailed test with $\alpha = 0.05$ direct entry into the second column of **Table 2.2** gives the corresponding $z_{0.975} = 1.9600$.

Table 2.3

Example 2.3

What value of $\theta(\alpha, \beta)$ would the investigator for the two-tailed situation described in *Example 2.2*, require?

For two-sided test $\alpha = 0.05$ and one-sided $\beta = 0.2$, direct entry into **Table 2.3** gives $\theta(\alpha, \beta) = \theta(0.05, 0.2) = 7.849$.

2.2 The Binomial distribution

In many studies the outcome is a particular response and the results are expressed as the proportion that achieve this response. As a consequence, the Binomial distribution plays an important role in the design and analysis of these trials.

For a specified probability of response π, the Binomial distribution quantifies the probability of observing exactly r (ranging from 0 to n) responses in n patients or

$$b(r; \pi, n) = \frac{n!}{r!(n-r)!}\pi^r(1-\pi)^{n-r}. \tag{2.8}$$

Here, $n! = n \times (n-1) \times (n-2) \times \ldots \times 2 \times 1$ and $0! = 1$.

For a fixed sample size n the shape of the Binomial distribution depends only on π. Suppose $n = 5$ patients are to be treated, and it is known that on average 0.25 will respond to this particular treatment. The number of responses actually observed can only take integer values between 0 (no responses) and 5 (all respond). The Binomial distribution for this case is illustrated in **Figure 2.3**. The distribution is not symmetric, it has a maximum at one response and the height of the blocks corresponds to the probability of obtaining the particular number of responses from the five patients yet to be treated. It should be noted that the mean or expected value for r, the number of successes yet to be observed if we treated n patients, is $n\pi$. The potential variation about this expectation is expressed by the corresponding standard deviation, $SD(r) = \sqrt{n\pi(1-\pi)}$.

Figure 2.3 illustrates the shape of the Binomial distribution for various n and $\pi = 0.25$. When n is small (here 5 and 10), the distribution is skewed to the right. The distribution becomes more symmetrical as the sample size increases (here 20 and 50). We also note that the width of the bars decreases as n increases since the total probability of unity is divided amongst more and more possibilities.

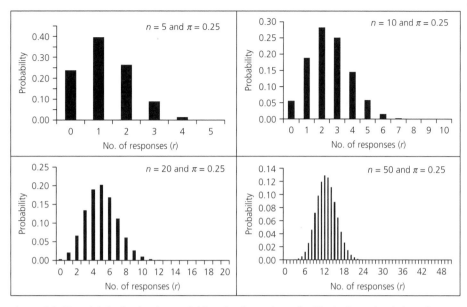

Figure 2.3 Binomial distribution for $\pi = 0.25$ and various values of n. The horizontal scale in each diagram shows the value of r the number of successes (from Campbell, Machin and Walters 2007).

If π were set equal to 0.5, then all the distributions corresponding to those of **Figure 2.3** would be symmetrical whatever the size of n. On the other hand, if $\pi = 0.75$ then the distributions would be skewed to the left.

The cumulative Binomial distribution is the sum of the probabilities of Equation 2.8 from $r = 0$ to a specific value of $r = R$, that is

$$B(R; \pi, n) = \sum_{r=0}^{r=R} \frac{n!}{r!(n-r)!} \pi^r (1 - \pi)^{n-r}. \tag{2.9}$$

The values given to r, R, π and n in Expressions 2.8 and 2.9 will depend on the context. This expression corresponds to the unshaded area of **Figure 2.1** and Equation 2.2 for the standardised Normal distribution.

2.3 The Poisson distribution

The Poisson distribution is used to describe discrete quantitative data such as counts that occur independently and randomly in time at some average rate. For example the number of deaths in a town from a particular disease per day, or the number of admissions to a particular hospital typically follow a Poisson distribution.

If the events happen with a rate of λ events per this unit, the probability of r events happening in this unit is

$$\text{Prob}(r \text{ events}) = \frac{\exp(-\lambda)\lambda^r}{r!} \tag{2.10}$$

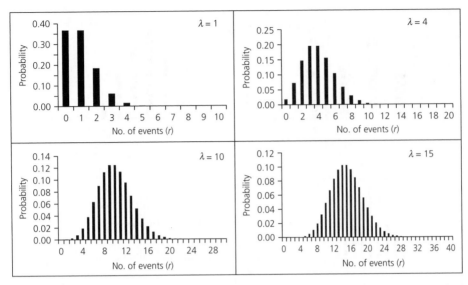

Figure 2.4 Poisson distribution for various values of λ. The horizontal scale in each diagram shows the value of r (from Campbell, Machin and Walters 2007).

where $\exp(-\lambda)$ is a convenient way of writing the exponential constant e raised to the power $-\lambda$. The constant e being the base of natural logarithms which is $2.718281\ldots$.

The mean of the Poisson distribution for the number of events per unit time is simply the rate, λ. The variance of the Poisson distribution is also equal to λ, and so $SD = \sqrt{\lambda}$.

Figure 2.4 shows the Poisson distribution for four different means $\lambda = 1, 4, 10$ and 15. For $\lambda = 1$ the distribution is very right skewed, for $\lambda = 4$ the skewness is much less and as the mean increases to $\lambda = 10$ or 15 it is more symmetrical, and looks more like the Binomial distribution in **Figure 2.3** and ultimately the Normal distribution.

2.4 The Beta distribution

Another distribution that we will utilise when discussing dose-finding studies and Phase II trials in **Chapters 15 and 16** is the Beta distribution. This distribution is similar to the Binomial distribution of Equation 2.8 but allows non-integer powers of the terms π and $(1 - \pi)$. It takes the form

$$beta(\pi; v, w) = \frac{1}{Beta(v, w)}\pi^{v-1}(1 - \pi)^{1-w}, \tag{2.11}$$

where v and w are usually > 1 for our purpose, and $Beta(v, w) = \int_0^1 u^{v-1}(1 - u)^{w-1}du$. This integral can be solved numerically for given v and w and its value ensures that the sum (strictly the integral) of all the terms of Equation 2.11 is unity. In contrast to Equation 2.8 the Beta distribution is that of the continuous variable π rather than of the integer r of the Binomial distribution.

In general when planning a study the Beta distribution may be used to encapsulate, our *prior* knowledge about π, the parameter we are trying to estimate with the trial. This prior knowledge may include relevant information from other sources such as the scientific literature or merely reflect the investigators' belief in the ultimate activity of the therapy under test. Once the study is completed, this prior information may be combined with the data generated using Bayesian methods to obtain a *posterior* distribution from which inferences are then made.

In particular, once trial recruitment is complete, and r responses from the n subjects entered are observed, the prior information is then combined with the study data to obtain a *posterior* distribution for π. This is formed from the product of Equations 2.11 and 2.8, that is, $\pi^{v-1}(1-\pi)^{1-w} \times \pi^{r}(1-\pi)^{n-r} = \pi^{r+v-1}(1-\pi)^{n-r+1-w}$. The Beta distribution is chosen as it combines easily with the Binomial distribution in this way. The posterior distribution (combining both our prior knowledge *and* the data) represents our overall belief at the close of the trial about the distribution of the population parameter, π. The combination of the prior and posterior distribution forms the basis of Bayesian methods.

Once we have obtained the posterior distribution, we can compute the probability that π falls within any pre-specified region of interest. For example, the investigator might wish to know the probability that the true response proportion exceeds a pre-specified target value. This contrasts with the confidence interval approach of the next section, which does not answer this question. Rather it provides an estimate of the true response proportion, along with the associated 95% confidence interval (termed Frequentist as opposed to Bayesian). When the main goal of, for example, a Phase II trial is not to obtain a precise estimate of the response rate of the new drug but rather to accept or reject the drug for further testing in a Phase III trial, then a Bayesian approach may seem best. However, the majority of studies are not designed using a Bayesian framework.

2.5 The Exponential distribution

In survival time studies such as those describing the survival experience of a group of patient with a cancer, if the death rate is constant then the pattern of their deaths follows an Exponential distribution. More generally the death rate is replaced by the hazard rate as the event of concern may not be death but (say) the healing time of an ulcer.

If the hazard rate is θ per unit time, then the proportion of subjects alive at time t is

$$S(t) = e^{-\theta t}. \tag{2.12}$$

This is often written $S(t) = \exp(-\theta t)$ and is termed the survival function of the exponential distribution. The constant hazard rate is a unique property of the Exponential distribution. Sample sizes for survival time studies are given in **Chapter 8**.

The shape of the exponential survival distribution of Equation 2.12 is shown in **Figure 2.5** for a particular value of the hazard rate $\theta = 0.25$ per month. It is clear from this graph that only about 0.2 (20%) of the population remain alive at 6 months, less than 10% at 12 months, and there are very few survivors beyond 18 months. This is not very surprising since the hazard rate tells us that one-quarter of those alive at a given time will die in the following month.

For a value of the hazard rate $\theta < 0.25$ the Exponential survival function will lie above that of **Figure 2.5** since the death rate is lower; for $\theta > 0.25$ it will fall below since, in this case, the death rate is higher.

A constant value of the hazard rate implies that the probability of death remains constant as successive days go by. This idea extends to saying that the probability of death in any time

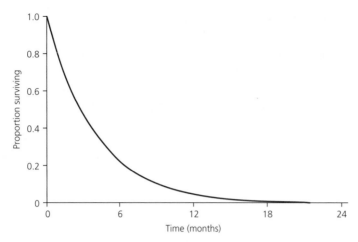

Figure 2.5 The Exponential survival function with a constant hazard $\theta = 0.25$.

interval depends only on the width of the interval. Thus the wider the time interval the greater the probability of death in that interval, but where the interval begins (and ends) has no influence on the death rate.

2.6 Confidence intervals

In any clinical study, the data collected are then used to estimate a summary statistic or statistics pertinent to the question under investigation. As such statistics are essentially obtained from samples there is some uncertainty as to how well they estimate the corresponding or underlying population value(s). This uncertainty is expressed by means of the standard error of the estimate and the associated confidence intervals (CI). We give below the expressions for standard errors and confidence intervals for three key summary statistics, the mean, proportion and rate corresponding to data obtained from the Normal, Binomial, Poisson and Exponential distributions.

Normal
Confidence interval for a mean
Large samples
The sample mean, proportion or rate is the best estimate we have of the true population mean, proportion or rate. We know that the distribution of these parameter estimates from many samples of the same size will roughly be Normal. As a consequence, we can construct a confidence interval—a range of values in which we are confident the true population value of the parameter will lie. Such an interval for the population mean μ_{Pop} is defined by

$$\bar{x} - [z_{1-\alpha/2} \times SE(\bar{x})] \text{ to } \bar{x} + [z_{1-\alpha/2} \times SE(\bar{x})], \tag{2.13}$$

where $\bar{x}$ is the mean from a sample of m subjects, and $SE(\bar{x}) = \sigma_{\mathrm{Pop}}/\sqrt{m}$. To calculate the confidence interval an estimate, s, of the standard deviation σ_{Pop} has to be obtained from the data. Values of $z_{1-\alpha/2}$ are found from **Table 2.2**, so that for a 95% CI, $\alpha = 0.05$ and we have $z_{0.975} = 1.9600$.

Example 2.4—birth weights of pre-term infants

Simpson (2004) reported the mean birth weight of 98 infants who were born prematurely as $\bar{x} = 1.31$ kg with $SE(\bar{x}) = 0.42/\sqrt{98} = 0.04$ kg. From these the 95% *CI* for the population mean is

$$1.31 - (1.96 \times 0.04) \text{ to } 1.31 + (1.96 \times 0.04)$$
or 1.23 to 1.39 kg.

Hence, loosely speaking, we are 95% confident that the true population mean birth weight for pre-term infants lies between 1.23 and 1.39 kg. Our best estimate is provided by the sample mean of 1.31 kg.

Strictly speaking, it is incorrect to say that there is a probability of 0.95 that the population mean birth weight lies between 1.23 and 1.39 kg as the population mean is a fixed number and not a random variable and therefore has no probability attached to it. Nevertheless most statisticians often describe confidence intervals in that way. The value of 0.95 is really the probability that the limits calculated from a random sample will include the population value. For 95% of the calculated confidence intervals it will be true to say that the population mean, μ_{Pop}, lies within this interval.

Small samples

Equation 2.13 for the $100(1 - \alpha)$% *CI* for a mean strictly only applies when the sample size is relatively large—a guide is if *m*, the number of subjects contributing to the mean, exceeds 25. When sample sizes are smaller, the following expression should be used instead,

$$\bar{x} - [t_{df,1-\alpha/2} \times SE(\bar{x})] \text{ to } \bar{x} + [t_{df,1-\alpha/2} \times SE(\bar{x})]. \tag{2.14}$$

Here $t_{df,1-\alpha/2}$ replaces the $z_{1-\alpha/2}$ of Equation 2.13.

Degrees of freedom (df)

Besides depending on α, $t_{df,1-\alpha/2}$ of Equation 2.14 also depends on the number of degrees of freedom, *df*, utilised to estimate the standard deviation, σ, in the final analysis of the study. For a single mean, there are $df = m - 1$ degrees of freedom. Values of $t_{df,1-\alpha/2}$ are found from **Table 2.4**. For example, for a sample mean based on $m = 10$ observations $df = 10 - 1 = 9$. The corresponding 95% *CI*, has $\alpha = 0.05$ and so $t_{df,1-\alpha/2} = t_{9,0.975} = 2.262$ whereas the corresponding $z_{0.975}$ (see the last row of **Table 2.4** and note that a *t*-distribution with $df = \infty$ is equivalent to a Normal distribution) is 1.960. Thus the small sample leads, for given α, to a wider confidence interval.

Example 2.5—birth weights of pre-term infants

Suppose the study of Simpson (2004) referred to in *Example 2.4* had reported the mean birth weight of infants born prematurely as $\bar{x} = 1.31$ kg with $SD = 0.42$ but on only $m = 16$ rather than the 98 actually weighed. In this situation the $SE(\bar{x}) = 0.42/\sqrt{16} = 0.105$ kg and $df = 16 - 1 = 15$. For a the 95% *CI*, **Table 2.4** gives $t_{df,1-\alpha/2} = t_{15,0.975} = 2.131$ so that Equation 2.14 leads to

$$1.31 - (2.131 \times 0.105) \text{ to } 1.31 + (2.131 \times 0.105)$$
or 1.09 to 1.53 kg.

Binomial

Confidence interval for a proportion

If r is the number of patients who respond out of m recruited to a trial, then the response proportion $p = r/m$ is the estimate of the true response rate π_{Pop}. The standard error of p is $SE(p) = \sqrt{\dfrac{p(1-p)}{m}}$ and the corresponding approximate $100(1-\alpha)\%$ CI for π_{Pop} is calculated using the 'traditional' method by analogy with Equation 2.13 as

$$p - [z_{1-\alpha/2} \times SE(p)] \text{ to } p + [z_{1-\alpha/2} \times SE(p)]. \tag{2.15}$$

Values of $z_{1-\alpha/2}$ are found from **Table 2.2**, so that for a 95% CI, $\alpha = 0.05$ and we have $z_{0.975} = 1.9600$.

The reason we can do this is provided by the distributions shown in **Figure 2.3** where, as m gets larger, the shape of the Binomial distribution comes closer and closer to that of the Normal distribution until they are almost indistinguishable. However, this 'traditional' approximation of Equation 2.15 should not be used if the proportion responding is either very low or very high, or the numbers of patients involved small. In these cases we advocate the use of the 'recommended' method described by Newcombe and Altman (2000) (see also Julious 2005) and which is computed as follows:

First calculate the three quantities

$$A = 2r + z_{1-\alpha/2}^2; B = z_{1-\alpha/2}\sqrt{z_{1-\alpha/2}^2 + 4r(1-p)} \text{ ; and } C = 2(n + z_{1-\alpha/2}^2).$$

The corresponding CI is then given by

$$(A - B)/C \text{ to } (A + B)/C. \tag{2.16}$$

This method can be used even when no responses occur, that is when $r = 0$, and hence $p = 0$. In which case the CI is

$$0 \text{ to } \frac{z_{1-\alpha/2}^2}{(n + z_{1-\alpha/2}^2)}. \tag{2.17}$$

Furthermore if all patients respond, $r = n$ so that $p = 1$, and the CI then becomes

$$\frac{n}{(n + z_{1-\alpha/2}^2)} \text{ to } 1. \tag{2.18}$$

A program for calculating the 'recommended' CIs is provided by Altman, Machin, Bryant and Gardner (2000). This warns against the use of the 'traditional' method when the data suggest it is inappropriate.

Example 2.6—dexverapamil and epirubicin for breast cancer

Lehnert, Mross, Schueller *et al.* (1998) used the Gehan (1961) (see **Chapter 16**) design for a Phase II trial of the combination dexverapamil and epirubicin in patients with breast cancer and observed a total of four responses from 23 patients, giving an estimated response rate of $p = 0.174$.

Using the 'traditional' method of Equation 2.13 gives a 95% CI for π_{Pop} of 0.019 to 0.329, whereas using the 'recommended' method of Equation 2.16 gives 0.070 to 0.371. These are quite different and only the latter is correct and should be quoted.

As it is usual to quote response rates in percentages, the corresponding trial report would quote for these data: '. . . the response rate observed was 17% (95% CI 7 to 37%).'

Poisson
Confidence interval for a rate

If r events are observed in a very large number of m subjects, then the rate is $R = r/m$ as with the Binomial proportion. However, for the Poisson distribution r is small relative to m, so the standard error of R, $SE(R) = \sqrt{\dfrac{R(1-R)}{m}}$, is approximately equal to $\sqrt{\dfrac{R}{m}}$. In this case, the approximate $100(1 - \alpha)\%$ CI for the population value of λ_{Pop} is calculated using the 'traditional' method, by

$$R - [z_{1-\alpha/2} \times SE(R)] \text{ to } \lambda + [z_{1-\alpha/2} \times SE(R)]. \tag{2.19}$$

Values of $z_{1-\alpha/2}$ are found from **Table 2.2**, so that for a 95% CI, $\alpha = 0.05$ and we have $z_{0.975} = 1.9600$. The reason we can do this is provided by the distributions shown in **Figure 2.4** where, as m gets larger, the shape of the Poisson distribution comes closer and closer to that of the Normal distribution until they are almost indistinguishable. However this 'traditional' approximation of Equation 2.19 should not be used if the rate is very low, or the numbers of patients involved small.

Example 2.7—standard error of a rate—cadaveric heart donors
The study of Wight, Jakubovic, Walters *et al.* (2004) gave the number of organ donations calculated over a 2-year period (731 days) as $R = 1.82$ per day. This is a rate with standard error $SE(R) = \sqrt{1.82/731} = 0.05$.

Therefore the 95% confidence interval for λ_{Pop} is $1.82 - 1.96 \times 0.05$ to $1.82 + 1.96 \times 0.05$ or 1.72 to 1.92 organ donations per day. This confidence interval is quite narrow suggesting that the true value of (strictly range for) λ_{Pop} is well established.

Exponential
Confidence interval for a hazard rate

It can be shown that if the number of events (deaths) is large, then an approximate 95% CI can be obtained for θ in the standard way, from

$$\theta - [1.96 \times SE(\theta)] \text{ to } \theta + [1.96 \times SE(\theta)]. \tag{2.20}$$

The expression for $SE(\theta)$ depends on whether or not censored observations are present. If they are not, that is, the critical event is observed in all n subjects, then an estimate of the $SE(\theta)$ is given by $SE(\lambda) = \lambda/\sqrt{n}$. In the presence of censoring a corresponding estimate of the SE is $SE(\lambda) = \lambda/\sqrt{(D-1)}$ where D is the number of events observed.

An alternative method of calculating a 95% CI is to use the expression

$$\log \theta - [1.96 \times SE(\log \theta)] \text{ to } \log \theta + [1.96 \times SE(\log \theta)], \tag{2.21}$$

since $\log \theta$ often follows more closely a Normal distribution than does θ itself. In this case $SE(\log \lambda) = 1/\sqrt{D}$.

Example 2.8—death rate—patients with colorectal cancer

Machin, Cheung and Parmar (2006) applying Equation 2.20 to an example of 24 patients with Dukes' C colorectal cancer in which $D = 12$ deaths are observed and $\theta = 0.0278$. These give $SE(\theta) = 0.0278/\sqrt{11} = 0.008395$. A 95% CI for θ is therefore $0.0278 - 1.96 \times 0.008395$ to $0.0278 + 1.96 \times 0.008395$ or 0.0113 to 0.0442 per month. On an annual basis this is 14–53%, which is extremely wide, as one might expect from such a small study. Also as the number of deaths here is quite small, the calculations of the SE are very approximate.

Alternatively, substituting $\theta = 0.0278$ in Equation 2.21 gives $\log \theta = -3.5827$, $SE(\theta) = 1/\sqrt{12} = 0.2887$ and the 95% CI for $\log \theta$ as $-3.5827 - 1.96 \times 0.2887$ to $-3.5827 + 1.96 \times 0.2887$ or -4.1485 to -3.0169. If we exponentiate both limits of this interval we obtain $\exp(-4.1485) = 0.0158$ to $\exp(-3.0169) = 0.0490$ for the 95% CI for θ. These are very similar to those obtained previously but the CI is no longer symmetric about $\theta = 0.0278$. It is preferable, however, to always to use this latter approach as Equation 2.20 can lead, for example, to negative values of the lower confidence limit.

Confidence intervals for some other situations are discussed in **Chapter 10**.

2.7 References

Altman DG, Machin D, Bryant TN and Gardner MJ (eds) (2000). *Statistics with Confidence*, 2nd edn. British Medical Journal, London.

Campbell MJ, Machin D and Walters SJ (2007). *Medical Statistics: A Textbook for the Health Sciences*, 4th edn. John Wiley & Sons, Chichester.

Gehan EA (1961). The determination of the number of patients required in a preliminary and follow-up trial of a new chemotherapeutic agent. *Journal of Chronic Diseases*, **13**, 346–353.

Julious SA (2005). Two-sided confidence intervals for the single proportion: comparison of seven methods. *Statistics in Medicine*, **24**, 3383–3384.

Lehnert M, Mross K, Schueller J, Thuerlimann B, Kroeger N and Kupper H (1998). Phase II trial of dexverapamil and epirubicin in patients with non-responsive metastatic breast cancer. *British Journal of Cancer*, **77**, 1155–1163.

Machin D, Cheung Y-B and Parmar MKB (2006). *Survival Analysis: A Practical Approach*, 2nd edn. John Wiley & Sons, Chichester.

Newcombe RG and Altman DG (2000). Proportions and their differences. In Altman DG, Machin D, Bryant TN and Gardner MJ (eds). *Statistics with Confidence*, 2nd edn. British Medical Journal Books, London, pp. 45–56.

Simpson AG (2004). A comparison of the ability of cranial ultrasound, neonatal neurological assessment and observation of spontaneous general movements to predict outcome in preterm infants. PhD Thesis, University of Sheffield.

Wight J, Jakubovic M, Walters S, Maheswaran R, White P and Lennon V (2004). Variation in cadaveric organ donor rates in the UK. *Nephrology Dialysis Transplantation*, **19**, 963–968.

Table 2.1 The Normal distribution function—probability that a Normally distributed variable is less than z.

z	0.00	0.01	0.02	0.03	0.04	0.05	0.06	0.07	0.08	0.09
0.0	0.50000	0.50399	0.50798	0.51197	0.51595	0.51994	0.52392	0.52790	0.53188	0.53586
0.1	0.53983	0.54380	0.54776	0.55172	0.55567	0.55962	0.56356	0.56749	0.57142	0.57535
0.2	0.57926	0.58317	0.58706	0.59095	0.59483	0.59871	0.60257	0.60642	0.61026	0.61409
0.3	0.61791	0.62172	0.62552	0.62930	0.63307	0.63683	0.64058	0.64431	0.64803	0.65173
0.4	0.65542	0.65910	0.66276	0.66640	0.67003	0.67364	0.67724	0.68082	0.68439	0.68793
0.5	0.69146	0.69497	0.69847	0.70194	0.70540	0.70884	0.71226	0.71566	0.71904	0.72240
0.6	0.72575	0.72907	0.73237	0.73565	0.73891	0.74215	0.74537	0.74857	0.75175	0.75490
0.7	0.75804	0.76115	0.76424	0.76730	0.77035	0.77337	0.77637	0.77935	0.78230	0.78524
0.8	0.78814	0.79103	0.79389	0.79673	0.79955	0.80234	0.80511	0.80785	0.81057	0.81327
0.9	0.81594	0.81859	0.82121	0.82381	0.82639	0.82894	0.83147	0.83398	0.83646	0.83891
1.0	0.84134	0.84375	0.84614	0.84849	0.85083	0.85314	0.85543	0.85769	0.85993	0.86214
1.1	0.86433	0.86650	0.86864	0.87076	0.87286	0.87493	0.87698	0.87900	0.88100	0.88298
1.2	0.88493	0.88686	0.88877	0.89065	0.89251	0.89435	0.89617	0.89796	0.89973	0.90147
1.3	0.90320	0.90490	0.90658	0.90824	0.90988	0.91149	0.91308	0.91466	0.91621	0.91774
1.4	0.91924	0.92073	0.92220	0.92364	0.92507	0.92647	0.92785	0.92922	0.93056	0.93189
1.5	0.93319	0.93448	0.93574	0.93699	0.93822	0.93943	0.94062	0.94179	0.94295	0.94408
1.6	0.94520	0.94630	0.94738	0.94845	0.94950	0.95053	0.95154	0.95254	0.95352	0.95449
1.7	0.95543	0.95637	0.95728	0.95818	0.95907	0.95994	0.96080	0.96164	0.96246	0.96327
1.8	0.96407	0.96485	0.96562	0.96638	0.96712	0.96784	0.96856	0.96926	0.96995	0.97062
1.9	0.97128	0.97193	0.97257	0.97320	0.97381	0.97441	0.97500	0.97558	0.97615	0.97670
2.0	0.97725	0.97778	0.97831	0.97882	0.97932	0.97982	0.98030	0.98077	0.98124	0.98169
2.1	0.98214	0.98257	0.98300	0.98341	0.98382	0.98422	0.98461	0.98500	0.98537	0.98574
2.2	0.98610	0.98645	0.98679	0.98713	0.98745	0.98778	0.98809	0.98840	0.98870	0.98899
2.3	0.98928	0.98956	0.98983	0.99010	0.99036	0.99061	0.99086	0.99111	0.99134	0.99158
2.4	0.99180	0.99202	0.99224	0.99245	0.99266	0.99286	0.99305	0.99324	0.99343	0.99361
2.5	0.99379	0.99396	0.99413	0.99430	0.99446	0.99461	0.99477	0.99492	0.99506	0.99520
2.6	0.99534	0.99547	0.99560	0.99573	0.99585	0.99598	0.99609	0.99621	0.99632	0.99643
2.7	0.99653	0.99664	0.99674	0.99683	0.99693	0.99702	0.99711	0.99720	0.99728	0.99736
2.8	0.99744	0.99752	0.99760	0.99767	0.99774	0.99781	0.99788	0.99795	0.99801	0.99807
2.9	0.99813	0.99819	0.99825	0.99831	0.99836	0.99841	0.99846	0.99851	0.99856	0.99861
3.0	0.99865	0.99869	0.99874	0.99878	0.99882	0.99886	0.99889	0.99893	0.99896	0.99900
3.1	0.99903	0.99906	0.99910	0.99913	0.99916	0.99918	0.99921	0.99924	0.99926	0.99929
3.2	0.99931	0.99934	0.99936	0.99938	0.99940	0.99942	0.99944	0.99946	0.99948	0.99950
3.3	0.99952	0.99953	0.99955	0.99957	0.99958	0.99960	0.99961	0.99962	0.99964	0.99965
3.4	0.99966	0.99968	0.99969	0.99970	0.99971	0.99972	0.99973	0.99974	0.99975	0.99976
3.5	0.99977	0.99978	0.99978	0.99979	0.99980	0.99981	0.99981	0.99982	0.99983	0.99983
3.6	0.99984	0.99985	0.99985	0.99986	0.99986	0.99987	0.99987	0.99988	0.99988	0.99989
3.7	0.99989	0.99990	0.99990	0.99990	0.99991	0.99991	0.99992	0.99992	0.99992	0.99992
3.8	0.99993	0.99993	0.99993	0.99994	0.99994	0.99994	0.99994	0.99995	0.99995	0.99995
3.9	0.99995	0.99995	0.99996	0.99996	0.99996	0.99996	0.99996	0.99996	0.99997	0.99997
z	0.00	0.01	0.02	0.03	0.04	0.05	0.06	0.07	0.08	0.09

Table 2.2 Percentage points of the Normal distribution for α and $1 - \beta$.

| α | | $1 - \beta$ | |
1-sided	2-sided	1-sided	z
0.0005	0.001	0.9995	3.2905
0.0025	0.005	0.9975	2.8070
0.005	0.01	0.995	2.5758
0.01	0.02	0.99	2.3263
0.0125	0.025	0.9875	2.2414
0.025	0.05	0.975	1.9600
0.05	0.1	0.95	1.6449
0.1	0.2	0.9	1.2816
0.15	0.3	0.85	1.0364
0.2	0.4	0.8	0.8416
0.25	0.5	0.75	0.6745
0.3	0.6	0.7	0.5244
0.35	0.7	0.65	0.3853
0.4	0.8	0.6	0.2533

Table 2.3 Values of $\theta(\alpha, \beta) = (z_{1-\alpha/2} + z_{1-\beta})^2$.

| Two-sided | One-sided β | | | | |
α	0.05	0.10	0.15	0.20	0.50
0.001	24.358	20.904	18.723	17.075	10.828
0.005	19.819	16.717	14.772	13.313	7.879
0.01	17.814	14.879	13.048	11.679	6.635
0.02	15.770	13.017	11.308	10.036	5.412
0.05	12.995	10.507	8.978	7.849	3.841
0.1	10.822	8.564	7.189	6.183	2.706
0.2	8.564	6.569	5.373	4.508	1.642
0.4	6.183	4.508	3.527	2.833	0.708

Table 2.4 The *t*-distribution.

df	α		
	0.10	**0.05**	**0.01**
1	6.314	12.706	63.657
2	2.920	4.303	9.925
3	2.353	3.182	5.841
4	2.132	2.776	4.604
5	2.015	2.571	4.032
6	1.943	2.447	3.707
7	1.895	2.365	3.499
8	1.860	2.306	3.355
9	1.833	2.262	3.250
10	1.812	2.228	3.169
11	1.796	2.201	3.106
12	1.782	2.179	3.055
13	1.771	2.160	3.012
14	1.761	2.145	2.977
15	1.753	2.131	2.947
16	1.746	2.120	2.921
17	1.740	2.110	2.898
18	1.734	2.101	2.878
19	1.729	2.093	2.861
20	1.725	2.086	2.845
21	1.721	2.080	2.831
22	1.717	2.074	2.819
23	1.714	2.069	2.807
24	1.711	2.064	2.797
25	1.708	2.060	2.787
26	1.706	2.056	2.779
27	1.703	2.052	2.771
28	1.701	2.048	2.763
29	1.699	2.045	2.756
30	1.697	2.042	2.750
∞	1.645	1.960	2.576

Comparing two independent groups for binary data

3

SUMMARY

This chapter considers sample-size calculations for comparisons between two groups where the outcome of concern is binary. The anticipated effect size between groups is expressed either as a difference between two proportions or by the odds ratio. The situation in which one of the proportions can be assumed known is described. Attention is drawn to difficulties that may arise if one of the proportions is anticipated to be close to zero or unity.

3.1 Introduction

A binary variable is one that only takes one of two values. For example, the outcome for patients receiving a treatment in a clinical trial may be regarded as a 'success' or 'failure'. Typical examples are alive/dead or disease-free/disease-recurrence.

Sometimes ordered categorical or continuous data may be dichotomised into binary form for ease of analysis. For example in a trial of diets in obese people, the outcome may be the body mass index (BMI) measured in kg/m^2. Nevertheless the design, and hence analysis, may be more concerned with the proportion of people no longer obese, where 'obesity' is defined as (say) a BMI greater than 30 kg/m^2 which is relevant to the population of concern.

However, it is not always a good idea to dichotomise an ordinal or continuous variable (see **Chapters 4 and 5**) since information is lost in this process and consequently a larger study may be required to answer the key question.

3.2 Comparing two proportions

The data necessary to estimate a proportion are often coded as 0 and 1 and so are essentially binary in form. If two groups are to be compared then the results can be summarised in a 2×2 table as shown in **Figure 3.1** in which $N = m + n$ patients are assigned at random to one of the treatments, m to Treatment 1 and n to Treatment 2. At the design stage, we may have the option either to randomise equally to the two alternative treatments, in which case the allocation ratio $\varphi = 1$ and $n = m$ in **Figure 3.1**, or to randomise with unequal allocation, in which case $\varphi \neq 1$ and $n = \varphi m$. Any analysis of the data compares the observed proportion of successes in the two treatment groups.

Sample Size Tables for Clinical Studies, 3rd edition. By David Machin, Michael J. Campbell, Say Beng Tan, and Sze Huey Tan. Published 2009 by Blackwell Publishing, ISBN: 978-1-4051-4650-0

Treatment or group	'Success' Code = 1	'Failure' Code = 0	Total	Observed proportion of successes	Anticipated proportion of successes
1	a	c	m	a/m	π_1
2	b	d	$n = \varphi m$	b/n	π_2
Total	r	s	N		

Figure 3.1 Notation for a clinical study comparing the proportion of treatment successes in two (independent) groups.

The standard tests for comparing two proportions are either the χ^2 test or Fisher's exact test. The latter is well approximated by the χ^2 test with Yates's continuity correction included which is termed χ^2_C. The choice of the appropriate test influences the sample size required to detect a difference in proportions. Clearly one should use the same test for the planning as for the analysis. At the analysis stage, χ^2_C is seldom used now as with modern statistical packages the Fisher's exact test can be readily computed. Here its close approximation to Fisher's test is useful for sample-size calculation purposes.

At the planning stage of a study we have to specify the anticipated effect size or anticipated difference in proportions $\delta_{\text{Plan}} = \pi_2 - \pi_1$. Here π_1 and π_2 are the anticipated proportion of successes under Treatment 1 and 2 respectively of **Figure 3.1**.

In some situations it may be difficult to propose a value for the effect size, δ_{Plan}, for which a trial is to be designed to detect. However, since the probability of success under Treatment 1 is π_1 the odds associated with it are $\pi_1/(1 - \pi_1)$. Similarly, the odds associated with success under Treatment 2 are $\pi_2/(1 - \pi_2)$. From these the ratio of these odds, termed the odds ratio, is $OR = \pi_2(1 - \pi_1) / [\pi_1(1 - \pi_2)]$. The OR can take any positive value and the corresponding value for the null hypothesis $H_{\text{Null}} : \pi_1 - \pi_2 = 0$ is $OR_{\text{Null}} = 1$. In this situation, if we are then given a plausible value of (say) π_1, then the value of π_2 is obtained from

$$\pi_2 = \frac{OR_{\text{Plan}}\pi_1}{(1 - \pi_1 + OR_{\text{Plan}}\pi_1)}. \tag{3.1}$$

Thus, rather than pre-specifying π_1 *and* π_2, an investigator may pre-specify an anticipated OR_{Plan} and (say) π_1 and use Equation 3.1 to obtain the anticipated π_2, after which the anticipated value for δ_{Plan} can be obtained.

Such a situation may arise if a previous study had used logistic regression for analysis (see Campbell, Machin and Walters 2007) and had quoted an OR that might then be regarded as a possible effect size for the study under design.

χ^2 **test**

Sample size

The required sample size m for Group 1, for a specified π_1, π_2, φ, two-sided test size α, power $1 - \beta$ and if the χ^2 test is to be used, is given by

$$m = \frac{\left\{z_{1-\alpha/2}\sqrt{[(1 + \varphi)\overline{\pi}(1 - \overline{\pi})]} + z_{1-\beta}\sqrt{[\varphi\pi_1(1 - \pi_1) + \pi_2(1 - \pi_2)]}\right\}^2}{\varphi\delta_{\text{Plan}}^2}, \tag{3.2}$$

where $\overline{\pi} = (\pi_1 + \varphi\pi_2) / (1 + \varphi)$. Values for $z_{1-\alpha/2}$ and $z_{1-\beta}$ can be obtained from **Table 2.2**.

The required sample size for Group 2 is $n = \varphi m$. Thus the total number of subjects required to compare the two groups is $N = m + n = m(1 + \varphi)$.

If the effect size is expressed as an odds ratio then the sample size can be determined from

$$m_{\text{Odds-Ratio}} = \left(\frac{1 + \varphi}{\varphi}\right)\frac{(z_{1-\alpha/2} + z_{1-\beta})^2}{(\log OR_{\text{Plan}})^2\overline{\pi}(1 - \overline{\pi})}. \tag{3.3}$$

In which case the total number of subjects required to compare the two groups is $N_{\text{Odds-Ratio}} = m_{\text{Odds-Ratio}} + n_{\text{Odds-Ratio}} = m_{\text{Odds-Ratio}}(1 + \varphi)$. This can be evaluated by using **Table 2.3** which gives $\theta(\alpha, \beta) = (z_{1-\alpha/2} + z_{1-\beta})^2$ for different values of α and β.

Equation 3.3, which is generalised in **Chapter 4** to the situation when the outcome data are ordered categorical rather than binary but $\varphi = 1$, is quite different in form to Equation 3.2. However, for all practical purposes, it gives very similar sample sizes, with divergent results only occurring for relatively large differences of the OR_{Plan} from unity. However, we would recommend the routine use of Equation 3.2.

Fisher's exact and χ_C^2 tests

Sample size

When using either the exact or the Yates's χ_C^2 test, the required sample size is obtained, after first determining m with Equations 3.2 or 3.3, from

$$m_{\text{Yates}} = Cm, \tag{3.4}$$

where

$$C = \frac{1}{4}\left\{1 + \sqrt{\left[1 + \frac{2(1 + \varphi)}{\varphi m \times |\delta_{\text{Plan}}|}\right]}\right\}^2, \tag{3.5}$$

and which is always > 1. This then gives the (larger) total number of patients required as $N_{\text{Yates}} = m_{\text{Yates}}(1 + \varphi)$.

Practical note

It is important to note that when either or both of the anticipated proportions are close to 0 or 1 then the design should anticipate that the Fisher's exact test will be used to compare the two groups. A rule-of-thumb is to be cautious if either one of the planning proportions results in the product $\pi(1 - \pi) < 0.15$.

Choice of allocation ratio

Although the majority of clinical trials allocate equal numbers of subjects to the two competing treatments, in many other situations there may be different numbers available for each group. If the choice of the relative sample sizes is within the control of the investigator it can be shown, if the study is to be large, that choosing the allocation ratio as

$$\varphi = \sqrt{\frac{\pi_2(1 - \pi_2)}{\pi_1(1 - \pi_1)}} \qquad (3.6)$$

maximises the possible power for the between groups comparison.

This is because the two proportions to be estimated from the study have variances proportional to $\pi_1(1 - \pi_1)$ and $\pi_2(1 - \pi_2)$ respectively. These are maximal when the success rate is 0.5 and so one would choose more subjects from the treatment whose anticipated success rate is nearer 0.5 as that treatment would have the higher variance. For example, in a situation in which the anticipated success rates were $\pi_1 = 0.3$ and $\pi_2 = 0.5$, then a design using an allocation ratio $\varphi = [(0.5 \times 0.5) / (0.3 \times 0.7)]^{1/2} = 1.09$ would provide the most powerful test.

However, the increased power obtained by unequal allocation is often rather small, particularly for φ between 0.5 and 2. In most practical situations π_1 and π_2 are not going to differ by so much as to make unequal allocation worthwhile. For a clinical trial any advantage is at the expense of greater complexity at the randomisation stage.

For observational studies, such as case-control studies however, there may be a limited number of cases available, and so collecting more controls is a suitable method of increasing the power of the study.

3.3 One proportion known

In some situations one may know, with a fair degree of certainty, the proportion of successes in one of the groups. For example, a large number of very similar clinical trials may have been conducted with a particular drug, showing that the success rate is about 20%. Thus, in a clinical trial to test a new product under identical conditions, it may not seem necessary to treat any patients with the standard drug. In this situation, we assume the success rate $\pi_1 (= \pi_{\text{Known}})$ is known. The object of the study is to estimate π_2, which is then compared with π_{Known}. Such designs are termed 'historical control studies' and care should be taken in their use.

χ^2 test
Sample size
The required number of subjects (now for a single group so $N = m$), for significance level α and power $1 - \beta$ for comparing the anticipated π_2 with the established success rate π_{Known} is

$$N = \frac{\left\{ z_{1-\alpha/2}\sqrt{[\pi_{\text{Known}}(1 - \pi_{\text{Known}})]} + z_{1-\beta}\sqrt{[\pi_2(1 - \pi_2)]} \right\}^2}{\delta^2} . \qquad (3.7)$$

Values for $z_{1-\alpha/2}$ and $z_{1-\beta}$ can be obtained from **Table 2.2**.

Unlike Equation 3.2, Equation 3.7 is not symmetrical in π_{Known} and π_2 unless $z_{1-\alpha/2} = z_{1-\beta}$ which is unlikely in practice. However, when π_{Known} and π_2 are not too different and $\varphi = 1$, we can ignore the lack of symmetry and halve the values given by Equation 3.2, which is tabulated in **Table 3.1**, to obtain m for this situation.

Further, since we now only have the *one* group in which we have to conduct the study, this implies that the *total* number of subjects is $N = m/2$ or 25% of that required for a trial in which *both* proportions are to be estimated.

3.4 Practicalities

In Equation 3.3 we give the necessary sample size to detect a given OR_{Plan}. However, in many studies, characteristics of the patients entering the study that are known to influence outcome are usually recorded. In the context of a clinical trial they may represent, for example, the stage of the disease with prognosis worsening with increasing stage. As a consequence, we may intend to run a logistic regression analysis to estimate the OR between the two groups but adjusting for such prognostic variables. Thus we are interested in the stability of the regression coefficient estimates of the ensuing logistic model.

At the design stage, the rule-of-thumb is to plan to observe at least $10(r + 1)$ events where r is the number of regression parameters to be estimated (excluding the constant term) in the logistic model. This formula is rather arbitrary, since there are no effect sizes or power considerations but can be useful if a preliminary study is needed.

The formula is based on the number of parameters in the model, not the number of variables. Thus if a single categorical variable with k categories was fitted, then $r = k - 1$ parameters would be included in the model. Thus if one had to estimate five parameters then one would need at least 60 events. If one assumed that the event rate was about 50% then this would translate into about $60/0.5 = 120$ subjects. In logistic regression the formula implies that events and non-events are treated symmetrically. Thus if the event rate is 90% (rather than 50%) then the non-event rate is 10% and thus one should try and get 60 non-events and so require $60/0.1 = 600$ subjects.

So, whatever the outcome of the sample size calculations arising from Equation 3.3, it should be cross-checked against the above rule.

3.5 Bibliography

Equation 3.2 appears in Fleiss, Levin and Paik (2003). Julious and Campbell (1996) discuss the approximation of Equation 3.3 while Demidenko (2007, Equation 14) gives an alternative expression but this gives similar sample sizes. Casagrande, Pike and Smith (1978) derived the approximate formulae for Equations 3.4 and 3.5 while Equation 3.7 was given by Fleiss, Tytun and Ury (1980). Campbell (1982) discusses sample-size calculations with unequal allocation to groups. Campbell, Julious and Altman (1995) and Sahai and Khurshid (1996) provide a comprehensive review of alternative sample-size formulae for testing differences in proportions. Hosmer and Lemeshow (2000) and Peduzzi, Concato, Kemper *et al.* (1996) give guidance on sample sizes when logistic regression is to be used to take account of baseline variables when making comparisons between groups.

3.6 Examples and use of the tables

Table 3.1 and Equation 3.2
Example 3.1—difference in proportions—treatment of severe burns
In a randomised trial by Ang, Lee, Gan *et al.* (2001), the standard wound covering (non-exposed) treatment was compared with moist exposed burns ointment (MEBO) in patients

with severe burns. One object of the trial was to reduce the methicillin-resistant *Staphylococcus aureus* (MRSA) infection rate at 2 weeks-post admission in such patients from 25 to 5%.

> Using **Table 2.2** with a 5% two-sided test size, $\alpha = 0.05$ gives $z_{0.975} = 1.96$ and for a power of 80% a one-sided $1 - \beta = 0.80$ gives $z_{0.80} = 0.8416$.

With planning values set at $\pi_1 = 0.25$, $\pi_2 = 0.05$, $\delta_{\text{Plan}} = \pi_2 - \pi_1 = -0.20$ and for a two-sided test size of 5% and power 80%, Equation 3.2 with $\varphi = 1$, gives $\bar{\pi} = [0.25 + (1 \times 0.05)] / (1 + 1) = 0.15$

$$\text{and} \quad m = \frac{\left\{ 1.96\sqrt{[(1+1)0.15(1-0.15)]} + 0.8416\sqrt{[1 \times 0.25(1-0.25) + 0.05(1-0.05)]} \right\}^2}{1 \times 0.20^2} = 48.84$$

or 50 per treatment group, that is $N = 100$ patients in total since $\varphi = 1$. Since $\delta_{\text{Plan}} < 0$, to use **Table 3.1** the labels for π_2 and π_1 are interchanged. Both **Table 3.1** and $\boxed{^S\!S_S}$ give $m = 49$.

Table 3.1, Equations 3.2, 3.4 and 3.5

Example 3.2—comparing two proportions—Fisher's exact test using Yates's correction

Had it been anticipated that the results of the trial planned in *Example 3.1* would be analysed using Fisher's exact test, what influence does this have on the number of patients to be recruited?

As previously $\pi_1 = 0.25$, $\pi_2 = 0.05$ and $\delta_{\text{Plan}} = \pi_2 - \pi_1 = -0.20$ and so $m = 49$. Further with allocation ratio $\varphi = 1$, Equation 3.5 gives the multiplying factor as

$$C = \frac{1}{4}\left\{ 1 + \sqrt{\left[1 + \frac{2(1+1)}{1 \times 49 \times |-0.20|} \right]} \right\}^2 = 1.195 . \quad \text{Hence from Equation 3.4,} \quad m_{\text{Exact}} = Cm =$$

$1.195 \times 49 = 58.6$ or 60 subjects, that is $N = 120$ patients in total. Direct use of $\boxed{^S\!S_S}$ gives $m_{\text{Yates}} = n_{\text{Yates}} = 59$ per treatment group.

As we have noted earlier, if either or both of the anticipated proportions are close to 0 or 1 then the design should anticipate that the Fisher's exact test will be used to compare the two groups. In this example, $\pi_1 = 0.05$ and is therefore close to 0 and so, in contrast to the calculations of *Example 3.1*, a more appropriate trial size is $N = 120$ rather than 100 for this proposed trial.

Table 3.2 and Equation 3.3

Example 3.3—comparing two groups—odds ratio

Suppose in the randomised trial by Ang, Lee, Gan *et al.* (2001), the design team had phrased their objectives as reducing the odds of MRSA by use of MEBO. In this case with the same MRSA infection rate at 2-weeks-post admission in such patients of 25% (odds 25% to 75% or 1 : 3) and they may have anticipated this would be reduced to as little as 1 : 5 by the use of MEBO.

> Using **Table 2.2** with a 5% two-sided test size, $\alpha = 0.05$ gives $z_{0.975} = 1.96$ and for a power of 80% a one-sided $1 - \beta = 0.80$ gives $z_{0.80} = 0.8416$. Alternatively from **Table 2.3**, $\theta(0.05, 0.2) = 7.849$.

Here the planning $OR_{Plan} = (1/5)/(1/3) = 0.6$, then with $\pi_1 = 0.25$ Equation 3.1 gives $\pi_2 = 0.1667$. Direct use of Equation 3.2 with these values in $^{SS}S_S$ with a two-sided test size of 5%, power 80% and $\varphi = 1$ gives $m = 372$. This suggests a trial of $N = 2m = 744$ or close to 750 patients.

Alternatively using $\bar{\pi} = (0.25 + 0.1667)/2 = 0.2084$ and $OR_{Plan} = 0.6$ in Equation 3.3 gives

$$m_{Odds-Ratio} = \frac{2 \times 7.849 / (\log 0.6)^2}{0.2084(1 - 0.2084)} = 364.67 \text{ or } 365. \text{ Thus } N_{Odds-Ratio} = 2 \times 365 = 730 \text{ which is}$$

14 fewer patients than the 744 derived from Equation 3.2 and indicates that Equation 3.3 underestimates slightly when the effect size is quite large.

To make use of **Table 3.2**, the inverse of the odds ratio needs to be used and in this case $1/0.6 = 1.67$. The nearest tabular entry, with test size of 5% and power 80%, is $1 - \bar{\pi} = 0.8$ and $OR = 1.7$ giving $m = 407$ patients or a total of approximately $N = 800$.

Whichever method used for the calculations, this sample size is markedly larger than that of *Example 3.1*, where the corresponding effect size was $OR_{Plan} = (0.05/0.95)/(0.25/0.75) = 0.1579$. This corresponds to a more extreme effect size than $OR_{Plan} = 0.6$ used previously as it further from the null hypothesis value of $OR_{Null} = 1$. Consequentially, since the effect size is much larger, the sample size of $N = 100$ in *Example 3.1* is *much smaller*.

This example underlines the need for the planning team to consider the anticipated effect size carefully as it has a profound effect on the ultimate study size.

Table 3.1 and Equation 3.7

Example 3.4—one proportion known—sample size
The rate of wound infection over 1 year in an operating theatre was 10%. This figure has been confirmed from several other operating theatres with the same scrub-up preparation. If an investigator wishes to test the efficacy of a new scrub-up preparation, how many operations does he need to examine in order to be 90% confident that the new procedure only produces a 5% infection rate?

Using **Table 2.2** with a 5% one-sided test size, $\alpha = 0.05$ gives $z_{0.95} = 1.6449$ and for a power of 90% a one-sided $1 - \beta = 0.90$ gives $z_{0.90} = 1.2816$.

Here $\pi_1 = 0.05$, $\pi_{Known} = 0.10$, power $1 - \beta = 0.90$ and if we set *one-sided* $\alpha = 0.05$ and

$$\text{Equation 3.7 yields } N = \frac{\left(1.6449\sqrt{0.1 \times 0.9} + 1.2816\sqrt{0.05 \times 0.95}\right)^2}{(0.1 - 0.05)^2} = 238.9 \text{ or } 239 \text{ operations.}$$

Alternatively the corresponding entry of **Table 3.1** gives 474 operations but since $\pi_{Known} (= \pi_2)$ is assumed *known*, we halve this to $474/2 = 237$ operations which is very close to 239. In practice, a final recruitment target for such a clinical study would be rounded to, say, $N = 250$ operations.

Since in this case, both $\pi_1 = 0.05$, $\pi_2 = 0.10$ are small, a more cautious approach would be to use the tabular values for Fisher's exact test in $^{SS}S_S$ which gives 513 (rather than 474) leading to $N = 513/2$ or approximately 260 operations in this case.

3.7 References

Ang ES-W, Lee S-T, Gan CS-G, See PG-J, Chan Y-H, Ng L-H and Machin D (2001). Evaluating the role of alternative therapy in burn wound management: randomized trial comparing moist exposed burn ointment with conventional methods in the management of patients with second-degree burns. *Medscape General Medicine*, 6 March 2001, 3, 3.

Campbell MJ (1982). The choice of relative group sizes for the comparison of independent proportions. *Biometrics*, **38**, 1093–1094.

Campbell MJ, Julious SA and Altman DG (1995). Sample sizes for binary, ordered categorical, and continuous outcomes in two group comparisons. *British Medical Journal*, **311**, 1145–1148.

Campbell MJ, Machin D and Walters SJ (2007). *Medical Statistics: A Textbook for the Health Sciences*, 4th edn. John Wiley & Sons, Chichester.

Casagrande JT, Pike MC and Smith PG (1978). An improved approximate formula for comparing two binomial distributions. *Biometrics*, **34**, 483–486.

Demidenko E (2007). Sample size determination for logistic regression revisited. *Statistics in Medicine*, **26**, 3385–3397.

Fleiss JL, Levin B and Paik MC (2003) *Statistical Methods for Rates and Proportions*. John Wiley & Sons, Chichester.

Hosmer DW and Lemeshow S (2000). *Applied Logistic Regression*, 2nd edn. John Wiley & Sons, Chichester.

Julious SA and Campbell MJ (1996). Sample size calculations for ordered categorical data (letter). *Statistics in Medicine*, **15**, 1065–1066.

Peduzzi P, Concato J, Kemper E, Holford TR and Feinstein AR (1996). A simulation study of the number of events per variable in logistic regression analysis. *Journal of Clinical Epidemiology*, **49**, 1372–1379.

Sahai H and Khurshid A (1996). Formulae and tables for the determination of sample sizes and power in clinical trials for testing differences in proportions for the two-sample design: A review. *Statistics in Medicine*, **15**, 1–21.

Table 3.1 Sample size for the comparison of two proportions. Each cell gives the number of subjects for each group, m. Hence, the total sample size for the study is $N = 2m$.

	Two-sided $\alpha = 0.05$; Power $1 - \beta = 0.8$									
	First proportion, π_1									
π_2	0.05	0.1	0.15	0.2	0.25	0.3	0.35	0.4	0.45	0.5
0.1	435	–	–	–	–	–	–	–	–	–
0.15	141	686	–	–	–	–	–	–	–	–
0.2	76	199	906	–	–	–	–	–	–	–
0.25	49	100	250	1094	–	–	–	–	–	–
0.3	36	62	121	294	1251	–	–	–	–	–
0.35	27	43	73	138	329	1377	–	–	–	–
0.4	22	32	49	82	152	356	1471	–	–	–
0.45	18	25	36	54	89	163	376	1534	–	–
0.5	15	20	27	39	58	93	170	388	1565	–
0.55	12	16	22	29	41	61	96	173	392	1565
0.6	11	14	17	23	31	42	62	97	173	388
0.65	9	11	14	18	24	31	43	62	96	170
0.7	8	10	12	15	19	24	31	42	61	93
0.75	7	8	10	12	15	19	24	31	41	58
0.8	6	7	8	10	12	15	18	23	29	39
0.85	5	6	7	8	10	12	14	17	22	27
0.9	4	5	6	7	8	10	11	14	16	20
0.95	4	4	5	6	7	8	9	11	12	15

	Two-sided $\alpha = 0.05$; Power $1 - \beta = 0.8$								
	First proportion, π_1								
π_2	0.5	0.55	0.6	0.65	0.7	0.75	0.8	0.85	0.9
0.55	1565	–	–	–	–	–	–	–	–
0.6	388	1534	–	–	–	–	–	–	–
0.65	170	376	1471	–	–	–	–	–	–
0.7	93	163	356	1377	–	–	–	–	–
0.75	58	89	152	329	1251	–	–	–	–
0.8	39	54	82	138	294	1094	–	–	–
0.85	27	36	49	73	121	250	906	–	–
0.9	20	25	32	43	62	100	199	686	–
0.95	15	18	22	27	36	49	76	141	435

Table 3.1 (*continued*): Sample size for the comparison of two proportions. Each cell gives the number of subjects for each group, *m*. Hence, the total sample size for the study is $N = 2m$.

π_2	\multicolumn{10}{c}{Two-sided $\alpha = 0.05$; Power $1 - \beta = 0.9$}
	\multicolumn{10}{c}{First proportion, π_1}									
	0.05	0.1	0.15	0.2	0.25	0.3	0.35	0.4	0.45	0.5
0.1	582	–	–	–	–	–	–	–	–	–
0.15	188	918	–	–	–	–	–	–	–	–
0.2	101	266	1212	–	–	–	–	–	–	–
0.25	65	133	335	1464	–	–	–	–	–	–
0.3	47	82	161	392	1674	–	–	–	–	–
0.35	36	57	97	185	440	1842	–	–	–	–
0.4	28	42	65	109	203	477	1969	–	–	–
0.45	23	33	47	72	118	217	503	2053	–	–
0.5	19	26	36	52	77	124	227	519	2095	–
0.55	16	21	28	39	54	81	128	231	524	2095
0.6	14	17	23	30	40	56	82	130	231	519
0.65	12	15	19	24	31	41	57	82	128	227
0.7	10	12	15	19	24	31	41	56	81	124
0.75	8	10	13	16	19	24	31	40	54	77
0.8	7	9	11	13	16	19	24	30	39	52
0.85	6	7	9	11	13	15	19	23	28	36
0.9	5	6	7	9	10	12	15	17	21	26
0.95	4	5	6	7	8	10	12	14	16	19

π_2	\multicolumn{9}{c}{Two-sided $\alpha = 0.05$; Power $1 - \beta = 0.9$}
	\multicolumn{9}{c}{First proportion, π_1}								
	0.5	0.55	0.6	0.65	0.7	0.75	0.8	0.85	0.9
0.55	2095	–	–	–	–	–	–	–	–
0.6	519	2053	–	–	–	–	–	–	–
0.65	227	503	1969	–	–	–	–	–	–
0.7	124	217	477	1842	–	–	–	–	–
0.75	77	118	203	440	1674	–	–	–	–
0.8	52	72	109	185	392	1464	–	–	–
0.85	36	47	65	97	161	335	1212	–	–
0.9	26	33	42	57	82	133	266	918	–
0.95	19	23	28	36	47	65	101	188	582

Table 3.2 Sample size for the comparison of two proportions using the odds ratio (OR). Each cell gives the number of subjects for each group, m. Hence, the total sample size for the study is $N = 2m$. The corresponding values for an OR < 1 are determined by entering the table with 1/OR and $(1 - \pi_1)$ replacing π_1.

| | Two-sided $\alpha = 0.05$, $1 - \beta = 0.8$ | | | | | | | | | |
| | | | | | π_1 | | | | | |
Odds ratio (OR)	0.05	0.1	0.15	0.2	0.25	0.3	0.35	0.4	0.45	0.5
1.2	9133	4870	3473	2795	2409	2171	2024	1936	1895	1893
1.3	4242	2274	1630	1318	1141	1034	968	930	914	917
1.4	2486	1340	965	784	682	621	583	563	555	559
1.5	1653	896	648	530	463	423	399	386	382	386
1.6	1190	648	472	387	340	311	295	287	285	289
1.7	904	495	362	299	263	242	230	225	224	227
1.8	715	394	289	240	212	196	187	183	183	186
1.9	582	322	238	198	176	163	156	153	153	157
2	486	270	201	168	149	139	133	131	132	135
3	154	91	70	61	56	54	53	53	54	56
4	83	51	41	36	34	33	33	34	35	36
5	54	35	29	26	25	25	25	25	26	28
10	19	14	13	12	12	12	13	13	14	15

| | Two-sided $\alpha = 0.05$, $1 - \beta = 0.8$ | | | | | | | | | |
| | | | | | π_1 | | | | | |
Odds ratio (OR)	0.5	0.55	0.6	0.65	0.7	0.75	0.8	0.85	0.9	0.95
1.2	1893	1930	2008	2137	2335	2637	3117	3944	5633	10 760
1.3	917	938	979	1046	1147	1300	1541	1956	2803	5369
1.4	559	574	601	644	709	805	958	1219	1750	3361
1.5	386	398	418	449	495	565	673	858	1235	2376
1.6	289	298	314	338	374	427	510	652	940	1811
1.7	227	235	249	268	297	340	407	521	752	1452
1.8	186	193	204	221	245	281	337	432	624	1207
1.9	157	163	173	187	208	239	287	368	533	1030
2	135	141	149	162	181	207	249	320	464	898
3	56	59	64	70	78	91	110	142	206	401
4	36	39	42	46	52	60	73	95	138	268
5	28	30	32	35	40	46	56	73	107	207
10	15	16	17	19	21	25	30	39	57	111

Table 3.2 (*continued*): Sample size for the comparison of two proportions using the odds ratio (OR). Each cell gives the number of subjects for each group, *m*. Hence, the total sample size for the study is $N = 2m$. The corresponding values for an OR < 1 are determined by entering the table with 1/OR and $(1 - \pi_1)$ replacing π_1.

Odds ratio (OR)	Two-sided $\alpha = 0.05$, $1 - \beta = 0.9$ π_1									
	0.05	0.1	0.15	0.2	0.25	0.3	0.35	0.4	0.45	0.5
1.2	12 226	6519	4649	3741	3224	2907	2709	2592	2537	2535
1.3	5678	3044	2182	1764	1528	1384	1295	1245	1223	1227
1.4	3327	1793	1292	1050	913	831	781	753	743	748
1.5	2212	1199	868	709	619	566	534	517	512	517
1.6	1592	867	631	518	454	417	395	384	381	386
1.7	1210	663	485	399	352	324	308	300	299	304
1.8	957	527	387	321	284	262	250	245	244	249
1.9	779	432	319	265	235	218	209	205	205	210
2	650	362	268	224	200	186	179	176	176	180
3	207	121	94	81	75	71	70	70	72	75
4	110	68	55	49	46	44	44	45	46	49
5	73	47	38	35	33	33	33	34	35	37
10	26	19	17	16	16	17	17	18	18	20

Odds ratio (OR)	Two-sided $\alpha = 0.05$, $1 - \beta = 0.9$ π_1									
	0.5	0.55	0.6	0.65	0.7	0.75	0.8	0.85	0.9	0.95
1.2	2535	2583	2688	2860	3126	3531	4172	5280	7541	14 404
1.3	1227	1255	1311	1400	1535	1740	2063	2619	3752	7187
1.4	748	768	805	862	949	1078	1282	1631	2343	4500
1.5	517	532	560	601	663	756	900	1149	1653	3181
1.6	386	399	420	453	500	572	683	872	1258	2424
1.7	304	315	333	359	398	455	545	697	1007	1943
1.8	249	258	273	296	328	376	451	578	836	1615
1.9	210	218	231	251	279	320	384	492	713	1379
2	180	188	200	217	242	278	333	429	621	1202
3	75	79	85	93	105	121	146	189	276	536
4	49	52	56	61	69	80	98	126	184	359
5	37	39	43	47	53	62	75	98	142	277
10	20	21	23	25	29	33	40	52	76	148

Comparing two independent groups for ordered categorical data

4

SUMMARY

This chapter extends the sample-size calculations for comparisons between two groups where the outcome of concern is binary to when the outcome is an ordered categorical variable. The anticipated effect size between groups is expressed by the odds ratio.

4.1 Introduction

Some endpoint variables in clinical studies simply assign categories to people, such as that they are of a particular blood group: O, A or AB. In some circumstances when there are more than two categories of classification it may be possible to order them in some logical way. For example, after treatment a patient may be either: (i) improved; (ii) the same; or (ii) worse. A woman may have either; (i) never conceived; (ii) conceived but spontaneously aborted; (iii) conceived but had an induced abortion; or (iv) given birth to a live infant. Outcomes such as these give what are known as *ordered categorical* or *ordinal* data. In some studies it may be appropriate to assign ranks to an outcome. For example, patients with rheumatoid arthritis may be asked to order their preference between four aids designed to assist their dressing. Here, although numerical values may be assigned to each dressing aid for convenience, one cannot treat them as being quantitative. They are in fact codes with 1 for best, 2 for second best, 3 for third and 4 for least preferable.

4.2 Ordered categorical data

Mann–Whitney U-test

A study may be undertaken where the outcome measure of interest is an ordered scale, such as a measure of opinion, say, which used a Likert scale with the ordered categories: Strongly disagree, disagree, agree and strongly agree. For an ordered variable it makes sense to describe one subject as being in a higher (or lower) category than another. The statistical test used to compare groups in this instance is the Mann–Whitney U-test with allowance for ties as described by, for example, Swinscow and Campbell (2002).

With only two categories in the scale we have the binary case described in **Chapter 3**. As always, we need to specify an anticipated effect size and it turns out to be easier to use an *OR* in this context. The experimenter may postulate that on the new therapy a patient is, say, twice as likely to have a higher score than on the standard treatment and so the anticipated *OR* = 2.

Sample Size Tables for Clinical Studies, 3rd edition. By David Machin, Michael J. Campbell, Say Beng Tan, and Sze Huey Tan. Published 2009 by Blackwell Publishing, ISBN: 978-1-4051-4650-0.

Playfullness	Category	Number of children		Proportion of children		Cumulative proportion		
		Control (A)	Paracet. (B)	Control (B)	Paracet. (B)	Control (B)	Paracet. (B)	
	i			$p_{Con,i}$	$p_{Par,i}$	$Q_{Con,i}$	$Q_{Par,i}$	OR
Normal	1	3	6	0.14	0.27	0.14	0.27	2.27
Slightly listless	2	5	9	0.24	0.41	0.38	0.68	3.47
Moderately listless	3	5	5	0.24	0.23	0.62	0.91	6.20
Very listless	4	8	2	0.38	0.09	1.00	1.00	–
	Total	21	22	1.00	1.00			

Figure 4.1 Playfulness in feverish children treated with (Paracetamol) and without (Control) paracetamol (data from Kinmonth, Fulton and Campbell 1992).

Alternatively, an experimenter may know the proportions expected for one group and speculate that, for a particular category, a clinically important difference would be for about 10% more patients to be in that category, or above, in the other group. From this an anticipated OR can be derived and hence all the anticipated proportions in the other group.

Example

In a randomised controlled trial of paracetamol for the treatment of feverish children, Kinmonth, Fulton and Campbell (1992) categorised playfulness on a scale from normal (1) to very listless (4). A total of 43 children were recruited and the results together with the proportions falling in each playfulness category and the corresponding cumulative proportions are given in **Figure 4.1**.

In this example, every child is categorised at the end of the trial and the numbers falling into the respective categories in each treatment noted. The individual proportions are then calculated by dividing these by the corresponding numbers in each treatment group.

To ease presentation below, we have relabelled the Control and Paracetamol groups of **Figure 4.1** as A and B respectively.

Sample size

The first requirement is to specify the proportion of subjects anticipated, in each category of the scale, for one of the groups (say A). Suppose we have κ ordered categories, for example in **Figure 4.1** $\kappa = 4$, and the anticipated proportions in group A are $\pi_{A1}, \pi_{A2}, \ldots \pi_{A\kappa}$ respectively with $\pi_{A1} + \pi_{A2} + \ldots + \pi_{A\kappa} = 1$. Further, let $Q_{A1}, Q_{A2}, \ldots, Q_{A\kappa}$ be the corresponding cumulative proportions, so that $Q_{A1} = \pi_{A1}, Q_{A2} = \pi_{A1} + \pi_{A2}$, and so on until $Q_{A\kappa} = \pi_{A1} + \pi_{A2} + \ldots + \pi_{A\kappa} = 1$. A similar notation applies for group B.

The OR is the chance of a subject being in a given category or higher in one group compared to the same categories in the other group. For category i, which takes values from 2 to κ, it is given by

$$OR_i = \frac{Q_{Ai}(1 - Q_{Bi})}{Q_{Bi}(1 - Q_{Ai})} \qquad (4.1)$$

The assumption of proportional odds specifies that the OR_i will be the same for all categories, from $i = 2$ to $i = \kappa$, and is equal to OR. In this case, if $\bar{\pi}_i$ is the average proportion of subjects anticipated in category i, that is, $\bar{\pi}_i = (\pi_{Ai} + \pi_{Bi})/2$, then the required sample size is

$$m_\kappa = \frac{1}{\left(1 - \sum_{i=1}^{\kappa} \bar{\pi}_i^3\right)} \frac{6(z_{1-\alpha/2} + z_{1-\beta})^2}{(\log OR)^2}. \tag{4.2}$$

This can be evaluated with the help of **Table 2.3** which gives $\theta(\alpha, \beta) = (z_{1-\alpha/2} + z_{1-\beta})^2$ for different values of α and β.

The assumption of constant OR implies that it is justified to use the Mann–Whitney U-test in this situation. It also means that one can use the anticipated OR from *any* pair of adjacent categories for planning purposes.

If the number of categories is large, it is clearly difficult to postulate the proportion of subjects who would fall into a given category.

Approximate formulae
Equation 4.2 is quite complex to evaluate but there are a number of ways that it can be simplified:
(i) $\bar{\pi}_i$ approximately equal
In particular, if the mean proportions $\bar{\pi}_i$ in each category are (approximately) equal, then

$$\Gamma = \left[1 - \sum_{i=1}^{\kappa} \bar{\pi}_i^3\right] \tag{4.3}$$

in the denominator of Equation 4.2 depends only on the number of categories, κ, concerned. In which case, $\Gamma = 1 - 1/\kappa^2$. For example, if $\kappa = 3$, and with all $\bar{\pi}_i$ approximating $1/3$, $\Gamma = 1 - (1/3)^2 = 8/9$.
(ii) $\kappa > 5$
If the number of categories *exceeds* five, then Γ is approximately unity so that

$$m \approx \frac{6(z_{1-\alpha/2} + z_{1-\beta})^2}{(\log OR)^2}. \tag{4.4}$$

(iii) $\kappa = 2$
For the special case of a binary variable, $\kappa = 2$ and Equation 4.4 becomes

$$\Gamma = 3\bar{\pi}(1 - \bar{\pi}). \tag{4.5}$$

Further in this situation, the worst-case scenario is when $\bar{\pi} = 0.5$ in which case $\Gamma = 3/4$.

Comment
From a practical perspective, if a simple dichotomy of the anticipated data had first been used to determine an *interim* value for the sample size, m_{Binary}, using Equation 3.3 of **Chapter 3** then we know that the *eventual* sample size chosen could be reduced by a factor of up to $\Gamma = 3/4$ or 0.75, if more categories are introduced.

Quick formula

For the situation of $\kappa > 5$ Equation 4.4 becomes, with a two-sided test size of $\alpha = 0.05$ and power $1 - \beta = 0.8$,

$$m = 47/(\log OR)^2.$$

(4.6)

This gives a speedy guide to the magnitude of the sample size that may be required.

4.3 Bibliography

Whitehead (1993) and Campbell, Julious and Altman (1995) describe sample-size calculations for ordered categorical data. They point out that there is little increase in power to be gained by increasing the number of categories beyond five. Julious and Campbell (1996) discuss some practical issues when determining sample size in this context.

4.4 Examples

Equation 4.2

Example 4.1—comparing two groups—odds ratio

Suppose a confirmatory trial is planned in which we wished to replicate the results of the randomised controlled trial of paracetamol for the treatment of feverish children conducted by Kinmonth, Fulton and Campbell (1992) and summarised in **Figure 4.1**. We will assume the distribution of children in the control group was anticipated to be about the same as found previously.

The *OR* in category $i = 1$ is calculated as $OR_1 = [0.27/(1 - 0.27)] / [0.14/(1 - 0.14)] = 2.272$. Similarly, using the corresponding cumulative proportions calculations for categories $i = 2$ and $i = 3$ give $OR_2 = 3.467$ and $OR_3 = 6.197$. The average $OR_{\text{Plan}} = (2.272 + 3.467 + 6.197)/3 = 3.98$ or approximately 4.

If an $OR_{\text{Plan}} = 4$ in favour of paracetamol were anticipated, then from the definition of the *OR* we can calculate the anticipated cumulative proportions in the paracetamol group by rearranging the equivalent of Equation 4.1. This gives

$$Q_{\text{Paracet},i} = \frac{OR_{\text{Plan}} \times Q_{\text{Control},i}}{[1 - Q_{\text{Control},i} + (OR_{\text{Plan}} \times Q_{\text{Control},i})]},$$

and so the proportion expected in the first category of the paracetamol group is $Q_{\text{Paracet},1} = 4 \times 0.14 / [1 - 0.14 + (4 \times 0.14)] = 0.3944$. The cumulative proportion expected in the second category of the paracetamol group is $Q_{\text{Paracet},2} = 4 \times 0.38 / [1 - 0.38 + (4 \times 0.38)] = 0.7103$; and similarly $Q_{\text{Paracet},3} = 0.8671$ and $Q_{\text{Paracet},4} = 1$. The actual proportions anticipated are therefore, 0.3944, $(0.7103 - 0.3944) = 0.3159$, $(0.8671 - 0.7103) = 0.1569$ and $(1 - 0.8671) = 0.1329$. The proportions averaged across treatment groups are then given by $(0.14 + 0.3944)/2 = 0.2672$, $(0.24 + 0.3159)/2 = 0.2780$, 0.1984 and 0.2564 respectively. From these, Equation 4.4 gives $(1 - \sum \bar{\pi}_i^3) = 1 - 0.0908 = 0.9092$.

> Using **Table 2.2** with a 5% two-sided test size, $\alpha = 0.05$ gives $z_{0.975} = 1.96$ and for a power of 80% a one-sided $1 - \beta = 0.80$ gives $z_{0.80} = 0.8416$. Alternatively from **Table 2.3**, $\theta(0.05, 0.2) = 7.849$.

For 80% power, 5% significance level and $OR_{\text{Plan}} = 4$, Equation 4.2 gives $m_4 = \dfrac{6 \times 7.849}{(\log 4)^2 \times 0.9092}$ = 26.95 or approximately 27. The planned total study size is therefore $N = 2 \times 27 = 54$ or approximately 60 patients.

Equations 4.2, 4.3 and 4.4

Example 4.2—comparing two groups—odds ratio—quick formula
How are the sample sizes of *Example 4.1* affected by the use of the quick formula?

Given that the proportions 0.2672, 0.2780, 0.1984 and 0.2564 in each of the $\kappa = 4$ categories, are approximately equal at 0.25, we can use Equation 4.3, to obtain $\Gamma = 1 - (1/4)^2 = 15/16 = 0.9375$. Then using this in Equation 4.2 the sample size can be obtained.

Equivalently, since the specified two-sided significance level is 5% and the power 80%, Equation 4.6 can be used to obtain $m_{\text{Interim}} = [47/(\log 4)^2] = 24.46$ from which $m_4 = 24.46 / 0.9375$ = 26.1 ≈ 27 patients. This is the same sample size as that given in *Example 4.1*.

Alternatively, if we had pooled subjects in categories 1–2 and those of categories 3–4, of **Figure 4.1**, rather than keeping them distinct, we would be designing a study with $\pi_{\text{Control}} = 0.38$ and $OR_{\text{Plan}} = 4$. Use of Equation 3.3 with SS would then result in $m = 33$ patients per group. Thus, use of all four categories, rather than simply pooling into two, yields a saving of $33 - 27 = 6$ patients per group. This might result in a substantial reduction in time and resources allocated to the study.

4.5 References

Campbell MJ, Julious SA and Altman DG (1995). Sample sizes for binary, ordered categorical, and continuous outcomes in two group comparisons. *British Medical Journal*, **311**, 1145–1148.

Julious SA and Campbell MJ (1996). Sample size calculations for ordered categorical data. *Statistics in Medicine*, **15**, 1065–1066.

Kinmonth A-L, Fulton Y and Campbell MJ (1992). Management of feverish children at home. *British Medical Journal*, **305**, 1134–1136.

Swinscow TDV and Campbell MJ (2002). *Statistics at Square One*, 10th edn. BMJ Books, London.

Whitehead J (1993). Sample size calculations for ordered categorical data. *Statistics in Medicine*, **12**, 2257–2272.

5 Comparing two independent groups for continuous data

SUMMARY

This chapter considers sample-size calculations for comparisons between two groups where the outcome of concern is continuous. The situations when the data can be assumed to have a Normal distribution form and when they do not are described.

5.1 Introduction

A continuous variable is one that, in principle, can take any value within a range of values. For example, in a trial comparing anti-hypertensive drugs one might record the level of blood pressure once a course of treatment has been completed and use this measure to compare different treatments. Continuous variables may be distributed Normally, meaning they have a characteristic bell-shaped curve which is completely determined by the mean and standard deviation. In such cases, groups are compared using the respective means and the corresponding t-test. In some situations, although the data may not be Normally distributed, they can be rendered Normal by a suitable transformation of the data. For example, by replacing the variable x by its logarithm, $y = \log x$, and regarding y as having a Normal distribution. If this is not possible then comparisons may be made using the Mann–Whitney U-test. Alternatively the data may be grouped into categories and sample size determined by the methods of **Chapter 4**.

5.2 Comparing two means

If continuous outcome variables are plausibly sampled from a Normal distribution, then the best summary statistic of the data is the mean, and the usual test to compare the (independent) groups is the two-sample t-test. If the observations are not Normally distributed, then a suitable test for a shift of location is the Mann–Whitney U-test.

Standardized effect size

In order to produce a set of sample-size tables for general use we need an index of treatment difference which is dimensionless, that is, one that is free of the original measurement units. Given two samples, we might postulate that they have different means, but the same standard

Sample Size Tables for Clinical Studies, 3rd edition. By David Machin, Michael J. Campbell, Say Beng Tan, and Sze Huey Tan. Published 2009 by Blackwell Publishing, ISBN: 978-1-4051-4650-0

deviation, σ. Thus, the alternative hypothesis might be that the two means are Δ standard deviations apart. Denoting the two alternative population means by μ_1 and μ_2 ($> \mu_1$) we have, the anticipated (standardised) effect size as

$$\Delta = \frac{\mu_2 - \mu_1}{\sigma}. \tag{5.1}$$

In many practical situations, one is more likely to have a feel for Δ than individual values of μ_1, μ_2 and σ. Cohen (1988) suggests a realistic range of Δ is from 0.1 to 1.0. A 'small' effect, that is a stringent criterion, might be $\Delta = 0.2$, a moderate one $\Delta = 0.5$ and a 'large' effect, that is a liberal criterion, $\Delta = 0.8$.

In other situations the investigator may know the likely range of the measurements, even though he or she does have a planning value for the standard deviation. On the assumption that the data will follow a Normal distribution one can find a ballpark figure for σ by dividing the likely range, that is, the largest likely observation minus the smallest likely observation, of the data by 4. This is because most (approximately 95%) of a Normal distribution is included within 2σ below the mean and 2σ above the mean.

Two-sample t-test

Sample size—equal variances in each group

Suppose we wished to detect an effect size Δ. Then, for two-sided test size α and power $1 - \beta$, the number of subjects in the first group is given by:

$$m = \left(\frac{1 + \varphi}{\varphi}\right) \frac{(z_{1-\alpha/2} + z_{1-\beta})^2}{\Delta^2} + \frac{z_{1-\alpha/2}^2}{2(1 + \varphi)}. \tag{5.2}$$

The number in the second group is given by $n = \varphi m$, where φ is the allocation ratio, and the total number of patients to be recruited is $N = m + n$. This can be evaluated with the help of **Table 2.3** which gives $\theta(\alpha, \beta) = (z_{1-\alpha/2} + z_{1-\beta})^2$ for different values of α and β.

It should be noted that when $\varphi = 1$, Equation 5.2 is simply the 'Fundamental Equation' 2.6 with an additional term which compensates for the fact that the usual test to compare two means is the Student's t-test since the variances are estimated from the data. If two-sided $\alpha = 0.05$, $z_{0.975} = 1.96$ and this last term is $(1.96)^2/4 \approx 1$, so that this extra term increases the total sample size by 2. This difference will only be of importance in small studies.

Quick formula

In many situations, it is useful to be able to obtain a quick idea of what sample size may be appropriate in a given situation and Lehr (1992) suggests two simple formulae. To detect an anticipated standardised difference Δ, with two-sided significance of 5% and a power of 80%, we have

$$m_{\text{Lehr}} = 16/\Delta^2. \tag{5.3}$$

For 90% power and two-sided significance of 5% this becomes

$$m_{\text{Lehr}} = 21/\Delta^2. \tag{5.4}$$

These approximations also provide a quick check that the sample size tables, of ^SS_S itself, have been used appropriately. They should not be used for the final calculation although in many circumstances the sample sizes obtained will be very similar.

Sample size—unequal variances

If it can be postulated that the variances in the two groups differ such that $\sigma_2^2 = \tau\sigma_1^2$, then one would use an unequal variance *t*-test such as that based on Satterthwaite's approximation described in Armitage, Berrry and Matthews (2002, p. 110) to compare groups. In this case the number of subjects required in the first group is

$$m_{\text{VariancesUnequal}} = \left(\frac{\tau + \varphi}{\varphi}\right)\frac{(z_{1-\alpha/2} + z_{1-\beta})^2}{\Delta_{\text{VariancesUnequal}}^2} + \frac{(\tau^2 + \varphi^3)z_{1-\alpha/2}^2}{2\varphi(\tau + \varphi)^2}. \tag{5.5}$$

Here $\Delta_{\text{VariancesUnequal}} = \dfrac{\mu_2 - \mu_1}{\sigma_1}$ differs from Equation 5.1 as it uses the anticipated standard deviation of Group 1 and not the value anticipated to be the same in both groups.

Allocation of subjects to treatment

Although Equations 5.2, and 3.2 of **Chapter 3**, give a general method for allowing for a difference in sample size between groups, maximum power is achieved by having equal numbers of subjects in the two groups. If group sizes are different, then the $SE(d)$ that we used in **Chapter 2** when deriving the Fundamental Equation 2.6, changes from $\sqrt{\dfrac{s^2}{m} + \dfrac{s^2}{m}}$ to $\sqrt{\dfrac{s^2}{m} + \dfrac{s^2}{\varphi m}} = s\sqrt{\dfrac{1}{m}\left(\dfrac{1+\varphi}{\varphi}\right)}$ for groups of size m and $n = \varphi m$. For a given total sample size $N = m + n$ this standard error is minimised when $m = n$, that is when $\varphi = 1$.

This standard error can also be written as $s\sqrt{\dfrac{2}{m}\left(\dfrac{1+\varphi}{2\varphi}\right)}$ and since, in general, the required sample size is directly proportional to the variance (the square of the standard error) this leads to a simple expression to modify the formula for a sample size for equal sized groups to give that for when the allocation ratio $\varphi \neq 1$. Thus if we define m_{Unequal} as the sample size in the first group and $n_{\text{Unequal}} (= \varphi m_{\text{Unequal}})$ the sample size in the second group, then

$$m_{\text{Unequal}} = \frac{(1 + \varphi)}{2\varphi}m_{\text{Equal}}. \tag{5.6}$$

Here m_{Equal} is the sample size calculated assuming equal-sized groups. This gives a total sample size $N_{\text{Unequal}} = m_{\text{Unequal}} + n_{\text{Unequal}} = m_{\text{Unequal}}(1 + \varphi)$, which will be larger than that for equal allocation.

Mann–Whitney U-test

Sample size

If the outcome variable is continuous but has a distribution which is not Normal, and a suitable transformation cannot be found, a Mann–Whitney U-test may be used to compare the two groups. If $F_1(x)$ and $F_2(x)$ are the probabilities of an outcome being less than a particular value (x) under treatments 1 and 2 respectively, then a non-parametric test has, as null hypothesis H_0, $F_1(x) = F_2(x)$. The alternative hypothesis H_1 is $F_1(x) \leq F_2(x)$ with strict inequality for at least one value of x. A simple alternative hypothesis is one which assumes that $F_1(x) = F_2(x - \delta)$ for some $\delta > 0$. Here δ represents a shift in location between the two alternative treatments or groups. It can be shown that an approximate formula for the sample size to give a two-sided significance level α and power $1 - \beta$ is given by

$$m = \frac{(z_{1-\alpha/2} + z_{1-\beta})^2}{6\delta^2 f^2}, \tag{5.7}$$

where f depends on the particular form of the distribution of $F_1(x)$ and $F_2(x)$.

To calculate f it is necessary to derive the cumulative distribution of the difference of two independent random variables under the null hypothesis assumption that $F_1(x) = F_2(x)$. The quantity f is the first derivative of the derived distribution evaluated at $x = 0$. If we assume the underlying distributions are Normal then $f = 1/(2\sigma\sqrt{\pi}) = 0.2821/\sigma$. Here the π here represents the irrational number 3.14159. . . . Equation 5.7 then becomes

$$m = \frac{2.09(z_{1-\alpha/2} + z_{1-\beta})^2}{\Delta^2} \tag{5.8}$$

which is a little larger than the Fundamental Equation 2.6. This implies that if a non-parametric analysis is conducted on data that have essentially a Normal distribution form, then to compensate for this $2.09/2 = 1.045$ or about 5% more patients are needed in the study.

If the formula for distribution of the data cannot be reliably obtained, then an alternative approach is to divide the outcome into (a maximum of five) categories, and use the methods for ordinal data described in **Chapter 4**.

5.3 One mean known

One-sample *t*-test
In this situation, we require the number of subjects, N, necessary to show that a given mean μ_2 differs from a target value $\mu_1 = \mu_{Known}$. Given a significance level α and a power $(1 - \beta)$ against the specified alternative μ_2 then the number of subjects in the group is

$$N = \frac{(z_{1-\alpha/2} + z_{1-\beta})^2}{\Delta^2} + \frac{z_{1-\alpha/2}^2}{2}, \tag{5.9}$$

where $\Delta = (\mu_2 - \mu_{Known})/\sigma$. Equation 5.9 can be evaluated with the help of **Table 2.3** which gives $\theta = (z_{1-\alpha/2} + z_{1-\beta})^2$ for different values of α and β.

Quick formula
A simple formula for the calculation of the number of observations required, for a two-sided significance level of 5% and power of 80%, is

$$N = \frac{8}{\Delta^2} + 2. \tag{5.10}$$

5.4 Bibliography

Schouten (1999) derived Equations 5.2 and 5.5 which extended equations given by Guenther (1981), who also gave Equations 5.9 and 5.10. Lehr (1992) gave the quick formula of Equations 5.3 and 5.4. Julious (2004) gives a comprehensive review of sample-size problems with Normal data.

5.5 Examples and use of the tables

Table 5.1 and Equations 5.2 and 5.5

Example 5.1—comparing two means—equal variances

An investigator compares the change in blood pressure due to placebo with that due to a drug. If the investigator is looking for a difference between groups of 5 mmHg, then, with a between-subject standard deviation (SD) of 10 mmHg, how many patients should the investigator recruit?

How is the calculation affected if the anticipated effect is 10 mmHg?

How is sample size affected if randomisation was conducted such that for every two patients who received placebo three patients would receive the drug?

In this case, a two-sided test is likely to be the most appropriate, because the investigator may not know if the drug effect is going to be less than or greater than the placebo effect.

> For a 5% two-sided test size, $\alpha = 0.05$ and the value from **Table 2.2** is $z_{0.975} = 1.96$ while for a power of 90% a one-sided $1 - \beta = 0.90$, $z_{0.90} = 1.2816$. Also **Table 2.3** gives $\theta(0.05, 0.1) = 10.507$.

Here, $\delta = \mu_2 - \mu_1 = 5$ mmHg, $\sigma = 10$ mmHg, therefore $\Delta = 5/10 = 0.5$. Assuming $\alpha = 0.05$ (two-sided) and $1 - \beta = 0.9$, **Table 5.1** gives $m = 86$ patients per group and therefore $N = 2m = 172$. Alternatively using Equation 5.2 directly we have $m = \left(\dfrac{1+1}{1}\right)\dfrac{10.507}{0.5^2} + \dfrac{1.96^2}{2(1+1)} = 85.02$

or 86 also.

If, on the other hand, $\Delta = 10/10 = 1.0$ he would have required only 22 patients per group or $N = 44$.

In the case when the randomisation ratio is no longer unity, $\varphi = 3/2 = 1.5$ and with $\Delta = 5/10 = 0.5$ $\boxed{SS_S}$ gives $m = 71$ and $n = 1.5 \times 71 = 106.5$ or approximately 107. Thus a total of $N = 71 + 107 = 178$ patients would be required. However, the total patient number should be divisible by five and so this suggests a trial of 180 patients. This is 4.6% more than if a 1 : 1 randomisation had been used.

Table 5.1 and Equation 5.2

Example 5.2—comparing two means—equal variances

In a clinical trial of the use of a drug in twin pregnancies, an obstetrician wishes to show a clinically important prolongation of pregnancy by use of the drug when compared to placebo. In the absence of any data on the standard deviation of pregnancy duration she argues that normal pregnancies range from 33 to 40 weeks, and so a rough guess for the standard deviation is $SD = (40 - 33)/4 = 1.75$ weeks. How many twin pregnancies must she observe if she decides that 1 week is a clinically important increase in the length of a pregnancy?

Note that she intends to use the t-test to compare means despite the fact that pregnancy duration is far from Normally distributed. However with reasonable sample sizes and equal numbers in the two groups, the t-test is sufficiently robust to give sensible answers.

> For a 5% two-sided test size, $\alpha = 0.05$ and the value from **Table 2.2** is $z_{0.975} = 1.96$ while for a power of 80% a one-sided $1 - \beta = 0.80$, $z_{0.80} = 0.8416$. Also **Table 2.3** gives $\theta(0.05, 0.2) = 7.849$.

Here, $\delta = \mu_2 - \mu_1 = 1$ week, $\sigma = 1.75$ weeks and $\Delta = 1/1.75 = 0.57 \approx 0.6$. Assuming a two-sided test with $\alpha = 0.05$ and power, $1 - \beta = 0.80$, **Table 5.1** gives, for $\Delta = 0.55$, $m = 53$ and for $\Delta = 0.60$, $m = 45$. Thus approximately $m = (53 + 45)/2 \approx 49$ mothers expecting twins would correspond to $\Delta = 0.57$. With equal numbers of mothers per group, the obstetrician would need to observe $N = 2 \times 49 \approx 100$ twin pregnancies for comparison between the drug and a placebo. $^{S}S_{S}$ gives $m = 50$ and hence $N = 100$ also.

Equations 5.3 and 5.4

Example 5.3—comparing two means—quick formula
Given an anticipated standardized effect size of $\Delta = 0.5$, what is the sample size per group using Lehr's quick method for two-sided significance of 5% and power 80%?

Lehr's formula (Equation 5.3) gives $m_{\text{Lehr}} = 16/0.5^2 = 64$ and agrees very closely with direct use of **Table 5.1** or $^{S}S_{S}$ which confirm $m = 64$. The approximate formula performs rather well in this example. A total of $N = 128$ or approximately 130 patients are required.

Table 5.2 and Equation 5.5

Example 5.4—comparing two means—unequal variances
Suppose the investigator of *Example 5.1* believed that although the effect of treatment would be to increase the change in blood pressure over that achieved by the use of placebo, it would also be likely to increase the between subject variability to an extent as to double the variance. Rather than find a transformation to stabilise the variance, the investigator wishes to analyse the outcome in its original units, and so use a t-test with unequal variances.

> For a 5% two-sided test size, $\alpha = 0.05$ and the value from **Table 2.2** is $z_{0.975} = 1.96$. Further with a power of 90% a one-sided $1 - \beta = 0.90$, $z_{0.90} = 1.2816$. **Table 2.3** gives $\theta(0.05, 0.1) = 10.507$.

In this case, $\sigma_2^2 = 2\sigma_1^2$ so we use Equation 5.5 with $\tau = 2$, $\varphi = 1.5$, $\delta = 5$ and $\sigma_1 = 10$ to

obtain $m_{\text{VariancesUnequal}} = \left(\dfrac{2 + 1.5}{1.5} \right) \dfrac{10.507}{0.5^2} + \dfrac{(2^2 + 1.5^3)1.96^2}{2 \times 1.5(2 + 1.5)^2} = 98.84$ or 100. From which

$n_{\text{VariancesUnequal}} = 1.5 \times 100 = 150$, giving a total of $N_{\text{VariancesUnequal}} = 250$ patients while $^{S}S_{S}$ gives 248. The large increase in sample size is mainly due to the increase in the overall variance of the outcome, rather than the unequal variance assumption per se.

Alternatively if, with a Group 1 variance $\sigma_1^2 = 10^2 = 100$ and a Group 2 variance of $\sigma_2^2 = 2\sigma_1^2 = 200$, we had averaged these to obtain $\sigma^2 = (\sigma_1^2 + \sigma_2^2)/2 = (100 + 200)/2 = 150$, then the average SD $= \sqrt{150} = 12.25$ mmHg. Using this in $^S\!S_S$ with $\Delta = (15 - 10)/12.25 = 0.408$, $\varphi = 1.5$ but with $\tau = 1$ gives $m = 107$ for Group 1 and $n = 1.5 \times 107 = 161$ for Group 2, a total of $N = 267$. This is more than the 248 patients estimated earlier. Thus, rather than assume an average SD in such cases, if we can specify separate SDs then we can achieve an overall sample size reduction.

Had the design proposed a 1:1 randomisation between placebo and the drug, then **Table 5.2**, which corresponds to $\varphi = 1$, with $\tau = 2$, $\delta = 5$, $\sigma_1 = 10$, hence $\Delta = 0.5$, two-sided test size 5% and power of 80%, gives $m = 96 \approx 100$ giving a total sample size of 200. This is less than the 250 when $\varphi = 1.5$.

Table 5.3, Equations 5.9, 5.11 and 5.10

Example 5.5—one mean

A psychologist wishes to test the IQ of a certain population and his null hypothesis is that the mean IQ is 100. However, he has no preconceived notion of whether the group is likely to be above or below this value. He wishes to be able to detect a fairly small difference, say, 0.2 standard deviations from 100, so that if he gets a non-significant result from his analysis, he can be sure the mean IQ from this population lies very close to 100. How many subjects should he recruit?

The test to use is the one-sample *t*-test. If the psychologist specifies $\alpha = 0.05$ for a two-sided test, and a power $1 - \beta = 0.8$, then, with $\Delta = 0.2$ from **Table 5.3** or $^S\!S_S$, he will require $N = 199$ or approximately 200 subjects in his sample. The quick formula of Equation 5.10 would suggest $N = 8/0.2^2 + 2 = 202$ which is very close to this number.

5.6 References

Armitage P, Berry G and Matthews JNS (2002). *Statistical Methods in Medical Research*, 4th edn. Blackwell Science, Oxford.

Guenther WC (1981). Sample size formulas for normal theory *t*-tests. *The American Statistician*, 35, 243–244.

Julious SA (2004). Sample sizes for clinical trials with Normal data. *Statistics in Medicine*, 23, 1921–1986.

Lehr R (1992). Sixteen s-squared over d-squared: a relation for crude sample size estimates. *Statistics in Medicine*, 11, 1099–1102.

Schouten HJA (1999). Sample size formula with a continuous outcome for unequal group sizes and unequal variances. *Statistics in Medicine*, 18, 87–91.

Table 5.1 Sample sizes for the two sample t-test with two-sided $\alpha = 0.05$. Each cell gives the number of subjects for each group, m. Hence, the total sample size for the study is $N = 2m$.

Standardised effect size	Power	
Δ	0.8	0.9
0.05	6281	8407
0.1	1571	2103
0.15	699	935
0.2	394	527
0.25	253	338
0.3	176	235
0.35	130	173
0.4	100	133
0.45	79	105
0.5	64	86
0.55	53	71
0.6	45	60
0.65	39	51
0.7	33	44
0.75	29	39
0.8	26	34
0.85	23	31
0.9	21	27
0.95	19	25
1.0	17	22
1.1	14	19
1.2	12	16
1.3	11	14
1.4	9	12
1.5	8	11

Table 5.2 Sample sizes for the two sample t-test with unequal variances. Each cell gives the number of subjects for each group, m. Hence, the total sample size for the study is $N = 2m$.

Δ	Two-sided $\alpha = 0.05$; Power $1 - \beta = 0.8$					
	Variance ratio, τ					
	1.5	**2**	**2.5**	**3**	**4**	**5**
0.05	7850	9420	10 990	12 560	15 700	18 839
0.1	1964	2356	2749	3141	3926	4711
0.15	874	1048	1223	1397	1746	2095
0.2	492	590	688	787	983	1179
0.25	315	378	441	504	630	755
0.3	220	263	307	351	438	525
0.35	162	194	226	258	322	386
0.4	124	149	173	198	247	296
0.45	98	118	137	157	196	234
0.5	80	96	112	127	159	190
0.55	66	79	92	105	132	158
0.6	56	67	78	89	111	133
0.65	48	57	67	76	95	113
0.7	42	50	58	66	82	98
0.75	36	43	50	58	72	86
0.8	32	38	45	51	63	75
0.85	29	34	40	45	56	67
0.9	26	31	36	40	50	60
0.95	23	28	32	36	45	54
1.0	21	25	29	33	41	49
1.1	18	21	24	28	34	41
1.2	15	18	21	24	29	35
1.3	13	15	18	20	25	30
1.4	12	14	16	18	22	26
1.5	10	12	14	16	19	23

Table 5.2 (*continued*): Sample sizes for the two sample *t*-test with unequal variances. Each cell gives the number of subjects for each group, *m*. Hence, the total sample size for the study is $N = 2m$.

Δ	Two-sided $\alpha = 0.05$; Power $1 - \beta = 0.9$					
	Variance ratio, τ					
	1.5	**2**	**2.5**	**3**	**4**	**5**
0.05	10 509	12 610	14 712	16 814	21 017	25 220
0.1	2628	3154	3679	4205	5256	6306
0.15	1169	1403	1636	1870	2337	2804
0.2	658	790	921	1052	1315	1578
0.25	422	506	590	674	842	1011
0.3	293	352	410	469	586	702
0.35	216	259	302	345	431	517
0.4	166	199	231	264	330	396
0.45	131	157	183	209	261	313
0.5	107	128	149	170	212	254
0.55	88	106	123	141	175	210
0.6	74	89	104	118	148	177
0.65	64	76	89	101	126	151
0.7	55	66	77	87	109	131
0.75	48	58	67	76	95	114
0.8	43	51	59	67	84	100
0.85	38	45	53	60	75	89
0.9	34	40	47	54	67	80
0.95	31	36	42	48	60	72
1.0	28	33	38	44	54	65
1.1	23	28	32	36	45	54
1.2	20	23	27	31	38	46
1.3	17	20	23	27	33	39
1.4	15	18	20	23	29	34
1.5	13	16	18	20	25	30

Table 5.3 Sample sizes for the one sample t-test with two-sided $\alpha = 0.05$.

Standardised effect size Δ	Power	
	0.8	0.9
0.05	3142	4205
0.1	787	1053
0.15	351	469
0.2	199	265
0.25	128	171
0.3	90	119
0.35	66	88
0.4	51	68
0.45	41	54
0.5	34	44
0.55	28	37
0.6	24	32
0.65	21	27
0.7	18	24
0.75	16	21
0.8	15	19
0.85	13	17
0.9	12	15
0.95	11	14
1.0	10	13
1.1	9	11
1.2	8	10
1.3	7	9
1.4	6	8
1.5	6	7

Cluster designs, repeated measures data and more than two groups

6

SUMMARY

We discuss sample size estimation for cluster-randomised trials and studies designed with repeated measures (of the same endpoint) over time included. **Chapters 3, 4 and 5** discussed sample-size estimation for the comparison of two groups for outcomes which were using different types of data. Here we describe how to extend these calculations for three or more group comparisons. Situations include those when there is no structure to the respective groups, when a dose–response relation might be expected and when a four-group study can be considered as a 2×2 factorial design. In some situations, it may be relevant to plan for unequal numbers of subjects in each group.

6.1 Cluster designs

In some circumstances the alternative interventions are allocated to groups of subjects, rather than to individuals. For example, one might be concerned to reduce the prevalence of some risk factor in patients attending their general practitioner (GP). The trial may be to evaluate the effectiveness of introducing an educational package for the GPs themselves which is intended to assist them in the way they help their patients to reduce their risk. Such a trial would randomly allocate some GPs (not the patients) to receive the package and others not. This implies that all the patients of a particular GP who receives the educational package will experience the consequences of that intervention. In contrast, all the patients of a particular GP who does not receive the educational package will not experience the consequences of the educational package in how they are advised concerning their risk. Similarly, in trials of two vaccines, for example, it might be more appropriate to randomise households, or even entire villages to the same vaccine rather than the two vaccines on a person-by-person basis.

Comparing two means

We will assume that the objective of the trial design is to compare two interventions and that several clusters have been identified. Each cluster is then assigned one of the alternative interventions at random. The endpoint is then determined in each individual from within the cluster. The analysis of the design will compare the two interventions taking into account both between and within cluster variation in each intervention. Subjects within the same cluster cannot be regarded as independent of each other and so the sample-size calculations

Sample Size Tables for Clinical Studies, 3rd edition. By David Machin, Michael J. Campbell, Say Beng Tan, and Sze Huey Tan. Published 2009 by Blackwell Publishing, ISBN: 978-1-4051-4650-0

must take this into account. Thus, if we denote the between-cluster variance by $\sigma^2_{\text{Between}}$ and the within-cluster variance by σ^2_{Within} the intra-class correlation is given by:

$$\rho_{\text{Intra}} = \frac{\sigma^2_{\text{Between}}}{\sigma^2_{\text{Between}} + \sigma^2_{\text{Within}}}. \tag{6.1}$$

The details of the appropriate analysis of clustered designs are given in Campbell, Donner and Klar (2007).

Sample size

We assume a continuous outcome measure and that there is a fixed number k of patients for each of c clusters which are to receive one of the two interventions. Thus $m_{\text{Cluster}} = ck$.

The sample size required first utilises the sample size, $m_{\text{Individual}}$, from the subject-by-subject randomisation design of **Chapter 5's** Equation 5.2. This assumes independent observations within each intervention group. To accommodate the clustering effect $m_{\text{Individual}}$ has to be inflated by the design effect (DE) where

$$DE = 1 + (k - 1)\rho_{\text{Intra}}, \tag{6.2}$$

and

$$m_{\text{Cluster}} = DE \times m_{\text{Individual}}. \tag{6.3}$$

This then leads to $n_{\text{Cluster}} = \varphi m_{\text{Cluster}}$, where φ is the allocation ratio, and the total number of subjects to be recruited is $N_{\text{Cluster}} = m_{\text{Cluster}} + n_{\text{Cluster}}$.

If the number of patients per intervention group, m_{Cluster}, is fixed and the number of subjects k of each cluster is also fixed, then the number of clusters required for one of the interventions is

$$c = \frac{m_{\text{Individual}}[1 + (k - 1)\rho_{\text{Intra}}]}{k}. \tag{6.4}$$

Thus the total number of clusters for the trial is $C = c(1 + \varphi)$.

On the other hand, if the number of clusters c is fixed, the number of subjects required per cluster is given by:

$$k = \frac{m_{\text{Individual}}(1 - \rho_{\text{Intra}})}{(c - \rho_{\text{Intra}} m_{\text{Individual}})}. \tag{6.5}$$

In order to design a cluster randomised trial one needs to provide a value of ρ_{Intra}. This may be obtained from cluster trials that have been done previously. However, there is a difficulty as intra-class correlation coefficients are not usually well estimated since the precision of the estimate of $\sigma^2_{\text{Between}}$, which is necessary for this calculation, is dependent on the number of clusters concerned and this number may be small. For this reason it is advisable that, before deciding on the eventual trial size, a sensitivity analysis with a range of values of the correlation is carried out. Typical values for ρ_{Intra} for clinical outcomes in primary care are about 0.05. Process outcomes (such as does the doctor always give analgesics for headache) will have higher values. Values in a public health context are typically very small, such as 0.001.

6.2 Repeated measures design

Analysis of covariance

Suppose in a two-group comparison trial we make v observations on each patient before randomisation to treatment and w observations afterwards. If the effect of the treatment is to change over the period of observation post-randomisation, then an efficient analysis is to compute the mean of the observations before randomisation and the mean of those after randomisation. The pre-randomisation mean from each patient are then used as a covariate in an analysis of covariance of the post-randomisation means. In this case, what is often assumed is that observations made at time t on a particular individual have a correlation ρ with observations made at time t'. This correlation is assumed the same for all values of t and t', provided $t \neq t'$. This type of correlation structure is termed 'compound symmetry'. Correlations of between 0.6 and 0.75 are commonly found.

Sample size

If two treatments are to be compared, and the observations come from a Normal distribution then, with the anticipated standardised effect size between them specified as Δ, the sample size in each treatment group for a two-sided test α and power $1 - \beta$ is

$$m_{\text{Repeated}} = R \left[\frac{2(z_{1-\alpha/2} + z_{1-\beta})^2}{\Delta^2} + \frac{z^2_{1-\alpha/2}}{4} \right]. \tag{6.6}$$

Equation 6.6 is the same as Equation 5.2 if $\varphi = 1$ except for the multiplying factor, R, where:

$$R = \left[\frac{1 + (w - 1)\rho}{w} - \frac{v\rho^2}{[1 + (v - 1)\rho]} \right]. \tag{6.7}$$

For the case of no pre-randomisation or baseline observations, $v = 0$ and Equation 6.7 becomes:

$$R = \left[\frac{1 + (w - 1)\rho}{w} \right]. \tag{6.8}$$

This is very similar in form to Equation 6.3 for the *DE* for clustered data except that k is replaced by w to distinguish the two situations and there is a divisor w. In the present situation the divisor arises because we are using the mean of the w observations as the unit of analysis of each patient.

6.3 More than two groups

Although there are many examples of studies conducted on three or more groups, they do pose difficulties at the design stage in relation to study size as more than one hypothesis is often under test. The approach to design will depend on the type of groups involved and the precise comparisons intended.

Several comparisons with placebo

In certain clinical trial situations there may be several potentially active treatments under consideration each of which it would be desirable to test against a placebo. The treatments considered may be entirely different formulations and one is merely trying to determine which, if any, are active relative to placebo rather than to make a comparison between them. In such cases a common minimum effect size to be demonstrated may be set by the clinical team for all the comparisons. Any treatment that demonstrates this minimum level would then be considered as 'efficacious' and perhaps then evaluated further in subsequent trials.

The conventional parallel group design would be to randomise these treatments and placebo (g options) equally, perhaps in blocks of size, $b = g$ or $2g$. However, it is statistically more efficient to have a larger number of patients receiving placebo than each of the other interventions. This is because every one of the $g - 1$ comparisons is made against placebo so that the placebo effect needs to be well established. The placebo group should have $\sqrt{(g - 1)}$ patients for every one patient of the other treatment options. For example, if $g = 5$, then $\sqrt{(g - 1)} = \sqrt{4} = 2$, thus the recommended randomisation is $2 : 1 : 1 : 1 : 1$ which can be conducted in blocks of size $b = 6$ or 12. However, if $g = 6$ for example, then $\sqrt{6} = 2.45$ which is not an integer but with convenient rounding this leads to a randomisation ratio of $2.5 : 1 : 1 : 1 : 1 : 1$ or equivalently $5 : 2 : 2 : 2 : 2 : 2$. The options can then be randomised in blocks of size, $b = 15$ or 30.

Trial size

If the variable being measured is continuous and can be assumed to have a Normal distribution then the number of subjects m, for the placebo treatment group can be calculated by suitably modifying Equation 5.2 to give

$$m = (1 + \sqrt{g - 1})\frac{(z_{1-\alpha/2} + z_{1-\beta})^2}{\Delta_{\text{Plan}}^2} + \frac{z_{1-\alpha/2}^2 \sqrt{g - 1}}{2(1 + \sqrt{g - 1})}, g \geq 2. \tag{6.9}$$

This leads to a total trial size of $N = m + (g - 1) \times n = [1 + \sqrt{(g - 1)}]\, m$ patients, where $n = m/\sqrt{g - 1}$ is the sample size of each of the $g - 1$ non-placebo groups.

If the endpoint is binary, and two proportions π_1 and π_2 are being compared, then the corresponding expression is

$$m = (1 + \sqrt{g - 1})\frac{\left\{z_{1-\alpha/2}\sqrt{[2\bar{\pi}(1 - \bar{\pi})]} + z_{1-\beta}\sqrt{[\pi_1(1 - \pi_1) + \pi_2(1 - \pi_2)]}\right\}^2}{\delta_{\text{Plan}}^2}, g \geq 2. \tag{6.10}$$

6.4 Bibliography

Randomisation by group has been discussed by Donner and Klar (2000). Campbell (2000) gives Equation 6.6 while Feng and Grizzle (1992) point out that estimates of the intra-class correlation coefficients have high variance. The relative efficiency of unequal versus equal cluster sizes is discussed by van Breukelen, Candel and Berger (2007).

Frison and Pocock (1992) describe how sample sizes for repeated measures designs comparing two means can be obtained. They also discuss the important topic of the relative merits of the use of analysis of covariance compared to change-from-baseline methods of analysis.

In the situation when comparing several options against placebo (or a standard control), Fleiss (1986, pp. 95–96) has shown that it is statistically more efficient to have a larger number of patients receiving placebo than each of the other interventions.

6.5 Examples and use of the tables

Equations 6.2, 6.3, 6.5 and Table 5.1

Example 6.1—comparing two means—clustered randomisation

Data from the Family Heart Study Group (1994) have shown that the intra-practice correlation for serum cholesterol is about 0.02. Suppose an investigator has designed an educational package for general practitioners, to try and improve the patients' lifestyle so as to reduce cholesterol levels. He believes that a reduction of about 0.2 mmol/L is achievable. The investigator intends to randomise 50 practices to either receive an educational package or not.

> Using **Table 2.2** with a 5% two-sided test size, $\alpha = 0.05$ gives $z_{0.975} = 1.96$ and for a power of 80% a one-sided $1 - \beta = 0.80$ gives $z_{0.80} = 0.8416$.

Lindholm, Ekbom, Dash *et al.* (1995) gives the between-subject standard deviation of serum cholesterol as about 0.65 mmol/L. Thus, we wish to detect an effect size of $\Delta = 0.2/0.65 \approx 0.3$. Use of **Table 5.1**, Equation 5.2 with $\varphi = 1$, or ^sS_s would suggest that under random allocation on a subject-by-subject basis, for a two-sided significance level 5% and a power 80% about $m_{\text{Individual}} = 176$ patients per group are required, which implies $N \approx 350$.

However, the corresponding design effect (DE) depends on the number of patients per cluster available k and $\rho_{\text{Intra}} = 0.02$. With $C = 50$ practices available equal practice allocation gives $c = 25$ for each intervention group and so, from Equation 6.5, $k = [176(1 - 0.02)]/[25 - (176 \times 0.02)] = 8.02$. Thus we would require $k = 8$ patients per practice to allow for clustering, rather than the $175/25 = 7$ patients under the independence assumption. Hence $DE = 1 + (8 - 1) \times 0.02 = 1.14$, so that from Equation 6.3, $m_{\text{Cluster}} = 176 \times 1.14 \approx 201$ and the final number of subjects required $N_{\text{Cluster}} = 2 \times 201$ or approximately 400.

If the intra-class correlation assumed were 0.015 or 0.025, then the number of practices suggested is 7.75 and 8.33 respectively, both suggesting $k = 8$.

Equation 6.5 and Table 3.1

Example 6.2—comparing two proportions—clustered randomisation

An investigator wishes to educate general practitioners into methods of persuading patients to give up smoking. The prevalence of middle-aged smokers is about 20% and the campaign would like to reduce it to 15%. A parallel group randomised trial is planned, and the investigator can recruit about 40 practices. How many patients per practice should be recruited, if the intra-class correlation for smoking in general practice is about 0.01, and we require 80% power and 5% two-sided significance?

> Using **Table 2.2** with a 5% two-sided test size, $\alpha = 0.05$ gives $z_{0.975} = 1.96$ and for a power of 80% a one-sided $1 - \beta = 0.80$ gives $z_{0.80} = 0.8416$.

From **Table 3.1**, Equation 3.2 or $\boxed{^S S_S}$ with $\pi_1 = 0.15$ and $\pi_2 = 0.20$ we find $m_{\text{Individual}} = 906$ patients. From Equation 6.5 with $\rho_{\text{Intra}} = 0.01$, $m_{\text{Individual}} = 906$, $c = 20$ we have $k = 82$ patients per practice. The clustering, therefore, increases the number of patients recruited per group from 906 to $20 \times 82 = 1640$ patients. If the intra-class correlation were 0.005 or 0.015, the respective sample sizes would be 1166 and 2785 showing how sensitive the calculation can be to the anticipated intra-class correlation coefficient.

Note that in this example, the sample size is more sensitive to the value of the intra-class correlation than the sample size in *Example 6.1*. This is because the number of patients per practice (cluster) is much higher at 82 against 8 in that case.

Table 6.1, Equations 6.6, 6.7 and Table 5.1

Example 6.3—repeated measures—post-randomization repeated measures only

Suppose we wished to design a study of a blood-pressure-reducing agent against a placebo control in which we had no pre-randomisation measure. How many subjects per group are required for 1, 2 or 3 post-randomisation assessments assuming an anticipated standardised effect size of 0.4, correlation 0.7 and test size 5% and power 80%?

> Using **Table 2.2** with a 5% two-sided test size, $\alpha = 0.05$ gives $z_{0.975} = 1.96$ and for a power of 80% a one-sided $1 - \beta = 0.80$ gives $z_{0.80} = 0.8416$.

Here $v = 0$, $w = 1, 2$ and 3, $\rho = 0.7$, $\Delta = 0.4$ and two-sided $\alpha = 0.05$, $1 - \beta = 0.80$. From **Table 5.1**, Equation 5.2, Equation 6.6 with $R = 1$, or $\boxed{^S S_S}$, without repeated measures, we would require $m = 100$ patients. **Table 6.1** with $v = 0$ and $\rho = 0.7$, gives the correction factors for $w = 1, 2$ and 3 as $R = 1.000, 0.850$ and 0.800 respectively. Thus, we require $m_{\text{Repeated}} = Rm = 1.00 \times 100 = 100$, 85 and 80 patients for $w = 1, 2$ and 3 repeated measures. In this example, by increasing the number of post-randomisation measures from 1 to 3 the necessary sample size has been reduced by $(100 - 80)/100 = 0.2$ or 20%. Thus, if the number of patients is limited, one can maintain the power of a study by increasing the number of repeat observations per individual. Use of $\boxed{^S S_S}$ directly gives the same sample sizes.

Table 6.1 and Equation 6.7

Example 6.4—repeated measures—pre- and post-treatment measures

Suppose, in the situation of *Example 6.3*, we also wished to have $v = 3$ pre-treatment measures. How will this affect the sample size?

In this case, **Table 6.1** gives the correction factor R as 0.387, 0.237 and 0.187, so $m_{\text{Repeated}} = 39$, 24 and 19 patients for $w = 1, 2$ and 3 repeated measures post-treatment. Thus the repeated pre-treatment observations also reduce the sample size. However, the final design of the study chosen will need to balance the cost of recruiting additional patients against the cost of recalling current patients on whom repeat measures are then taken.

Equation 6.9

Example 6.5—comparisons with placebo—continuous data—prophylaxis following myocardial infarction

Wallentin, Wilcox, Weaver *et al.* (2003) include in a randomised trial placebo and four doses of a thrombin inhibitor ximelagatran to test for its possible use for secondary prophylaxis after myocardial infarction. Patients were randomly allocated to Placebo or 24, 36, 48 and 60 mg twice daily of ximelagatran for 6 months on a $2 : 1 : 1 : 1 : 1$ basis.

Suppose we intend to run a trial with a similar design, but with a continuous outcome such as a liver enzyme concentration. Assuming liver enzyme concentration has an approximately Normal distribution at each dose, how large should the trial be?

> Using **Table 2.2** with a 5% two-sided test size, $\alpha = 0.05$ gives $z_{0.975} = 1.96$ and for a power of 80% a one-sided $1 - \beta = 0.80$ gives $z_{0.80} = 0.8416$. Also from **Table 2.3**, $\theta(0.05, 0.20) = 7.849$.

For this trial $g = 5$, and suppose the minimal standardised effect size of clinical interest has been set at $\Delta_{\text{Plan}} = 0.5$, then with two-sided test size $\alpha = 0.05$ and power, $1 - \beta = 0.8$, $^{S}S_{S}$ or Equation 6.9 give $m_{\text{Placebo}} = \left(1 + \sqrt{5 - 1}\right)\dfrac{7.849}{0.5^{2}} + \dfrac{1.96^{2}\sqrt{5 - 1}}{2(1 + \sqrt{5 - 1})} = 95.7$ or 96. This implies that each of the other $g - 1$ treatments will be given to $n = m_{\text{Placebo}}/\sqrt{(g - 1)} = 96/2 = 48$ patients. Thus a total trial size of $N = 96 + (5 - 1) \times 48 = 288$ or approximately 300 patients would seem appropriate. The trial could then be conducted either in $r = 50$ replicate randomised blocks of size $b = 6$ patients or with $r = 25$ and $b = 12$.

Equation 6.10

Example 6.6—comparisons with placebo—binary data—prophylaxis following myocardial infarction

Wallentin, Wilcox, Weaver *et al.* (2003) expected a myocardial infarction rate of about 20% with placebo in their trial and expected the biggest reduction with active treatment to give an infarction rate of about 14%.

> Using **Table 2.2** with a 5% two-sided test size, $\alpha = 0.05$ gives $z_{0.975} = 1.96$ and for a power of 80% a one-sided $1 - \beta = 0.80$ gives $z_{0.80} = 0.8416$.

Using $^{S}S_{S}$, or Equation 6.10 directly, with $g = 5$, $\pi_{\text{Placebo}} = \pi_{1} = 0.14$ and $\pi_{2} = 0.20$ gives, with two-sided test size $\alpha = 0.05$ and power, $1 - \beta = 0.8$, $m = 1843$. This implies that each of the other $g - 1$ treatments will be given to $n = m_{\text{Placebo}}/\sqrt{(g - 1)} = 1843/2$ or 922 patients. Thus a total trial size of $N = 1843 + (5 - 1) \times 922 = 5531$ or approximately 2800 patients would seem appropriate. The trial could then be conducted in $r = 461$ replicate randomised blocks of size $b = 12$ patients to give 5532 patients.

The important feature here is that each dose is considered in isolation whereas Walletin Wilcox, Weaver *et al.* (2003) consider a more sensitive dose-response design and estimated they needed 1800 subjects in all

6.6 References

Campbell MJ (2000). Cluster randomized trials in general (family) practice research. *Statistical Methods in Medical Research*, **9**, 81–94.

Campbell MJ, Donner A and Klar N (2007). Developments in cluster randomized trials and *Statistics in Medicine*. *Statistics in Medicine*, **26**, 2–19.

Donner A and Klar N (2000). *Design and Analysis of Cluster Randomised Trials*. Edward Arnold, London.

Family Heart Study Group (1994). Randomized controlled trial evaluating cardiovascular screening and intervention in general practice: principal results of British family heart study. *British Medical Journal*, **308**, 313–320.

Feng Z and Grizzle JE (1992). Correlated binomial variates: Properties of estimator of intraclass correlation and its effect on sample size calculation. *Statistics in Medicine*, **11**, 1607–1614.

Fleiss JL (1986). *The Design and Analysis of Clinical Experiments*. John Wiley & Sons, New York.

Frison L and Pocock SJ (1992). Repeated measures in clinical trials: analysis using mean summary statistics and its implications for design. *Statistics in Medicine*, **11**, 1685–1704.

Lindholm LH, Ekbom T, Dash C, Eriksson M, Tibblin G and Schersten B (1995). The impact of health care advice given in primary care on cardiovascular risk. *British Medical Journal*, **310**, 1105–1109.

Van Breukelen GJP, Candel MJJM and Berger MPF (2007). Relative efficiency of unequal *versus* equal cluster sizes in cluster randomized and multicentre trials. *Statistics in Medicine*, **26**, 2589–2603.

Wallentin L, Wilcox RG, Weaver WD, Emanuelsson H, Goodvin A, Nyström P and Bylock A (2003). Oral ximelagatran for secondary prophylaxis after myocardial infarction: the ESTEEM randomised controlled trial. *Lancet*, **362**, 789–797.

Table 6.1 Multiplying factor for repeated measures designs. *v* is the number of pre-intervention observations, *w* the number of post-intervention observations and ρ is the anticipated correlation between successive (equally spaced in time) observations.

						ρ				
v	*w*	0.1	0.2	0.3	0.4	0.5	0.6	0.7	0.8	0.9
0	1	1.000	1.000	1.000	1.000	1.000	1.000	1.000	1.000	1.000
	2	.0.550	0.600	0.650	0.700	0.750	0.800	0.850	0.900	0.950
	3	0.400	0.467	0.533	0.600	0.667	0.733	0.800	0.867	0.933
	4	0.325	0.400	0.475	0.550	0.625	0.700	0.775	0.850	0.925
	5	0.280	0.360	0.440	0.520	0.600	0.680	0.760	0.840	0.920
1	1	0.990	0.960	0.910	0.840	0.750	0.640	0.510	0.360	0.190
	2	0.540	0.560	0.560	0.540	0.500	0.440	0.360	0.260	0.140
	3	0.390	0.427	0.443	0.440	0.417	0.373	0.310	0.227	0.123
	4	0.315	0.360	0.385	0.390	0.375	0.340	0.285	0.210	0.115
	5	0.270	0.320	0.350	0.360	0.350	0.320	0.270	0.200	0.110
2	1	0.982	0.933	0.862	0.771	0.667	0.550	0.424	0.289	0.147
	2	0.532	0.533	0.512	0.471	0.417	0.350	0.274	0.189	0.097
	3	0.382	0.400	0.395	0.371	0.333	0.283	0.224	0.156	0.081
	4	0.307	0.333	0.337	0.321	0.292	0.250	0.199	0.139	0.072
	5	0.262	0.293	0.302	0.291	0.267	0.230	0.184	0.129	0.067
3	1	0.975	0.914	0.831	0.733	0.625	0.509	0.388	0.262	0.132
	2	0.525	0.514	0.481	0.433	0.375	0.309	0.238	0.162	0.082
	3	0.375	0.381	0.365	0.333	0.292	0.242	0.188	0.128	0.065
	4	0.300	0.314	0.306	0.283	0.250	0.209	0.163	0.112	0.057
	5	0.255	0.274	0.271	0.253	0.225	0.189	0.148	0.102	0.052
4	1	0.969	0.900	0.811	0.709	0.600	0.486	0.368	0.247	0.124
	2	0.519	0.500	0.461	0.409	0.350	0.286	0.218	0.147	0.074
	3	0.369	0.367	0.344	0.309	0.267	0.219	0.168	0.114	0.058
	4	0.294	0.300	0.286	0.259	0.225	0.186	0.143	0.097	0.049
	5	0.249	0.260	0.251	0.229	0.200	0.166	0.128	0.087	0.044
5	1	0.964	0.889	0.795	0.692	0.583	0.471	0.355	0.238	0.120
	2	0.514	0.489	0.445	0.392	0.333	0.271	0.205	0.138	0.070
	3	0.364	0.356	0.329	0.292	0.250	0.204	0.155	0.105	0.053
	4	0.289	0.289	0.270	0.242	0.208	0.171	0.130	0.088	0.045
	5	0.244	0.249	0.235	0.212	0.183	0.151	0.115	0.078	0.040

7 Comparing paired groups for binary, ordered categorical and continuous outcomes

SUMMARY

The purpose of this chapter is to describe methods for calculating sample sizes for studies which yield paired data for the situations where outcomes are binary, ordered categorical or continuous. Common designs are comparisons using matched pairs in either case-control or before and after studies, and two-period two-treatment cross-over trials.

7.1 Introduction

Chapters **3, 4** and **5** describe sample-size calculations for the comparison of two groups for binary, ordered categorical and continuous outcomes respectively. Those calculations assume that the data for one group are independent of that of the other; that is, whatever the results in one group they would not influence the results obtained from the other and vice-versa. However, a common situation is when the data are linked in some way and so the assumption of independence no longer holds. Linked data arise in a number of ways, for example each treatment in a cross-over trial is evaluated in every patient so the two endpoint observations, one following each treatment, from each subject form a pair. Similarly in a case-control study design, each case with the disease in question may be matched, for example for age and gender, with a disease-free control. In other situations, patients may be assessed before and after an intervention.

The basic endpoint unit for analysis is now the difference between these pairs of observations. Here we describe sample-size calculations for the comparison of paired data when these differences have a binary, ordered categorical or continuous form.

7.2 Designs

Cross-over trial

Suppose a cross-over trial is planned in which patients are to be asked whether they obtain relief of symptoms on each of two medications, termed A and B. For expository purposes, we summarise the results of such a trial in the format of **Figure 7.1** and indicate 'Yes' as implying a response or success and 'No' a lack of response or failure.

Sample Size Tables for Clinical Studies, 3rd edition. By David Machin, Michael J. Campbell, Say Beng Tan, and Sze Huey Tan. Published 2009 by Blackwell Publishing, ISBN: 978-1-4051-4650-0

Response to treatment A	Response to treatment B			Anticipated proportions
	No	Yes	Total	
No	r	s	$r+s$	π_A
Yes	t	u	$t+u$	$1-\pi_A$
Total	$r+t$	$s+t$	N_{Pairs}	
Anticipated proportions	π_B	$1-\pi_B$		

Figure 7.1 Notation for a 2 × 2 cross-over trial comparing treatments A and B with a binary endpoint.

Cases	Controls		Total
	Exposed	Not exposed	
Exposed	r	s	$r+s$
Not exposed	t	u	$t+u$
Total	$r+t$	$s+t$	N_{Pairs}

Figure 7.2 Notation for a 1 to 1 matched case-control study with a binary endpoint.

In **Figure 7.1**, r is the number of patients whose response was 'No' with both treatments and u is the number whose response is 'Yes' with both treatments. In contrast, s patients failed to respond to treatment A but responded to treatment B. Finally, t patients responded to treatment A but failed on treatment B. The anticipated proportions of patients who will respond on A is π_A and on B is π_B.

Matched case-control study

Figure 7.2 illustrates the paired situation for a matched case-control study in which each index case of interest is matched to a control. In this case the matching variables chosen are potential confounders which, unless accounted for in some way, may obscure the true difference between cases and controls. Once the matching is made, the relevant exposure history to the risk of concern is ascertained so that each case-control pair can then be assigned to one of the four categories of **Figure 7.2**.

Before-and-after Design

A 'before-and-after' design is a variation of the matched pairs design. In such a design, the pair (of observations) is completed by a second measurement on the same subject. Thus observations are made on each subject, once before (at baseline) and once after—perhaps post an intervention. However, this design is not suitable for evaluation of alternative therapies. To illustrate this, suppose a trial is planned to compare the current standard therapy (*S*) against a test therapy (*T*). Patients in Period I of the design are first recruited to *S*, then when a new therapy comes along all subsequent patients are switched to *T* during Period II of the design. In contrast with a crossover trial, only the sequence *ST* is tested and not also *TS*. Thus, although the differences between the before-and-after observations may measure the effect of the intervention, any observed changes (or their apparent absence) may also be attributed to changes that are temporal in nature. Such changes may be outside the control of the investigator, so that the true benefit of the intervention cannot be estimated.

7.3 Binary data

McNemar's test

The data arising from the designs of either **Figures** 7.1 or 7.2 are often summarised using the odds ratio, calculated as $\psi = s/t$, while the corresponding test of significance is the McNemar's test.

For illustration we focus on a cross-over trial, where ψ is a measure of how much more likely it is that a patient will respond 'Yes' with Treatment B and 'No' on Treatment A as opposed to 'Yes' on A and 'No' on B. We note that the $(r + u)$ patients who respond to both A and B in the same way (that is, they either fail on both treatments or respond to both treatments) do not enter this calculation. This odds ratio and the corresponding McNemar's test are often termed 'conditional' as they are calculated using only the discordant data, that is, they are 'conditional' on the discordance.

Effect size

In order to calculate the required sample size N_{Pairs}, which implies treating each individual twice and therefore making $2 \times N_{\text{Pairs}}$ observations, we need to specify the anticipated values of *s* and *t*. Equivalently, we can specify their anticipated total $(s + t)$, often expressed by means of $\pi_{\text{Discordant}} = \dfrac{s + t}{N_{\text{Pairs}}}$, together with the anticipated value of $\psi = s/t$.

An investigator may have difficulty in anticipating the values of *s* and *t*, but may be able to specify π_A and π_B, the marginal probabilities of response to treatments A and B. In this case, we estimate the anticipated values with $\dfrac{s}{N_{\text{Pairs}}} = \pi_A(1 - \pi_B)$ and $\dfrac{t}{N_{\text{Pairs}}} = \pi_B(1 - \pi_A)$, and from these obtain the anticipated values for $\pi_{\text{Discordant}} = \pi_A(1 - \pi_B) + \pi_B(1 - \pi_A)$ and $\psi = \dfrac{\pi_A(1 - \pi_B)}{\pi_B(1 - \pi_A)}$.

These calculations assume that the response to treatment A is *independent* of the response to treatment B in each subject although this may not be the case. However, we have to make assumptions of some kind for sample size calculation purposes and this may be considered as reasonable.

Sample size

For a two-period two-treatment cross-over trial or a $1:1$ matched case-control study for two-sided test size α and power $1 - \beta$, the number of pairs required is

$$N_{\text{Pairs}} = \frac{\left(z_{1-\alpha/2}(\psi + 1) + z_{1-\beta}\sqrt{[(\psi + 1)^2 - (\psi - 1)^2 \pi_{\text{Discordant}}]}\right)^2}{(\psi - 1)^2 \pi_{\text{Discordant}}}. \tag{7.1}$$

An alternative approach is first to consider the number of discordant pairs required as it is this that is used in estimating ψ and conducting the statistical test. This sets $\pi_{\text{Discordant}} = 1$ in Equation 7.1 to give the number of discordant pairs required as

$$N_{\text{Discordant}} = \frac{\left(z_{1-\alpha/2}(\psi + 1) + 2z_{1-\beta}\sqrt{\psi}\right)^2}{(\psi - 1)^2}. \tag{7.2}$$

The attraction of this method is that the investigator only has to provide an anticipated value of the effect size ψ of interest.

When designing a study therefore one could use Equation 7.2 to estimate the discordant sample size and then recruit subject-by-subject until $N_{\text{Discordant}}$ discordant paired observations are observed at which point recruitment stops.

Unfortunately this strategy implies that the total number to be recruited is not known in advance. So even though we can base enrolment into a study on the discordant sample size there still has to be some estimate of the total sample size for planning and budgetary purposes. Thus to calculate the total sample size we divide the discordant sample size by the anticipated proportion of pairs that will be discordant to obtain a sample size, that is,

$$N_{\text{Pairs}} = \frac{N_{\text{Discordant}}}{\pi_{\text{Discordant}}}. \tag{7.3}$$

Thus a combination of Equations 7.2 and 7.3 provides an alternative means of deriving a sample size. This method is termed a *conditional* approach in that we first calculate a discordant sample size and then dependent on this the total sample size is calculated.

A case-control study may be designed in such a way that the number of controls matched to a given case is greater than one. This may arise when the number of cases available is not numerous, but controls are relatively easy to find. This device can be useful way to maintain sufficient power in a study when cases are scarce—at the expense of requiring more controls.

In this situation a matched unit comprises of a single case together with the corresponding C controls, thus the matched unit consists of $(1 + C)$ individuals. To determine the number of units required, the study size is first calculated from Equations 7.1, or 7.2 with 7.3, which assumes one control for each case, to obtain N_{Equal}. The number of units required in a $1:C$-matching is then given by

$$N_{\text{Units}} = \frac{N_{\text{Equal}}(1 + C)}{2C}. \tag{7.4}$$

Thus the number of cases required is $N_{Cases} = N_{Units}$ and the number of controls required is $N_{Controls} = CN_{Cases}$. Finally the total number of subjects recruited to the study will be $N_{Total} = N_{Cases} + N_{Controls}$.

This method can retain the same power as a design with 1 : 1 matching, but the number of cases now required is then *reduced* at the expense of an *increased* number of controls. However as a consequence, the total number of subjects recruited to the study is correspondingly larger.

In practice, there is little benefit in having more than $C = 4$ cases for each control as the additional *gain* in power diminishes with each extra control so that the benefit of further imbalance adds little to the statistical efficiency of the design.

7.4 Ordered categorical data

Wilcoxon signed rank test

Paired ordered categorical data arise in a number of clinical situations, such as in trials that compare a scored symptom or component of quality of life before and after treatment or a study to compare visual acuity measured before and after surgery. Alternatively, we may have a continuous variable for which the assumption of a Normal distribution does not hold and so we then regard it as categorical data but with many categories. In either case, the Wilcoxon signed rank test would be the most appropriate statistical test for analysis.

The format of data resulting from such studies extends the number of rows (and columns) of **Figure** 7.2 from 2 to κ, where κ represents the number of ordered categories. Observations which then lie along the diagonal of such a $(\kappa \times \kappa)$ contingency table, correspond to those whose category has not changed following the intervention, and they do not contribute information on the comparison.

Effect size

For pairs in different categories, the largest difference possible is $\kappa - 1$ categories apart. To calculate the sample size, it is necessary to specify the distribution of differences, that is, what proportion of subjects are likely to differ by one category, by two categories and so on until by $\kappa - 1$ categories.

For example, with a three-point scale the design team may suspect that the new treatment will be an improvement over the control so the difference in pairs will tend to be positive. They then anticipate that, conditional on the overall difference being positive, proportions ξ_2 and ξ_1 of subjects will improve by $c_2 = +2$ and $c_1 = +1$ categories respectively. Similarly they then anticipate the proportions for $c_0 = 0$, $c_{-1} = -1$ and $c_{-2} = -2$ as ξ_0, ξ_{-1} and ξ_{-2}. These anticipated values may be based on a pilot study, published data or the collective views of the design team.

In general, once the $2(\kappa - 1) + 1$ anticipated probabilities ξ_j have been specified the next step is to calculate the anticipated proportions in each of the $2(\kappa - 1)$ non-zero difference groups, that is, $v_i = \xi_j / (1 - \xi_0)$. From these the planning effect size

$$\eta = \sum_{j=-(\kappa-1)}^{(\kappa-1)} v_j c_j \tag{7.5}$$

and the corresponding standard deviation

$$\sigma_{\text{Discordant}} = \sqrt{\sum_{j=-(k-1)}^{k-1} v_j c_j^2 - \eta^2} \qquad (7.6)$$

are obtained. The appropriate standardised difference for comparing groups is then

$$\Delta_{\text{Categorical}} = \frac{\eta}{\sigma_{\text{Discordant}}}. \qquad (7.7)$$

Sample size
The required number of pairs, for two-sided test size α and power $1 - \beta$, if the Wilcoxon signed rank sum test is to be used is given by

$$N_{\text{Pairs}} = \frac{2(z_{1-\alpha/2} + z_{1-\beta})^2}{\Delta_{\text{Categorical}}^2} + \frac{z_{1-\alpha/2}^2}{2}. \qquad (7.8)$$

This equation can be evaluated with the help of **Table 2.2** together with **Table 2.3** the latter which gives $\theta(\alpha, \beta) = (z_{1-\alpha/2} + z_{1-\beta})^2$ for different values of α and β.

Practical note
In practice, there may be little information to base the anticipated probabilities required to quantify the standardised effect size and hence make the sample size calculations of Equation 7.8. In this instance a recommendation would be to ignore the distribution of the individual scores in the discordant categories (for three-point scales -2, -1, 1 and 2) and merely provide the anticipated ratio of the number of positives over the number of negatives. In effect we have then dichotomised the scores to be either positive or negative (ignoring their magnitude) and anticipated the odds ratio ψ of positives over negatives.

Once we have ψ we can then use Equation 7.2 to calculate the discordant sample size, $N_{\text{Discordant}}$ and then use Equation 7.3, with a corresponding $\pi_{\text{Discordant}}$, to estimate the total sample size N_{Pairs}. However, by increasing the number of categories (over the binary situation) the appropriate total sample size will be nearer to the discordant sample. So a sample size mid-way between $N_{\text{Discordant}}$ and N_{Pairs} may be a practical compromise.

7.5 Continuous data

Within and between subject variation
If only one measurement is made per individual it is impossible to separate the *within* from the *between* subjects sources of variation. In such cases the usual variance formula summarises a composite of both the within *and* between subject sources so that the total variation comprises $\sigma_{\text{Total}}^2 = \sigma_{\text{Between}}^2 + \sigma_{\text{Within}}^2$. The *within*-subject variance quantifies the anticipated variation among repeated measurements on the *same* individual. It is a compound of true variation

in the individual and any measurement error. The *between*-subject variance quantifies the anticipated variation *between* subjects.

Paired *t*-test

As we have indicated, when the units of observation are paired, or matched, essentially the end-point observations from the two members of each unit are linked and the difference between them is used as the endpoint for analysis. However, in the case of a continuous variable, the tabulations similar to **Figures 7. 1 and 7.2** cannot in general be constructed except in the unusual case when many of the paired observations are tied, that is they have the same numerical value, and the number of different values actually observed is very limited.

Suppose in a case-control study cases with a particular disease are matched perhaps, by age and gender to healthy controls, then the endpoint for analysis for pair i is $d_i = (x_i - y_i)$ where x_i is the continuous observation from the case and y_i the continuous observation from the control and there are N pairs. For the situation of C controls for every case in a matched case-control study, the unit for analysis becomes $d_i = (x_i - \bar{y}_i)$ where $\bar{y}_i$ is the mean of the C continuous observations from the controls of matched group i.

The analysis of such a design involves calculating the mean difference $\bar{d} = \sum d_i / N$ and the corresponding standard deviation of the differences, $s = \dfrac{\sum (d_i - \bar{d})^2}{N - 1}$. These allow a paired t-test of the null hypothesis of no difference between cases and control as well as a confidence interval to be constructed.

Effect size

This is simply the anticipated difference of means between cases and controls or between before and after intervention means. We denote this by δ_{Plan}.

Planning standard deviation of the difference

If we consider one individual for a moment then, for example, their blood pressure will vary over time even if the underlying average value remains constant. An individual measurement may depart from this 'average' level but were we to take successive readings we would hope that their mean would estimate the underlying level and that their standard deviation gives an estimate of the within-subject standard deviation, σ_{Within} which essentially quantifies the random variation. We clearly cannot determine σ_{Within} from a single measure in an individual. In a matched case-control design we assume that σ_{Within} (were we able to estimate it) will be the same for both the case and the control whose individual measures are independent of each other even though they are linked as a pair.

In this case, the variance of the paired difference is $\sigma^2_{\text{Difference}} = \text{Var}(d_i) = \text{Var}(x_i - y_i) = \sigma^2_{\text{Within}} + \sigma^2_{\text{Within}} = 2\sigma^2_{\text{Within}}$.

In such a case-control study for pair i the value of x_i observed from the case, and y_i observed from the control, may differ in value from each other through three ways:

1 due to random variation alone;

2 because there is a difference between cases and controls in their 'average' levels; and

3 for both reasons.

Sample size

For planning purposes, the standardized effect size is

$$\Delta_{\text{Continuous}} = \frac{\delta_{\text{Plan}}}{\sigma_{\text{Difference}}}, \tag{7.9}$$

where the planning value for $\sigma_{\text{Difference}}$ itself can be provided directly or from values of its component σ_{Within}. However, in many circumstances, the investigators will provide a direct planning value for $\Delta_{\text{Continuous}}$ itself rather than specifying its components.

The formula to calculate the total sample size required to detect an anticipated standardised difference $\Delta_{\text{Continuous}}$ at two-sided significance level α and power $1 - \beta$ is

$$N_{\text{Pairs}} = \frac{2(z_{1-\alpha/2} + z_{1-\beta})^2}{\Delta_{\text{Continuous}}^2} + \frac{z_{1-\alpha/2}^2}{2}. \tag{7.10}$$

This can be evaluated with the help of **Table 2.2** and **Table 2.3**. The latter gives $\theta(\alpha, \beta) = (z_{1-\alpha/2} + z_{1-\beta})^2$ for different values of α and β.

Note Equation 7.10 is the same algebraic expression as Equation 7.8. The difference being in the way the effect size, here $\Delta_{\text{Continuous}}$, there $\Delta_{\text{Categorical}}$, is obtained.

A simple formula for the calculation of the number of paired observations required for a two-sided significance level of 5% and power of 80%, is

$$N_{\text{Pairs}} = 2 + \frac{8}{\Delta_{\text{Continuous}}^2}. \tag{7.11}$$

An equivalent result for two-sided significance of 5% and 90% power is

$$N_{\text{Pairs}} = 2 + \frac{10.5}{\Delta_{\text{Continuous}}^2}. \tag{7.12}$$

Analysis of variance

For a 2×2 cross-over trial comparing two treatments A and B, patients will be randomised in equal numbers, $m \,(= N_{\text{Pairs}}/2)$ per sequence, between the two treatment sequences AB and BA. Treatment A will be given in the first period (Period I) of the design, then, usually after a washout period, B will be given in the Period II. Thus for patient i in sequence AB, the observation following treatment A belongs to Period I and is denoted x_{1Ai}, while that following B belongs to Period II and is denoted x_{2Bi}. Thus the difference $d_{1A2Bi} = x_{1Ai} - x_{2Bi}$ reflects a difference between A and B. Similarly for the sequence BA for patient j (say) we have $d_{1B2Aj} = x_{1Bj} - x_{2Aj}$ while the respective means are: $\bar{d}_{1A2B} = \bar{x}_{1A} - \bar{x}_{2B}$ and $\bar{d}_{1B2A} = \bar{x}_{1B} - \bar{x}_{2A}$. The corresponding estimate of δ, the effect of treatment, is,

$$\bar{d} = \frac{\bar{d}_{1B2A} - \bar{d}_{1A2B}}{2} = \frac{(\bar{x}_{1B} - \bar{x}_{2A}) - (\bar{x}_{1A} - \bar{x}_{2B})}{2} = \frac{(\bar{x}_{1B} + \bar{x}_{2B}) - (\bar{x}_{1A} + \bar{x}_{2A})}{2} \tag{7.14}$$

The analysis of variance (ANOVA) for a cross-over trial partitions the total variation into components due to treatment, period (each with 1 degree of freedom) and a within subjects (residual) term with $(N_{Pairs} - 2)$ degrees of freedom.

In some situations, the period effect is assumed negligible, see Senn (2002) for more details, in which case the ANOVA omits this calculation and the within subjects degrees of freedom becomes $(N_{Pairs} - 1)$. For design purposes however it is usual to assume there is a period effect.

Effect size
As for the general paired *t*-test, for the planned cross-over trial, the anticipated difference of means between treatments is denoted δ_{Plan}.

The planning within subject standard deviation
In the case of a cross-over trial, there are two observations taken from the experimental unit (a patient) and these are correlated to a degree determined by the magnitude of the Pearson correlation coefficient, ρ between the values of the outcome measure obtained on the two occasions. In this case it can be shown that $\sigma^2_{Within} = \sigma^2_{Total}(1 - \rho)$.

The correlation could be estimated if, for example, a baseline value was collected and then correlated with the post-treatment values of one of the treatment groups. Thus if a planning value of σ_{Total} is available and ρ can be anticipated, then these combined can provide a planning value for σ_{Within}.

Standardised effect size
The standard deviation corresponding to δ_{Plan} takes two forms depending on whether a period effect is allowed for or not. If no period effect is planned for then, $\sigma_{Plan} = \sqrt{2}\,\sigma_{Within}$ whereas if a period effect is anticipated, and is to be taken account of in the analysis, then $\sigma_{Plan} = \sigma_{Within}$. In both cases the standardized effect size is $\Delta = \delta_{Plan}/\sigma_{Plan}$.

Sample size
Assuming a period effect is anticipated, then ANOVA will be used for analysis, and for sample-size calculations purposes the anticipated standardised effect is

$$\Delta_{ANOVA} = \delta_{Plan}/\sigma_{Within}. \tag{7.15}$$

This is then used in Equation 7.10 to obtain the corresponding sample size N_{Pairs}.

Practice
Since the planning value used for σ_{Within} may depend on a choice of ρ, an exploratory approach to determining the chosen sample size is to try out various values of ρ to see what influence this will have on the proposed sample size.

For example, it is unlikely that ρ would be negative since paired studies are designed to exploit the positive association within pairs. Consequently, if we set $\rho = 0$ we obtain a conservative estimate of the required sample size. In this worst-case scenario, the sample size for the cross-over trial would be half that of the corresponding two-group trial. On the other hand, if one could be sure of a positive correlation, then the sample size would be smaller.

Cases (High out-of-hours)	Controls (Low out-of-hours attendance)		
	Single/divorced	Married/cohabiting	Total
Single/divorced	3	12	15
Married/cohabiting	1	24	25
Total	4	36	40

Figure 7.3 Case-control status by whether a child's mother was single/divorced or married/cohabiting (after Morrison, Gilmour and Sullivan 1991).

7.6 Bibliography

Connett, Smith and McHugh (1987) derived Equation 7.1 which they compared with the discordant pairs approach of Equations 7.2 and 7.3 derived by Schlesseman (1982). They concluded that their approach is 'preferable overall' but that Equation 7.3 is an adequate approximation provided the power is not too large or $\pi_{\text{Discordant}}$ not close to 0 or 1. Royston (1993) describes a modification to Equation 7.1 which requires an iterative procedure to obtain the corresponding sample size. Julious and Campbell (1998) discuss paired ordinal data, Julious (2004) discusses paired continuous data, while Julious, Campbell and Altman (1999) give some practical hints.

7.7 Examples and use of tables

Table 7.1 and Equations 7.1, 7.2 and 7.3

Example 7.1—paired binary data—case-control study
Using 40 case-control pairs, Morrison, Gilmour and Sullivan (1991) wished to identify the reasons why some children received more out-of-hours visits by general practitioners (GP) than others. The cases were children aged under 10 who were identified as high out-of-hours users and the controls, who were not high out-of-hours users, matched by age and gender. It was postulated that the marital status of the child's mother might be a determinant of referral and their data are summarized in **Figure 7.3**.

The estimated odds ratio for a single/divorced mother with respect to 'High out-of-hours visiting' as compared to the married/cohabiting mothers is, $\psi = 12/1 = 12$, which is large, and $\pi_{\text{Discordant}}$ is estimated as $(12 + 1)/40 = 0.325$.

Suppose a similar study is planned but in GP practices from another geographical area. However, the effect size for a single/divorced mothers compared to married/cohabiting is anticipated to be close to $\psi = 3$, much less than experienced previously. In addition, the research team expects that around 40% of cases will differ from their controls in terms of their out-of-hours utilisation. Thus the anticipated value of $\pi_{\text{Discordant}} = 0.4$.

> Using **Table 2.2** with a 5% two-sided test size, $\alpha = 0.05$ gives $z_{0.975} = 1.96$ and for a power of 90% a one-sided $1 - \beta = 0.90$ gives $z_{0.90} = 1.2816$.

From Equation 7.1, assuming a two-sided significance level of 5%, power 90%, $\psi = 3$ and $\pi_{\text{Discordant}} = 0.4$, the number of pairs required is

$$N_{\text{Pairs}} = \frac{\left(1.96 \times (3+1) + 1.2816\sqrt{[(3+1)^2 - (3-1)^2 \times 0.4]}\right)^2}{(3-1)^2 \times 0.4} = 100.9.$$

Utilising either **Table 7.1** with $\psi = 3$ and $\pi_{\text{Discordant}} = 0.4$, or $\boxed{^S S_S}$ with the same input values, gives $N_{\text{Pairs}} = 101$.

Alternatively from Equation 7.2, assuming a two-sided significance level of 5%, power 90% and $\psi = 3$, we anticipate that

$$N_{\text{Discordant}} = \frac{\left[1.96 \times (3+1) + 2 \times 1.2816 \times \sqrt{3}\right]^2}{(3-1)^2} = \frac{150.79}{4} = 37.7 \text{ or } 38 \text{ discordant pairs are}$$

required. With $N_{\text{Discordant}} = 38$ discordant case-control pairs necessary, the use of Equation 7.3 implies $N_{\text{Pairs}} = 38/0.4 = 95$ or approximately 100 pairs would be required. $\boxed{^S S_S}$ with the same input values gives $N_{\text{Discordant}} = 38$ and then with $\pi_{\text{Discordant}} = 0.4$ gives $N_{\text{Pairs}} = 101$.

Table 7.1 and Equation 7.1

Example 7.2—paired binary data—case-control study

Suppose the investigators of *Example 7.1* did not have a very clear view of the proportion of discordant pairs but believed for the marginal totals that about 10% of controls would be single/divorced mothers compared to 30% of cases. How many matched-pairs need to be recruited assuming again two-sided $\alpha = 0.05$, $1 - \beta = 0.9$?

> Using **Table 2.2** with a 5% two-sided test size, $\alpha = 0.05$ gives $z_{0.975} = 1.96$ and for a power of 90% a one-sided $1 - \beta = 0.90$ gives $z_{0.90} = 1.2816$.

Using the notation of **Figure 7.1** we have $\pi_A = 0.3$ and $\pi_B = 0.1$. Under the assumption of independence of response for each subject, we anticipates therefore, that $\dfrac{s}{N_{\text{Pairs}}} = \pi_A(1 - \pi_B)$ $= 0.3 \times 0.9 = 0.27$ and $\dfrac{t}{N_{\text{Pairs}}} = \pi_B(1 - \pi_A) = 0.1 \times 0.7 = 0.07$. These give $\pi_{\text{Discordant}} = 0.27 + 0.07 = 0.34$ and $\psi = 0.27/0.07 = 3.86$. Using either Equation 7.1 or $\boxed{^S S_S}$ with input values $\pi_{\text{Discordant}} = 0.34$ and $\psi = 3.86$, gives $N_{\text{Pairs}} = 86$.

However, a cautious investigator may also consider a reduced ψ of (say) 3.0 and values of $\pi_{\text{Discordant}}$ perhaps ranging from 0.3 to 0.4. These options suggest with **Table 7.1** or $\boxed{^S S_S}$ sample sizes of 136 and 80 respectively. Thus a sensible (compromise) sample size may be $N_{\text{Pairs}} = 100$.

C	GP more important than midwife		No difference	Midwife more important than GP		
	−2	−1	0	+1	+2	Total
Anticipated proportions	0.05	0.15	0.20	0.45	0.15	1
Discordant proportions						
ξ	0.0625	0.1875	–	0.5625	0.1875	1
$\xi \times c$	−0.1250	−0.1875	–	0.5625	0.3750	0.625
$\xi \times c^2$	0.2500	0.1875	–	0.5625	0.7500	1.75

(Discordant category spans the five category columns above)

Figure 7.4 The anticipated proportions of responses from trainee general Practitioners (TGPs) in the different categories.

Table 7.1, Equations 7.1 and 7.4

Example 7.3—paired binary data—multiple controls

Suppose a researcher wished to repeat the results of Morrison, Gilmour and Sullivan (1991) and believed that he would be able to obtain four controls for every case in the study. How does this affect the sample size if we presume, as in *Example 7.1*, that $\pi_{\text{Discordant}} = 0.4$ and $\psi = 3$?

In this case, use of Equation 7.1, **Table 7.1** or $^S S_S$ give $N_{\text{Equal}} = 101$ and so with $C = 4$, use of Equation 7.4 gives $N_{\text{Units}} = \dfrac{101 \times (1 + 4)}{2 \times 4} = 63.1 \approx 64$. This implies that $N_{\text{Cases}} = 64$ (1 per unit) and hence $N_{\text{Controls}} = C \times N_{\text{Cases}} = 4 \times 64 = 256$ controls (4 per unit). Thus the 64 units of size 5 imply $64 + 256 = 310$ mothers in total would be involved.

Table 7.2 and Equation 7.8

Example 7.4—paired ordered categorical data

Smith (1992) describes a survey in which 765 trainee general practitioners (TGP), ranked from 1 to 3 (unimportant, neutral, important), the importance of midwives and GPs in providing care during normal birth. Suppose a repeat study is planned and the endpoint is the difference in assessments allocated by each TGP, that is, the rank for midwife minus the rank given to the GP. For design purposes, the anticipated proportions in the five possible response categories are as given in **Figure 7.4**.

Assuming the two-sided test size is 5% and power 80%, how many responses from TGPs would be required from a new survey?

Using **Table 2.2** with a 5% two-sided test size, $\alpha = 0.05$ gives $z_{0.975} = 1.96$ and for a power of 80% a one-sided $1 - \beta = 0.80$ gives $z_{0.80} = 0.8416$. Additionally from **Table 2.3**, $\theta(0.05, 0.2) = 7.849$.

The calculations necessary to evaluate Equations 7.5 and 7.6 are summarised in **Figure 7.4** from which planning values of $\eta = 0.625$ and $\sigma_{\text{Discordant}} = \sqrt{1.75 - (0.625)^2} = 1.1659$ are obtained.

The corresponding standardised effect size of Equation 7.7 is $\Delta_{\text{Categorical}} = \dfrac{0.625}{1.166} = 0.5361$.

Finally use of Equation 7.8 gives $N_{\text{Pairs}} = \dfrac{7.849}{0.5361^2} + \dfrac{1.96^2}{2} = 29.2 \approx 30$ pairs. **Table 7.2** gives

for $\Delta_{\text{Categorical}} = 0.5, N_{\text{Pairs}} = 34$.

Alternatively, if we had ignored the ordinal nature of the data and simply taken the ratio of the proportion positive over the proportion negative in **Figure 7.4** we would

have $\psi = \dfrac{0.5625 + 0.1875}{0.0635 + 0.1875} = 3$. If we then use $\psi = 3$ in Equation 7.2 we obtain $N_{\text{Discordant}} =$

$\dfrac{\left(1.96 \times (3+1) + 2 \times 0.8416\sqrt{3}\right)^2}{(3-1)^2} = 28.9$ or approximately 30. Thus the two methods give

approximately the same sample size in this instance.

Table 7.2 and equation (7.10)

Example 7.5 Paired continuous data—Before and after study

Cruciani, Dvorkin, Homel *et al.* (2006) gave 27 patients with known carnitine deficiency a 1-week supplementation of L-Carnitine. They measured their baseline (pre) and post supplementation cartinine levels. Both measures were taken in all but one patient. On the basis of the difference between the logarithms of these matched measures the mean log carnitine value was raised by 0.4651 with a standard deviation of 0.4332.

If a repeat before-and-after study is planned how many patients would need to be recruited, assuming a two-sided test size of 5% and a power of 80%?

> Using **Table 2.3** with a 5% two-sided test size, $\alpha = 0.05$ and for a power of 80% a one-sided $1 - \beta = 0.80$ gives $\theta(0.05, 0.2) = 7.849$.

From the above, the design standardised effect size is $\Delta_{\text{Plan}} = 0.4651/0.4332 = 1.07 \approx 1$ which is a large effect size by the standards set by Cohen (1988). Using equation (7.10) directly, we

obtain $N_{\text{Pairs}} = \dfrac{7.849}{1^2} + \dfrac{1.96^2}{2} = 9.77$ or 10 patients.

A more cautious investigator may question the magnitude of the assumptions or perhaps wish to recruit patients with less evidence of carnitine deficiency. In which case different scenarios for a range of values for Δ_{Plan} would be investigated.

Thus, for the above test size and power and Δ_{Plan} equal to 0.4, 0.6 and 0.8, the corresponding sample sizes from **Table 7.2** are 51, 24 and 15. These can also be obtained from $\boxed{^{S}S_{S}}$ by setting $\delta = \Delta_{\text{Plan}}$ and $\sigma = 1$. With the original specification of $\delta = 0.4651$ and $\sigma_{\delta} = 0.4332$, $\boxed{^{S}S_{S}}$ gives $N_{\text{Pairs}} = 9$.

Table 7.2, Equations (7.10) and (7.12)

Example 7.6—paired continuous data—cross-over trial

Suppose we wished to design a placebo controlled cross-over trial of a possible new treatment (T) for refractory dyspnoea against a placebo (P). The primary outcome is to be morning dyspnoea scores as measure by visual analogue scale and an effect of interest is a reduction in this of 6 mm over placebo. We will design the new trial under the assumption of no carry-over effects. A similar trial had been conducted by Abernethy, Currrow, Frith *et al.* (2003) which has a reported standard deviation of the difference of 15.

For a 5% two-sided test size, $\alpha = 0.05$ and the value from **Table 2.2** is $z_{0.975} = 1.96$ and for a power of 90% a one-sided $1 - \beta = 0.90$ gives $z_{0.90} = 1.2816$. Additionally from **Table 2.3**, $\theta(0.05, 0.1) = 10.507$.

The standardised effect size is therefore 6/15 or 0.40. From Equation 7.10, for a two-sided significance level of 5% and 90% power, $N_{\text{Pairs}} = \dfrac{10.507}{0.4^2} + \dfrac{1.96^2}{2} = 67.6$ or 68 pairs. Direct use of **Table 7.2** or SS also gives the total sample size required as 68. Alternatively, using the simple formula Equation 7.12 gives $N = 2 + 10.5/(0.4^2) = 67.6$ or 34 patients on each sequence.

In a cross-over trial it is preferable to recruit an even number of subjects so that equal numbers can be allowed in each sequence, in this case, 34 would be randomised to receive the sequence PT and the same number TP.

7.8 References

Abernethy AP, Currow DC, Frith P, Fazekas BS, McHugh A and Bui C (2003). Randomised, double blind, placebo controlled crossover trial of sustained release morphine for the management of refractory dyspnoea. *British Medical Journal*, **327**, 523–528.

Cohen J (1988). *Statistical Power Analysis for the Behavioral Sciences*, 2nd edn. Lawrence Earlbaum, New Jersey.

Connett JE, Smith JA and McHugh RB (1987). Sample size and power for pair-matched case-control studies. *Statistics in Medicine*, **6**, 53–59.

Cruciani RA, Dvorkin E, Homel P, Malamud S, Culliney B, Lapin J, Portenoy RK and Esteban-Cruciani N (2006). Safety, tolerability and symptom outcomes associated with L-carnitine supplementation in patients with cancer, fatigue, and carnitine deficiency: a Phase I/II study. *Journal of Pain and Symptom Management*, **32**, 551–559.

Julious SA and Campbell MJ (1998). Sample sizes for paired or matched ordinal data. *Statistics in Medicine*, **17**, 1635–1642.

Julious SA, Campbell MJ and Altman DG (1999). Estimating sample sizes for continuous, binary and ordinal outcomes in paired comparisons: practical hints. *Journal of Biopharmaceutical Statistics*, **9**, 241–251.

Julious SA (2004). Sample sizes for clinical trials with Normal data. *Statistics in Medicine*, **23**, 1921–1986.

Morrison JM, Gilmour H and Sullivan F (1991). Children seen frequently out of hours in one general practice. *British Medical Journal*, **303**, 1111–1114.

Royston P (1993). Exact conditional and unconditional sample size for pair-matched studies with binary outcome: a practical guide. *Statistics in Medicine*, **12**, 699–712.

Schlesseman JJ (1982). *Case-control Studies*. Oxford University Press, Oxford.

Senn S (2002). *Cross-over Trials in Clinical Research*, 2nd edn. John Wiley & Sons, Chichester.

Smith LFP (1992). Roles, risks and responsibilities in maternal care: trainees' beliefs and the effects of practice obstetric training. *British Medical Journal*, **304**, 1613–1615.

Table 7.1 Sample sizes for paired binary data. Each cell gives the number of pairs of patients, N_{Pairs}, that should be entered into the study.

Odds Ratio	Two-sided $\alpha = 0.05$; Power $1 - \beta = 0.8$									
	Proportion of discordant pairs, π_D									
ψ	0.1	0.2	0.3	0.4	0.5	0.6	0.7	0.8	0.9	1
1.5	1960	979	652	489	391	325	278	243	216	194
1.6	1472	735	489	367	293	244	209	182	162	146
1.7	1166	582	387	290	232	193	165	144	128	115
1.8	960	479	319	239	190	158	135	118	105	94
1.9	813	406	270	202	161	134	115	100	89	80
2.0	705	351	234	175	139	116	99	86	77	69
2.1	622	310	206	154	123	102	87	76	67	60
2.2	556	277	184	138	110	91	78	68	60	54
2.3	504	251	167	125	99	82	70	61	54	49
2.4	461	230	152	114	91	75	64	56	50	44
2.5	425	212	141	105	84	69	59	51	46	41
3.0	312	155	103	77	61	50	43	37	33	29
4.0	216	107	71	53	42	34	29	25	22	20
5.0	175	86	57	42	33	27	23	20	18	16

Odds Ratio	Two-sided $\alpha = 0.05$; Power $1 - \beta = 0.9$									
	Proportion of discordant pairs, π_D									
ψ	0.1	0.2	0.3	0.4	0.5	0.6	0.7	0.8	0.9	1
1.5	2623	1310	872	653	522	434	372	325	288	259
1.6	1969	983	654	490	391	325	278	243	216	194
1.7	1560	778	517	387	309	257	220	192	170	153
1.8	1284	640	425	318	254	211	180	157	139	125
1.9	1087	542	360	269	215	178	152	133	118	105
2.0	942	469	312	233	185	154	131	114	101	91
2.1	831	414	274	205	163	135	116	101	89	80
2.2	744	370	245	183	146	121	103	90	79	71
2.3	673	335	222	166	132	109	93	81	71	64
2.4	616	306	203	151	120	100	85	74	65	58
2.5	568	282	187	139	111	92	78	68	60	53
3.0	417	206	136	101	80	66	56	49	43	38
4.0	288	142	94	69	55	45	38	33	29	25
5.0	233	114	75	55	43	36	30	26	22	20

Table 7.2 Sample sizes for paired continuous data with two-sided $\alpha = 0.05$. Each cell gives the number of pairs, N_{pairs}, of patients that should be entered into the study.

Standardised effect size	Power	
Δ	0.8	0.9
0.05	3142	4205
0.1	787	1053
0.15	351	469
0.2	199	265
0.25	128	171
0.3	90	119
0.35	66	88
0.4	51	68
0.45	41	54
0.5	34	44
0.55	28	37
0.6	24	32
0.65	21	27
0.7	18	24
0.75	16	21
0.8	15	19
0.85	13	17
0.9	12	15
0.95	11	14
1.0	10	13
1.1	9	11
1.2	8	10
1.3	7	9
1.4	6	8
1.5	6	7

Comparing survival curves

8

SUMMARY

The purpose of this chapter is to describe methods for calculating sample sizes for studies in which a survival time is the outcome event of primary concern and censored observations are probable. The main summary statistic utilised is the hazard ratio and the Logrank test is used to compare groups. We emphasise that it is the number of events observed, rather than the total number of subjects recruited, that is critical. Also included is the situation of competing risks in which, for example, the main event is time-to-death (index death) from a certain disease but other causes of death may intercede before the index death can occur. These prevent the index death time from ever being observed. Adjustment for these interceding events needs to be made when calculating the number of subjects to be recruited.

8.1 Introduction

There are many clinical trials in which patients are recruited and randomised to receive a particular treatment, then followed up until some critical event occurs. The length of follow-up for each patient is then used in comparing the efficacy of the two treatments by use of, so called survival techniques, in particular the Logrank test. The basic difference between this type of study and those described in **Chapter 3** is that, in the latter, success or failure of treatment is determined at some 'fixed' time, say 5 years, after randomisation. Whereas here, if patients with a particular cancer are recruited to a trial, one might record the individual survival experience of each patient rather than merely record how many are dead 5 years post-randomisation. The more detailed information will usually lead to a more sensitive comparison of the treatments.

If the endpoint of interest is a 'survival', then this may be the actual duration of time from the date of randomisation (to treatment) to the date of death of a cancer patient, or the time from hospital admission to some event such as contracting methicillin-resistant *Staphylococcus aureus* (MRSA) infection. In these cases, the 'events' are death and MRSA infection respectively. The number of subjects to be recruited to a study is set so that the requisite number of 'events' may be observed.

It should be emphasised that it is not essential in such studies that all patients are followed until the critical event occurs; indeed in many cancer trials some patients will survive for many years after randomisation, so observation of all their deaths would not be possible in a reasonable time-frame. It is usual, in such circumstances, to fix a date beyond which no

Sample Size Tables for Clinical Studies, 3rd edition. By David Machin, Michael J. Campbell, Say Beng Tan, and Sze Huey Tan. Published 2009 by Blackwell Publishing, ISBN: 978-1-4051-4650-0

further information is to be collected on any patient. Any patient still alive at that date will nevertheless be used in the treatment comparison. Such an observation is called 'censored'. For this reason in such trials, it is the number of events observed rather than the number of subjects recruited that is important.

For subjects in whom the 'events' occur, the actual survival time, t, is observed. The remainder of the subjects concerned have censored survival times, $T+$, as for them the 'event' has not (yet) occurred up to this point in their observation time. The eventual analysis of these data, which involves either t or $T+$ for every subject, will involve Kaplan–Meier estimates of the corresponding cumulative survival curves. Comparisons between groups can be made using the Logrank test and the summary statistic used is the hazard ratio (HR). Survival endpoints in the context of early (Phase II) trial designs are discussed in **Chapter 16**.

8.2 Theory and formulae

The hazard ratio (*HR*)

Suppose the critical event of interest is death and that two treatments give rise to survival distributions with instantaneous death rates, λ_1 and λ_2. The instantaneous death rate is the probability of death in a unit of time, and is often called the hazard. The ratio of the risks of death in the two groups is the hazard ratio (HR), that is,

$$HR = \frac{\lambda_2}{\lambda_1}. \tag{8.1}$$

Possible values of the HR range from 0 to ∞ with those < 1 corresponding to $\lambda_1 > \lambda_2$ and vice-versa for those > 1. The test of the null hypothesis of equality of event rates between the groups with respect to the endpoint event concerned provides the basis for the sample size calculations. This is expressed as $H_{\text{Null}} : HR = 1$.

In the situation where the survival can be assumed to follow an Exponential distribution, the relationships between the hazard rate, λ, the proportion alive, π, at a fixed point of time, T, and the median survival time, M, can be summarised by

$$\lambda = \frac{-\log \pi_T}{T} = \frac{-\log 0.5}{M}. \tag{8.2}$$

Then, if the two treatments give rise to survival proportions π_1 and π_2 at some chosen time-point, for example at 1-year after diagnosis,

$$HR = \frac{\log \pi_2}{\log \pi_1}. \tag{8.3}$$

In planning a study, therefore, it may be easier to provide anticipated values of π_1 and π_2, rather than λ_1 and λ_2 of Equation 8.1, and then use Equation 8.3 to obtain an anticipated HR. It is also useful to note that Equation 8.3 can be rearranged to give:

$$\pi_2 = \exp(HR \times \log \pi_1). \tag{8.4}$$

Thus, if the planning values of π_1 and HR are provided, an anticipated value of π_2 can be determined.

In other circumstances it may be easier to think of median survival times, in which case, if M_1 and M_2 are the anticipated median survival times for the two groups, then

$$HR = \frac{M_1}{M_2}. \tag{8.5}$$

Note that it is M_1 (not M_2) that is in the numerator. If the median survival time M_1 of one of the groups is given rather than a survival proportion at a fixed time then this implies that, at that time, $\pi_1 = 0.5$. Further if M_2 is given, then since $HR = M_1/M_2$, use of Equation 8.4, gives $\pi_2 = \exp(\log 0.5 \times HR) = \exp(-0.6932\, HR)$.

Equations 8.1, 8.3 and 8.5 are equivalent expressions for the HR at least in the circumstances where the hazards can be assumed to be proportional (PH). PH occurs when the instantaneous death rates within each group are constant over time or if they are not constant but their *ratio* remains so.

Events

A primary concern in any survival type study is the presence of censored observations whose presence implies that the reliability of a study does not depend on the total study size, N, but rather on the total number of events observed, E. This in turn implies, that a study should recruit the N subjects and then wait until the required E events are observed before conducting the analysis and reporting the results. In a study without censored survival times N and E will be equal but such a situation will not usually occur.

Logrank test

Number of events

If we assume that patients are to be entered into a clinical trial and randomised to receive one of two treatments in the ratio $1 : \varphi$, then for an anticipated HR the number of events to be observed in Group 1 that is required for a two-sided test size α and power $1 - \beta$ is approximately

$$e_1 = \frac{1}{(1+\varphi)\varphi} \left(\frac{1 + \varphi HR_{\text{Plan}}}{1 - HR_{\text{Plan}}} \right)^2 (z_{1-\alpha/2} + z_{1-\beta})^2. \tag{8.6}$$

For Group 2, $e_2 = \varphi e_1$ events giving a total of $E = e_1 + e_2$ for the study as a whole.

The equation can be evaluated by using **Table 2.3** which gives $\theta(\alpha, \beta) = (z_{1-\alpha/2} + z_{1-\beta})^2$ for different values of α and β.

Number of subjects

It should be noted that Equation 8.6 contains the effect size as expressed by the single summary HR_{Plan} and leads to the total number of events required. However, in order to calculate the number of subjects needed for this number of events to be observed, it is necessary to specify the anticipated values for π_1 and π_2.

The number of subjects required in order to observe the specified number of events for Group 1 is

$$m = \frac{1}{\varphi} \left(\frac{1 + \varphi HR_{\text{Plan}}}{1 - HR_{\text{Plan}}} \right)^2 \frac{(z_{1-\alpha/2} + z_{1-\beta})^2}{[(1 - \pi_1) + \varphi(1 - \pi_2)]}. \tag{8.7}$$

For Group 2, $n = \varphi m$, leading to $N = m + n = m(1 + \varphi)$ subjects in all.

Exponential survival

In certain situations, it is possible to postulate an Exponential distribution for the distribution of survival times. In which case the survivor function is given, see Equation 2.2, by

$$S(t) = \exp(-\lambda t), t \geq 0, \tag{8.8}$$

where λ is the constant hazard rate and therefore does not change with time, t. In this case the hazard λ and the median survival time M are related by

$$M = \log 2/\lambda. \tag{8.9}$$

This is the basis for Equation 8.5 above.

Number of events

If we assume that patients are to be entered into a clinical trial and randomised to receive one of two treatments in the ratio $1 : \varphi$ then, with anticipated HR_{Plan}, the number of events to be observed in Group 1 for a two-sided size α and power $1 - \beta$ is approximately

$$e_1 = \frac{2(z_{1-\alpha/2} + z_{1-\beta})^2}{\varphi(\log HR_{\text{Plan}})^2}. \tag{8.10}$$

For Group 2, $e_2 = \varphi e_1$ events giving a total of $E = e_1 + e_2$ for the trial as a whole.

Sample size

The number of subjects required in order to observe the specified number of events for Group 1 is

$$m = e_1 \times \frac{(1 + \varphi)}{[(1 - \pi_1) + \varphi(1 - \pi_2)]} = \frac{2(z_{1-\alpha/2} + z_{1-\beta})^2}{\varphi(\log HR_{\text{Plan}})^2} \frac{(1 + \varphi)}{[(1 - \pi_1) + \varphi(1 - \pi_2)]}. \tag{8.11}$$

For Group 2, $n = \varphi m$, leading to $N = m + n = m(1 + \varphi)$ subjects in all.

Equations 8.10 and 8.11 can be evaluated by using **Table 2.3** which gives $\theta(\alpha, \beta) = (z_{1-\alpha/2} + z_{1-\beta})^2$ for different values of α and β.

Study duration

We have noted earlier that it is the total number of events that determines the power of the study or equivalently the power of the subsequent Logrank test. For any study with a survival time endpoint there is clearly a period of accrual during which subjects are recruited to a study and a further period of follow-up beyond the end of accrual during which time more events are observed. To observe a pre-specified number of events we can either: (i) keep the accrual period as short as possible and extend follow-up; or (ii) have the accrual period as long as practicable and have a short post-recruitment follow-up; or (iii) achieve a balance between accrual and follow-up. The approach taken depends on the scarcity of subjects available for study, the event rate in the control arm and practical considerations, such as the costs of accrual and follow-up. For example, in rare diseases it may be considered best to minimise the number of patients required while maximising the follow-up period. Alternatively, in a more common disease it may be more appropriate to minimise the total study time, which comprises the sum of the accrual and follow-up periods.

In the case of $\varphi = 1$, one method of estimating the number of patients corresponding to the required number of events E is to assume that the number of patients who enter the trial in a given time period can be regarded as a Poisson random variable with average entry rate per unit of time R. If we define D as the duration of patient entry, after which patient recruitment is stopped and follow-up is closed, then this is determined by the solution of the following equation

$$\left(D - \frac{E}{R}\right)\left(\frac{1}{\lambda_1} + \frac{1}{\lambda_2}\right) - \frac{[1 - \exp(-\lambda_1 D)]}{\lambda_1^2} - \frac{[1 - \exp(-\lambda_2 D)]}{\lambda_2^2} = 0. \tag{8.12}$$

The median survival time, M_1, of control group C, is used as the unit of time for calculating both D and R. Since, for the Exponential distribution, $M = \log 2/\lambda$ then knowledge of M_1 and M_2 can be used to provide values for λ_1 and λ_2 for Equation 8.12.

There is no explicit solution to this equation and the value for D has to be found using an iterative method. Nevertheless, a lower limit for D is provided by

$$D_{\text{Lower}} = E/R. \tag{8.13}$$

Thus D will always be at least as large as D_{Lower}. Having calculated D from Equation 8.12 or 8.13 the number of subjects required is

$$N = RD. \tag{8.14}$$

Consequently the number per group is $m = n = N/2$.

Although this section specifically relates to comparisons of survival times both following the Exponential distribution the estimates can be used as approximations to other PH situations such as comparisons using the Logrank test. This is because λ_1 and λ_2 remain constant under the Exponential distribution, so their ratio has PH.

Loss to follow-up

One aspect of a study, which will affect the number of subjects recruited, is the anticipated proportion who are subsequently lost to follow-up. Since these subjects are lost, we will never observe and record the date of the critical event, even though it may have occurred. Such subjects have censored observations, in the same way as those for whom the event of interest has still not occurred by the time of analysis of the study. Such lost subjects however do not, and will never, contribute events for the analysis and, therefore, we need to compensate for their loss.

If the anticipated loss or withdrawal rate is w or $100w\%$, then the required number of patients, N, derived from either Equations 8.7 or 8.11 as appropriate should be increased to

$$N_{\text{Adjusted}} = N/(1 - w). \tag{8.15}$$

The estimated size of w can often be obtained from reports of studies conducted by others. If there is no such experience to hand, than a pragmatic value may be to take $w = 0.1$. We are assuming that the loss to follow-up is occurring at random and is not related to the current (perhaps health) status of the subject. If this cannot be assumed then the basis of the Logrank analysis is brought into question.

8.3 Competing risks

In certain types of study, there may be many alternative causes leading to the event of concern. For example, suppose a study is conducted in workers at a nuclear installation who are exposed to the risk of dying from leukaemia, which is the *main* risk. However, they may also die from *competing risks* (CR) such as accident, cardiovascular disease, diabetes, and so on. These causes can be regarded as all competing within each individual to be responsible for their ultimate death. Thus, in a sense, we can think of these causes all racing to be the first and hence to be 'the' cause of the death and thereby preventing the 'other' causes from being responsible. This implies that if the death is caused by a cardiovascular accident (CVA), then t_{CVA} is observed while, for example, t_{Accident}, t_{Cancer} and t_{Diabetes} will never be observed but have the corresponding censored survival times T^+_{Accident}, T^+_{Cancer}, and T^+_{Diabetes}, censored at t_{CVA}.

In the presence of CRs, the cumulative incidence method (CIM) estimates the cumulative probability for each cause of failure, in the presence of all risks acting on the index population.

Suppose in a clinical trial an intrauterine device (IUD) is to be used in a group of women for fertility regulation for 1 year and there are just two causes of failure, expulsions and removals for medical reasons. Thus in this period 'expulsion' and 'removal' are competing to be the first (failure) event to occur. Further suppose at time t in the trial an expulsion occurs, then its incidence is estimated as

$$I_{\text{Expulsion}}(t) = h_{\text{Expulsion}}(t) \times EFS(t\text{-}),$$

where $(t\text{-})$ is the time immediately preceding t. Here $EFS(t\text{-})$ is the Kaplan–Meier estimate of the event-free (neither expulsion nor removal) survival proportion and $h_{\text{Expulsion}}(t)$ is the risk of an expulsion. The risk of 'removal' as the competing failure to 'expulsion' is taken into account in the calculation of $EFS(t\text{-})$. Finally, the *CIM* at time t is

$$CIM_{\text{Expulsion}}(t) = \sum I_{\text{Expulsion}}(t).$$

Here the summation is over all previous failure times observed from the commencement of the trial. Similar calculations give $CIM_{\text{Removal}}(t)$. Whatever the number of competing events, the sum of all the *CIM*s equals $(1 - EFS)$. The necessary calculations can be made using, for example, Stata (StataCorp, 2007) as described by Coviello and Boggess (2004).

If we assume an Exponential survival distribution of survival times, then if no CRs are present, the cumulative incidence curve is given by

$$F(t) = 1 - \exp(-\lambda_{EV} t), \tag{8.16}$$

whereas in the presence of a CR, it becomes

$$F_{EV}(t) = \frac{\lambda_{EV}}{\lambda_{EV} + \lambda_{CR}} \{1 - \exp[-(\lambda_{EV} + \lambda_{CR})t]\}. \tag{8.17}$$

Here λ_{EV} and λ_{CR} are the hazards for the main outcome event and for the CRs respectively.

The corresponding cumulative incidence curve for the CR is

$$F_{CR}(t) = \frac{\lambda_{CR}}{\lambda_{EV} + \lambda_{CR}} \{1 - \exp[-(\lambda_{EV} + \lambda_{CR})t]\}. \tag{8.18}$$

It follows from Equations 8.17 and 8.18 that

$$\lambda_{EV} = F_{EV}(t) \times \frac{-\log[1 - F_{EV}(t) - F_{CR}(t)]}{t[F_{EV}(t) + F_{CR}(t)]} \tag{8.19}$$

and

$$\lambda_{CR} = F_{CR}(t) \times \frac{-\log[1 - F_{EV}(t) - F_{CR}(t)]}{t[F_{EV}(t) + F_{CR}(t)]}. \tag{8.20}$$

Sample size

To compare two groups with respect to the main event, the hazard ratio of interest is the ratio of the hazards for that event in the individual groups, that is $HR = \lambda_{EV,2} / \lambda_{EV,1}$ and a planning value for this is provided at the design stage.

The corresponding number of subjects to recruit when comparing two groups in the ratio $1 : \varphi$, with two-sided test size α and power $1 - \beta$ is given, using Equation 8.10, by

$$N = \frac{E}{P_{EV}} = \frac{2(1 + \varphi)(z_{1-\alpha/2} + z_{1-\beta})^2}{\varphi(\log HR)^2 P_{EV}}. \tag{8.21}$$

where E is the total number of events to be observed and

$$P_{EV} = \frac{\lambda_{EV}}{\lambda_{EV} + \lambda_{CR}} \times \left[1 - \frac{\exp[-f(\lambda_{EV} + \lambda_{CR})] - \exp[-(f + D)(\lambda_{EV} + \lambda_{CR})]}{D(\lambda_{EV} + \lambda_{CR})} \right]. \tag{8.22}$$

As previously defined, D is the accrual time while f is the extra follow-up time after ending accrual.

8.4 Bibliography

Theory, formulae and tables corresponding to Equations 8.10 and 8.12 are given by George and Desu (1974) while those for the calculation of sample sizes for the Logrank test were first given by Freedman (1982), who also gives guidelines for their use. Pintilie (2002) describes the adjustment to sample sizes necessary in the presence of competing risks. Ahn and Anderson (1995) discuss sample size determination for comparing more than two groups while Barthel, Babiker, Royston and Parmar (2006) additionally examine, and provide software for, the implications of non-uniform accrual, non-proportional hazards, loss to follow-up and dilution due to treatment changes including cross-over between treatment arms. Machin, Cheung and Parmar (2006) provide more details of both the Exponential distribution and the Logrank test.

8.5 Examples and use of the tables

Table 8.1 and Equation 8.6

Example 8.1 Logrank test—number of events
An adjuvant study of the drug Levamisole is proposed for patients with resectable cancer of the colon (Dukes' C). The primary objective of the study is to compare the efficacy of Levamisole against placebo control with respect to relapse-free survival. How many relapses need to be observed in the trial if a decrease in relapse rates at 1 year, from 50 to 40% is anticipated, and a power of 80% is required?

> Using **Table 2.2** with a 5% two-sided test size, $\alpha = 0.05$ gives $z_{0.975} = 1.96$ while for a power of 80%, one-sided $1 - \beta = 0.80$ and $z_{0.80} = 0.8416$. Direct use of **Table 2.3** gives $\theta(0.05, 0.2) = 7.849$.

Here we wish to increase the success rate, that is, failure to relapse, from 50 to 60%, so $\pi_1 = 0.5$, $\pi_2 = 0.6$ and so from Equation 8.3 $HR = \log 0.6 / \log 0.5 = 0.7369$. With $1 - \beta = 0.8$, assuming a two-sided test with $\alpha = 0.05$ and $\varphi = 1$, then Equation 8.6 gives

$$e_1 = \frac{1}{(1+1) \times 1} \left(\frac{1 + 1 \times 0.7369}{1 - 0.7369} \right)^2 \times 7.849 = 171.0 \text{ or } 172.$$ Thus a total of $E = 2 \times 172 = 344$

relapses would have to be observed. Alternatively this can be obtained directly from $^{S}S_{S}$ or from **Table 8.1** with $\pi_1 = 0.5$, $\pi_2 = 0.6$ to give $e_1 = 172$.

Table 8.2 and Equation 8.7

Example 8.2—Logrank test—sample size
The Multicenter Study Group (1980) describe a double-blind controlled study of long-term oral acetylcysteine against placebo in chronic bronchitis. Their results gave the percentage of exacerbation-free subjects with placebo at 6 months as 25%. They also observed a doubling of median exacerbation-free times with the active treatment. A repeat trial is planned. How many subjects should be recruited if the power is to be set at 90% and the two-sided test size at 5%?

> Using **Table 2.2** with a 5% two-sided test size, $\alpha = 0.05$ gives $z_{0.95} = 1.96$ while for a power of 90%, $1 - \beta = 0.90$ and $z_{0.90} = 1.2816$. Direct use of **Table 2.3** gives $\theta(0.05, 0.1) = 10.507$.

The doubling of the median time implies $M_2 = 2M_1$, hence from Equation 8.5 $HR_{Plan} = M_1/M_2 = 0.5$. Further $\pi_1 = 0.25$ and so Equation 8.4 gives $\pi_2 = \exp[0.5 \times (\log 0.25)] = 0.50$.

In addition, two-sided $\alpha = 0.05$, power $1 - \beta = 0.9$ and if we assume $\varphi = 1$, then Equation 8.7 gives $m = \dfrac{1}{1}\left(\dfrac{1 + 1 \times 0.5}{1 - 0.5}\right)^2 \times \dfrac{10.507}{[(1 - 0.25) + 1 \times (1 - 0.50)]} = 75.7$ or 76. Thus a total of $N = 2 \times 76 = 152$ or approximately 160 patients should therefore be recruited to the trial. Alternatively this can be obtained directly from $\boxed{^S S_S}$ or from **Table 8.2** with $\pi_1 = 0.25$, $\pi_2 = 0.5$ to give $N = 2 \times 77 = 154$.

Table 8.2, Equations 8.7 and 8.15

Example 8.3—differences in survival—withdrawals—gastric cancer
In the trial of Cuschieri, Weeden, Fielding *et al.* (1999), the investigators compared two forms of surgical resection for patients with gastric cancer and the anticipated 5-year survival rate of D_1 surgery was 20%, while an improvement in survival to 34% (14% change) with D_2 resection was anticipated. If it is assumed that there will be a 10% withdrawal of patients beyond the control of the investigator, how does this affect the planned trial size?

Using **Table 2.2** with a 5% two-sided test size, $\alpha = 0.05$ gives $z_{0.95} = 1.6449$ while for a power of 90% $1 - \beta = 0.90$, $z_{0.90} = 1.2816$. Direct use of **Table 2.3** gives $\theta(0.05, 0.1) = 10.507$.

Here $\pi_1 = 0.2$, $\pi_2 = 0.34$ and so from Equation 8.3 the anticipated $HR_{\text{Plan}} = \log 0.34 / \log 0.2 = 0.67$. The authors set $1 - \beta = 0.9$ and apply a two-sided test size $\alpha = 0.05$ and a randomisation in equal numbers to each group, hence $\varphi = 1$. Substituting all the corresponding values in Equation 8.7 gives $m = \left(\dfrac{1 + 0.67}{1 - 0.67}\right)^2 \times \dfrac{10.507}{[(1 - 0.2) + 1 \times (1 - 0.34)]} = 184.3 \approx 185$ per surgical group. This implies a trial including at least 370 patients. Alternatively this can be obtained directly from $\boxed{^S S_S}$ with $\pi_1 = 0.2$, $\pi_2 = 0.34$ to give $N = 370$ or from **Table 8.2** using $\pi_2 = 0.35$ rather than 0.34 to give $N = 2 \times 165 = 330$. Note that the change from the planning value of 0.34 to 0.35 has quite a considerable influence on the resulting sample size.

Allowing for a withdrawal rate of 10% or $w = 0.1$ and using Equation 8.15 we obtain $N_{\text{Adjusted}} = 370/0.9 = 412$. Thus a total of approximately 420 subjects should be recruited to the trial.

Table 8.2 and Equation 8.7

Example 8.4—cystic fibrosis
Suppose in a confirmatory trial of that reported by Valerius, Koch and Hoiby (1991), using the anti-pseudomonas therapy in patients with cystic fibrosis, the investigators had decided that, since the proposed therapy, T, is new and had an 85% response, they would like to gain some experience with the therapy itself whereas they are very familiar with the (no treatment) control option, C with 50% response. In such a situation it may be appropriate to randomise patients in a ratio of 2 : 3 in favour of the test treatment, that is, $\varphi = 3/2 = 1.5$. This implies 2 patients receive C for every 3 receiving T. In such circumstances it is usual to randomise patients in blocks of size, $b = 5$ (or size $2b$), each block containing 2 (or 4) C and 3 (or 6) T patients receiving the respective allocation.

Using **Table 2.2** with a 5% two-sided test size, $\alpha = 0.05$ gives $z_{0.95} = 1.96$ while for a power of 80%, $1 - \beta = 0.80$, $z_{0.80} = 0.8416$. Direct use of **Table 2.3** to give $\theta = 7.849$.

With $\alpha = 0.05$ and $1 - \beta = 0.8$ and substituting these together with $\varphi = 1.5$ and $HR = \dfrac{\log \pi_T}{\log \pi_C} = \dfrac{\log 0.85}{\log 0.5} = 0.2345$ in Equation 8.6 gives $e_C = \dfrac{1}{(1 + 1.5) \times 1.5} \left(\dfrac{1 + 1.5 \times 0.2345}{1 - 0.2345} \right)^2 \times 7.849$

$= 6.5 \approx 7$ events implying $E = 7 + 1.5 \times 7 \approx 18$ in total.

Substituting this in Equation 8.7 with $\pi_C = 0.50$ and $\pi_T = 0.85$ gives a total of

$$m = 7 \times \frac{(1 + 1.5)}{[(1 - 0.50) + 1.5 \times (1 - 0.85)]} = 7 \times 3.4483 = 24.1 \text{ or } 25, \text{ thus } N = 25 + 1.5 \times 25 = 62.5.$$

Rounding this to the nearest but larger integer divisible by the block size of five gives $N = 65$. Then, dividing these in a ratio of $2 : 3$, gives 26 to receive C and 39 T.

Alternatively this can be obtained directly from $^S\!S_S$ with $\pi_1 = 0.5$, $\pi_2 = 0.85$ and $\varphi = 1.5$ to give $E = 17$, $m = 26$ and $n = 38$. It is important to note that $^S\!S_S$ rounds numbers upwards at key stages to give integer values for the number of events and for the final group sizes.

Table 8.3, Equations 8.10 and 8.11

Example 8.5—exponential survival—number of events—duration of pyrexia

Two drugs, Ampicillin and Metronidazole are to be compared for their differing effects on the post-operative recovery of patients having an appendectomy as measured by duration of post-operative pyrexia. A previous trial of Chant, Turner and Machin (1983) suggested the median duration of pyrexia with Metronidazole to be approximately 80 hours. Duration of post-operative pyrexia is assumed to follow an exponential distribution. How many patients should be recruited to a trial to demonstrate a clinically worthwhile reduction of 15 hours in post-operative pyrexia by use of Ampicillin at two-sided test size $\alpha = 0.05$ and power $1 - \beta = 0.90$?

Using **Table 2.2** with a 5% two-sided test size, $\alpha = 0.05$ gives $z_{0.975} = 1.96$ while for a power of 90% $1 - \beta = 0.90$, $z_{0.90} = 1.2816$. Direct use of **Table 2.3** gives $\theta(0.05, 0.9) = 10.507$.

Here $M_1 = 80$, $M_2 = 80 - 15 = 65$ and $HR_{Plan} = 80/65 = 1.23$, with two-sided $\alpha = 0.05$, $1 - \beta = 0.90$

and $\varphi = 1$. Equation 8.10 then gives $e_1 = \dfrac{2 \times 10.507}{1 \times (\log 1.23)^2} = 490.4$. Thus the total number of

events to be observed is $E = 2e_1 = 982$.

To obtain the sample size, the corresponding proportions π_1 and π_2 have to be provided. The median time of 80 hours for the control group corresponds to $\pi_1 = 0.5$. Thus, from Equation 8.4, $\pi_2 = \exp(1.23 \times \log 0.5) = 0.426$ or 0.43 and use of Equation 8.11 with these values gives $m = 916.6 \approx 950$ or a total sample size of $N = 1900$.

Calculations using $^S\!S_S$ with $M_1 = 80$, $M_2 = 65$ (implying $\pi_1 = 0.5$ and $\pi_2 = 0.569$) and an entry rate of $R = 1$ (in this case 1 patient every 80 hours) gives $E = 975$ events for a total sample size of $N = 2 \times 541 = 1082$ or approximately 1100 patients with the trial schedule to continue for 1080.7/24 = 45 days. Increasing the entry rate to $R = 5$ decreases the number to recruit to $N = 294$ but the trial can be closed (and analysed) by 294.9/24 = 12 days!

It should be noted that such a trial does not require prolonged follow up of patients as the event of interest, that is, return to normal temperature, will be observed in almost all patients. There will also be very few patient losses as the follow-up time is only a few days and the patients are hospitalised during this period.

Table 8.3, Equations 8.10, 8.13 and 8.15

Example 8.6—exponential survival—recruitment period—sample size
In the study described in *Example 8.1*, assuming relapse times have an exponential distribution, how many relapses need to be observed in the trial if it is anticipated that the median relapse free time is likely to be increased from 1 to 1.3 years. Suppose that a two-sided test size of 5% and a power of 80% are required, and it is anticipated that the recruitment rate will be approximately 80 patients per year. For what period should the trial be conducted and how many patients should be recruited?

> Using **Table 2.2** with a 5% two-sided test size, $\alpha = 0.05$ gives $z_{0.975} = 1.96$ while for a power of 80% a one-sided $1 - \beta = 0.80$, $z_{0.80} = 0.8416$. Direct use of **Table 2.3** gives $\theta(0.05, 0.2) = 7.849$.

Here $M_1 = 1$, $M_2 = 1.3$ and therefore the anticipated $HR = 1 \,/\, 1.3 = 0.77$. Now with the two-sided $\alpha = 0.05$ and $1 - \beta = 0.8$, Equation 8.10 gives $e_1 = \dfrac{2 \times 7.849}{1 \times (\log 0.77)^2} = 229.8 \approx 230$.

Thus a total of $E = 2e_1 = 460$ relapses would need to be observed.

Since **Table 8.3** only gives the total number of events for situations when $HR > 1$, in situations where $HR_{Plan} < 1$ the inverse should be entered in its place. Thus the value to be entered in **Table 8.3** is $1/0.77 = 1.3$ giving $E = 457$ events required.

Thus with entry rate $R = 80$ patients per M_1 of time (in this case per year), the total duration of the trial from Equation 8.13 is as $D_{Lower} = 460/80 = 5.75$ time units or years.

A lower limit to the total number of subjects required is obtained from Equation 8.14, with $D = D_{Lower}$, as $N_{Lower} = 80 \times 5.75 = 460$ or approximately 500 patients would need to be recruited to the trial.

In contrast, calculations using $\boxed{SS}$ give $D = 7.4$ (> 5.75) and so from Equation 8.14 a more realistic estimate of the required total sample size is $N = 7.4 \times 80 = 592.0$ or 600 patients.

Equations 8.16, 8.17 and 8.18

Example 8.7—competing risks—myocardial infarction in breast cancer survivors
Pintille (2002) alludes to a clinical trial in which the main question was to investigate whether the incidence of myocardial infraction (MI) in survivors of breast cancer was affected by tangential radiation treatment which was known to irradiate the heart when given to the left (Left) breast but not to the right (Right). In the population of women considered, the probability of CRs is large since only a small minority will live long enough to experience MI.

It was anticipated that the incidence of MI is 1.5% at 10 years for patients treated on the right side and double this for those treated on the left. The incidence of CR was considered equal for both as 68% at 10 years. Assuming a two-sided test size of 5% and power 80% how many breast cancer patients would be needed for such a study? Accrual was anticipated to take 9 years with an additional 10 years of follow up.

> Using **Table 2.2** with a 5% two-sided test size, $\alpha = 0.05$ gives $z_{0.975} = 1.96$ while for a power of 80% a one-sided $1 - \beta = 0.80$, $z_{0.80} = 0.8416$. Direct use of **Table 2.3** to gives $\theta = 7.849$.

For Right the anticipated cumulative incidence for MI is $F_{Right,MI}(10) = 0.015$ and for the CR $F_{Right,CR}(10) = 0.68$. Thus from Equations 8.19 and 8.20, at $t = 10$ years, $\lambda_{Right,EV} = 0.015 \times$ $\dfrac{-\log[1 - 0.015 - 0.68]}{10 \times [0.015 + 0.68]} = 0.00256$ and $\lambda_{Right,CR} = 0.11618$. The corresponding values for Left are $F_{Left,MI}(10) = 0.03$ and $F_{Left,CR} = 0.68$ giving $\lambda_{Left,EV} = 0.00523$ and $\lambda_{Left,CR} = 0.11856$.

These give the planning hazard ratio for MI as $HR_{Plan,MI} = \lambda_{Right,MI}/\lambda_{Left,MI} = 0.00256/0.00523 = 0.49$ or approximately 0.5.

Further $D = 9$ and $f = 10$ years so that from Equation 8.22 $P_{Right,MI} = \dfrac{0.00256}{0.00256 + 0.00512} \times$
$\left[1 - \dfrac{\exp[-10 \times (0.00256 + 0.00512)] - \exp[-(10 + 9)(0.00256 + 0.00512)]}{9 \times (0.00256 + 0.00512)} \right] = 0.01754$ and similarly $P_{Left,MI} = 0.03486$. Thus the mean event rate, $P_{Event} = (0.01754 + 0.03486)/2 = 0.02620$ and so from one component of Equation 8.21, $E = \dfrac{2 \times (1 + 1) \times 7.849}{1 \times (\log 0.5)^2} = 65.3$ or a total of 66 events from both breast groups. Thus $N = 66/0.02620 = 2519.1$ or approximately 2600 women would need to be recruited, or 1300 radiated to the Right and 1300 to the Left breast.

Alternatively use of $^{S}S_{S}$ with two-sided $\alpha = 0.05$, $1 - \beta = 0.8$, and the anticipated values summarized below give the required number of events $E = 62$, and $N = 2367$. So a study of 2500 women might be contemplated.

Time of interest	t	10 years
Main event	$F_{Right,MI}(t)$	0.015
	$FL_{Left,MI}(t)$	0.03
Competing risk	$F_{Right,CR}(t)$	0.68
	$F_{Left,CR}(t)$	0.68
Accrual time	D	9 years
Follow-up	f	10 years

The discrepancy arises as $^{S}S_{S}$ uses the calculated $HR_{Plan,MI} = 0.49$, which is more extreme than the rounded 0.5, and so the number of events required and consequently the sample size are reduced.

8.6 References

Ahnn S and Anderson SJ (1995). Sample size determination for comparing more than two survival distributions. *Statistics in Medicine*, **14**, 2273–2282.

Barthel FM-S, Babiker A, Royston P and Parmar MKB (2006). Evaluation of sample size and power for multi-arm survival trials allowing for non-uniform accrual, non-proportional hazards, loss to follow-up and cross-over. *Statistics in Medicine*, **25**, 2521–2542.

Chant ADB, Turner DTL and Machin D (1983). Metronidazole v Ampicillin: differing effects on the post-operative recovery. *Annals of the Royal College of Surgeons of England*, **66**, 96–97.

Coviello V and Boggess M (2004). Cumulative incidence estimation in the presence of competing risks. *The Stata Journal*, **4**, 103–112.

Cuschieri A, Weeden S, Fielding J, Bancewicz J, Craven J, Joypaul V, Sydes M and Fayers P (1999). Patient survival after D_1 and D_2 resections for gastric cancer: long-term results of the MRC randomized surgical trial. *British Journal of Cancer*, **79**, 1522–1530.

Freedman LS (1982). Tables of the number of patients required in clinical trials using the logrank test. *Statistics in Medicine*, **1**, 121–129.

George SL and Desu MM (1974). Planning the size and duration of a clinical trial studying the time to some critical event. *Journal of Chronic Diseases*, **27**, 15–24.

Machin D, Cheung Y-B and Parmar MKB (2006). *Survival Analysis: A Practical Approach*, 2nd edn. John Wiley & Sons, Chichester.

Multicenter Study Group (1980). Long-term oral acetycysteine in chronic bronchitis. A double-blind controlled study. *European Journal of Respiratory Diseases*, **61** (Suppl.111), 93–108.

Pintilie M (2002). Dealing with competing risks: testing covariates and calculating sample size. *Statistics in Medicine*, **21**, 3317–3324.

StataCorp (2007). *Stata Statistical Software: Release 10*. College Station, TX.

Valerius NH, Koch C and Hoiby N (1991). Prevention of chronic *Pseudomonas aeruginosa* colonisation in cystic fibrosis by early treatment. *Lancet*, **338**, 725–726.

Table 8.1 Number of critical events for comparison of survival rates (Logrank test). Each cell gives the number of events for each group, e_1. Hence, the total number of events for the study is $E = 2e_1$.

π_2	Two-sided $\alpha = 0.05$; Power $1 - \beta = 0.8$ First proportion, π_1									
	0.05	0.1	0.15	0.2	0.25	0.3	0.35	0.4	0.45	0.5
0.1	230	–	–	–	–	–	–	–	–	–
0.15	78	422	–	–	–	–	–	–	–	–
0.2	44	126	584	–	–	–	–	–	–	–
0.25	30	64	163	708	–	–	–	–	–	–
0.3	22	40	79	189	793	–	–	–	–	–
0.35	17	29	48	89	206	839	–	–	–	–
0.4	14	22	33	53	95	214	851	–	–	–
0.45	12	17	24	35	55	96	213	832	–	–
0.5	11	14	19	25	36	55	94	205	787	–
0.55	9	12	15	19	25	35	53	89	191	721
0.6	8	10	12	15	19	25	33	49	82	172
0.65	8	9	10	12	15	18	23	31	44	73
0.7	7	8	9	10	12	14	17	21	27	39
0.75	6	7	8	9	10	11	13	15	18	23
0.8	6	6	7	7	8	9	10	11	13	15
0.85	5	6	6	6	7	7	8	9	9	11
0.9	5	5	5	6	6	6	6	7	7	8
0.95	5	5	5	5	5	5	5	5	6	6

π_2	Two-sided $\alpha = 0.05$; Power $1 - \beta = 0.8$ First proportion, π_1								
	0.5	0.55	0.6	0.65	0.7	0.75	0.8	0.85	0.9
0.55	721	–	–	–	–	–	–	–	–
0.6	172	638	–	–	–	–	–	–	–
0.65	73	149	544	–	–	–	–	–	–
0.7	39	62	125	444	–	–	–	–	–
0.75	23	32	51	99	343	–	–	–	–
0.8	15	19	26	39	74	246	–	–	–
0.85	11	12	15	20	29	51	159	–	–
0.9	8	9	10	11	14	19	31	87	–
0.95	6	6	6	7	8	9	11	15	33

Table 8.1 (*continued*): Number of critical events for comparison of survival rates (Logrank test). Each cell gives the number of events for each group, e_1. Hence, the total number of events for the study is $E = 2e_1$.

	Two-sided $\alpha = 0.05$; Power $1 - \beta = 0.9$									
	First proportion, π_1									
π_2	0.05	0.1	0.15	0.2	0.25	0.3	0.35	0.4	0.45	0.5
0.1	307	–	–	–	–	–	–	–	–	–
0.15	105	564	–	–	–	–	–	–	–	–
0.2	58	168	781	–	–	–	–	–	–	–
0.25	39	86	218	947	–	–	–	–	–	–
0.3	29	54	106	253	1061	–	–	–	–	–
0.35	23	38	64	119	276	1124	–	–	–	–
0.4	19	29	44	70	127	286	1139	–	–	–
0.45	16	23	32	47	73	129	285	1114	–	–
0.5	14	19	25	34	48	73	126	274	1054	–
0.55	12	16	20	26	34	47	70	119	255	964
0.6	11	13	16	20	25	33	45	66	109	230
0.65	10	12	14	16	19	24	31	41	59	97
0.7	9	10	12	13	16	18	22	28	36	52
0.75	8	9	10	11	13	14	17	20	24	31
0.8	8	8	9	10	11	12	13	15	17	20
0.85	7	7	8	8	9	10	10	11	12	14
0.9	7	7	7	7	8	8	8	9	9	10
0.95	6	6	6	6	7	7	7	7	7	8

	Two-sided $\alpha = 0.05$; Power $1 - \beta = 0.9$								
	First proportion, π_1								
π_2	0.5	0.55	0.6	0.65	0.7	0.75	0.8	0.85	0.9
0.55	964	–	–	–	–	–	–	–	–
0.6	230	853	–	–	–	–	–	–	–
0.65	97	200	728	–	–	–	–	–	–
0.7	52	83	167	594	–	–	–	–	–
0.75	31	43	68	133	459	–	–	–	–
0.8	20	26	35	53	100	330	–	–	–
0.85	14	17	20	26	38	68	213	–	–
0.9	10	11	13	15	18	25	41	116	–
0.95	8	8	8	9	10	11	14	20	45

Table 8.2 Number of subjects for comparison of survival rates (Logrank test). Each cell gives the number of subjects for each group, m. Hence, the total sample size for the study is $N = 2m$.

π_2	\multicolumn{10}{c	}{Two-sided $\alpha = 0.05$; Power $1 - \beta = 0.8$}

	\multicolumn{10}{c	}{First proportion, π_1}
π_2	0.05	0.1	0.15	0.2	0.25	0.3	0.35	0.4	0.45	0.5
0.1	249	–	–	–	–	–	–	–	–	–
0.15	87	483	–	–	–	–	–	–	–	–
0.2	51	149	708	–	–	–	–	–	–	–
0.25	36	78	204	914	–	–	–	–	–	–
0.3	27	51	102	253	1094	–	–	–	–	–
0.35	22	38	64	123	295	1243	–	–	–	–
0.4	19	30	46	76	141	330	1362	–	–	–
0.45	16	24	35	52	85	154	355	1447	–	–
0.5	16	21	29	39	58	92	164	373	1500	–
0.55	13	18	24	31	42	61	97	170	382	1518
0.6	12	16	20	26	34	46	63	99	173	383
0.65	13	15	17	21	28	35	46	66	98	172
0.7	12	14	16	19	23	28	36	47	64	98
0.75	11	13	15	18	20	24	29	36	45	62
0.8	11	11	14	15	17	21	24	28	35	43
0.85	10	12	13	13	16	17	21	25	26	34
0.9	10	10	11	14	15	15	16	20	22	27
0.95	10	11	12	12	13	14	15	16	20	22

π_2	\multicolumn{9}{c	}{Two-sided $\alpha = 0.05$; Power $1 - \beta = 0.8$}

	\multicolumn{9}{c	}{First proportion, π_1}
π_2	0.5	0.55	0.6	0.65	0.7	0.75	0.8	0.85	0.9
0.55	1518	–	–	–	–	–	–	–	–
0.6	383	1502	–	–	–	–	–	–	–
0.65	172	373	1451	–	–	–	–	–	–
0.7	98	166	358	1367	–	–	–	–	–
0.75	62	92	157	330	1248	–	–	–	–
0.8	43	59	87	142	296	1094	–	–	–
0.85	34	41	55	80	129	256	909	–	–
0.9	27	33	40	49	70	109	207	696	–
0.95	22	24	27	35	46	60	88	151	440

Table 8.2 (*continued*): Number of subjects for comparison of survival rates (Logrank test). Each cell gives the number of subjects for each group, *m*. Hence, the total sample size for the study is $N = 2m$.

	Two-sided $\alpha = 0.05$; Power $1 - \beta = 0.9$									
	First proportion, π_1									
π_2	0.05	0.1	0.15	0.2	0.25	0.3	0.35	0.4	0.45	0.5
0.1	332	–	–	–	–	–	–	–	–	–
0.15	117	645	–	–	–	–	–	–	–	–
0.2	67	198	947	–	–	–	–	–	–	–
0.25	46	105	273	1222	–	–	–	–	–	–
0.3	36	68	137	338	1464	–	–	–	–	–
0.35	29	50	86	165	395	1666	–	–	–	–
0.4	25	39	61	101	189	441	1823	–	–	–
0.45	22	32	46	70	113	207	475	1938	–	–
0.5	20	28	38	53	77	122	220	499	2008	–
0.55	18	24	31	42	57	82	128	227	510	2030
0.6	17	21	26	34	44	61	86	133	230	512
0.65	16	20	24	28	35	46	62	87	132	229
0.7	15	17	21	24	31	36	47	63	85	130
0.75	14	16	19	21	26	30	38	48	60	83
0.8	14	15	18	21	24	27	31	38	46	58
0.85	13	14	17	17	21	24	26	30	35	44
0.9	14	14	15	16	19	20	22	26	28	34
0.95	12	13	14	15	18	19	20	22	24	30

	Two-sided $\alpha = 0.05$; Power $1 - \beta = 0.9$								
	First proportion, π_1								
π_2	0.5	0.55	0.6	0.65	0.7	0.75	0.8	0.85	0.9
0.55	2030	–	–	–	–	–	–	–	–
0.6	512	2008	–	–	–	–	–	–	–
0.65	229	500	1942	–	–	–	–	–	–
0.7	130	222	478	1828	–	–	–	–	–
0.75	83	123	210	444	1670	–	–	–	–
0.8	58	81	117	193	400	1467	–	–	–
0.85	44	57	73	104	169	341	1218	–	–
0.9	34	40	52	67	90	143	274	928	–
0.95	30	32	36	45	58	74	112	201	600

Table 8.3 Number of critical events for comparison of two exponential survival distributions with two-sided $\alpha = 0.05$. Each cell gives the total number of events for the comparison of two exponential survival distributions.

	Power $1 - \beta$	
HR	0.8	0.9
1.1	3457	4627
1.2	945	1265
1.3	457	611
1.4	278	372
1.5	191	256
1.6	143	191
1.7	112	150
1.8	91	122
1.9	77	103
2	66	88
2.1	58	77
2.2	51	68
2.3	46	61
2.4	41	55
2.5	38	51
2.6	35	47
2.7	32	43
2.8	30	40
2.9	28	38
3	27	35
3.5	21	27
4	17	22
4.5	14	19
5	13	17

Equivalence

9

SUMMARY

In previous chapters we have been concerned with situations that, if the null hypothesis is rejected in a two-group clinical trial, then superiority is claimed for one of the groups. Here we are concerned with situations in which we may wish to claim equivalence (embracing both therapeutic equivalence of the alternatives as well as non-inferiority of a test against a standard) of the two treatments and not superiority. In these situations, if the difference between groups is less than a certain magnitude it may be inferred that one group is effectively as good as the other. We discuss the concept of bioequivalence which is of particular relevance at the early development stage of a new therapy.

9.1 Introduction

Implicit in a comparison between two groups is the presumption that if the null hypothesis is rejected then a difference between the groups being compared is claimed. Thus, if this comparison involves two treatments for a particular condition, the conclusion drawn by rejecting the null hypothesis is that one treatment is superior to the other irrespective of the magnitude or clinical relevance of the difference observed. For this reason, they are termed 'Superiority' trials. However in some situations, a new therapy may bring certain advantages over the current standard, possibly in a reduced side-effects profile, easier administration or lower cost but it may not be anticipated to be better with respect to the primary efficacy variable. Under such conditions, the new approach may be required to be at least 'equivalent', or more usually 'non-inferior', to the standard in relation to efficacy if it is to replace it in future clinical use. This implies that 'equivalence' is a pre-specified maximum difference between two groups which if observed to be less, after the clinical trial is conducted, would render the two groups equivalent. The implication being that the test could replace the standard for routine clinical use. It is important to emphasize that failure to find a statistically significant difference after conducting a superiority trial, does not mean that two treatments are equivalent but rather that there is insufficient evidence to distinguish between them.

In designing an equivalence trial, the 'effect size' of a superiority trial is replaced by the 'equivalence limit'.

In this chapter, we use the term 'equivalence' to include studies which aim to show that two compounds are bioequivalent, two treatments are therapeutically equivalent, and that one treatment is not inferior to the other (non-inferiority).

Sample Size Tables for Clinical Studies, 3rd edition. By David Machin, Michael J. Campbell, Say Beng Tan, and Sze Huey Tan. Published 2009 by Blackwell Publishing, ISBN: 978-1-4051-4650-0

9.2 Theory and formulae

Confidence intervals

In general, having conducted a study to compare groups with respect to a particular outcome, the investigator calculates the observed difference between groups, d, and the corresponding $100(1 - \alpha)\%$ confidence interval (CI) for the true difference, δ, between them. This CI covers the true difference, δ, with a given probability, $1 - \alpha$. The difference may result from a comparison of means, proportions or hazard rates depending on the context.

The concept of equivalence is illustrated in **Figure 9.1** by considering the range of options possible for the confidence intervals that might result at the end of a trial comparing a Test with a Standard approach to treatment. The 'equivalence' limit, ε, is set above and below $\delta = 0$ which corresponds to the null hypothesis of no true difference between treatments. These limits therefore define a region within which, if d were to fall, then this would be indicative of equivalence—the Test could replace the Standard—but outside of which would be regarded as a clinically important divergence from equivalence—the Test would not replace the Standard.

If we examine the confidence intervals of **Figure 9.1,** then CI: A, clearly demonstrates an important difference between groups since even the lower limit of this confidence interval is beyond $+\varepsilon$. If a confidence interval crosses a boundary (CI: B and F) then one would be uncertain as to whether or not the treatments were equivalent, whereas if it were totally between the limits $-\varepsilon$ to $+\varepsilon$ (CI: C, D, E) then equivalence would be claimed. The uncertain outcome of CI: H would correspond to a trial of inadequate sample size, as the confidence interval is so wide.

It is quite possible to show a statistically significant difference between two treatments yet also demonstrate therapeutic equivalence (CI: C and E: neither cut the vertical line through the null hypothesis value of $\delta = 0$ nor the $\delta = -\varepsilon$ or $+\varepsilon$ lines). These are not contradictory statements but simply a realisation that although there is evidence that one treatment works better than another, the size of the benefit is so small that it has little or no practical advantage.

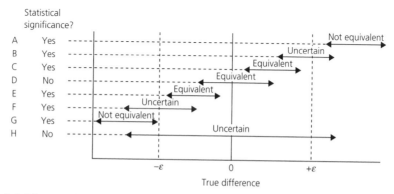

Figure 9.1 Schematic diagram to illustrate the concept of equivalence by using a series of possible comparative trial outcomes of a Test against a Standard therapy as summarised by their reported (two-sided) confidence intervals (after Jones, Jarvis, Lewis and Ebbutt 1996).

Associated hypotheses

When comparing two means, proportions or hazards in the *superiority* context of earlier chapters, we specified the null hypothesis by $H_{\text{Null}}: \delta = \mu_1 - \mu_2 = 0$, $\delta = \pi_1 - \pi_2 = 0$ or $\delta = \lambda_1 - \lambda_2 = 0$ as appropriate. Thus, in the conventional test of statistical significance, we seek to test if $\delta = 0$, using the test statistic of the form:

$$z = \frac{d}{SE_0(d)}. \qquad (9.1)$$

where the observed difference between treatments, d, is the estimate of δ and $SE_0(d)$ is the corresponding standard error estimated as if the null hypothesis were true. Essentially we commence by assuming the two groups are the *same* and seek to demonstrate they are *different*.

However in the case of an equivalence trial the null hypothesis H_{Null} has two components of non-equivalence that is: $\delta \leq -\varepsilon$ and $\delta \geq \varepsilon$, whereas the alternative hypothesis of equivalence H_{Alt} is: $-\varepsilon < \delta < \varepsilon$ (equivalence). Here we commence by assuming the two groups are *different* and seek to demonstrate they are the *same*.

These hypotheses lead to a change in the test statistic of Equation 9.1 to a test statistic of the form

$$z_{\text{Equivalence}} = \frac{|d| - \varepsilon}{SE_{\text{NE}}(d)}, \qquad (9.2)$$

where $SE_{\text{NE}}(d)$ is now calculated under the *modified* null hypothesis of non-equivalence (NE). In this situation, if the test statistic is significant we conclude that the treatments are equivalent.

9.3 Bioequivalence

Often as a drug or vaccine is developed for clinical use small adjustments are necessary to their formulation, for example, a change in formulation from that used in early phase trials to one more suitable for routine clinical use. Thus, although these may be minor changes, they may require appropriate investigation to assess whether the new formulation is indeed equivalent to the old. This assessment is done by examination of the pharmacokinetics of the two formulations with the assumption that if there are equal pharmacokinetic properties then this implies equal clinical effect in terms of both safety and efficacy.

Cross-over design

Bioequivalence of different formulations of the same drug is usually taken to mean equivalence with respect to rate and extent of drug absorption. The area under the concentration/time curve, AUC, serves to measure the extent of absorption whereas, in the case of fast-releasing formulations, the maximum concentration, C_{max}, and the time of its occurrence, t_{max}, may characterise the rate of absorption.

For many drug substances, a large between-subject variation is known to exist and so cross-over designs are recommended for bioequivalence studies. It is usual to employ a balanced two-period design as described by Machin and Campbell (2005). In such a cross-over trial, if a test (T) formulation is to be compared with a reference (R) formulation, then the subjects

Type of trial	Hypotheses		Error		Confidence interval
	Null	Alternative	Type I α	Type II β	
Superiority	$\delta = 0$	$\delta \neq 0$ Superiority	2-sided	1-sided	2-sided
Usual			5%	10 or 20%	95%
Bioequivalence	$\delta \leq -\varepsilon$ or $\delta \geq \varepsilon$ Not bioequivalent	$-\varepsilon < \delta < \varepsilon$ Bioequivalent	1-sided	2-sided	2-sided
FDA recommended			5%	20%	90%
Equivalence	$\delta \leq -\varepsilon$ or $\delta \geq \varepsilon$ Not equivalent	$-\varepsilon < \delta < \varepsilon$ Equivalent	1-sided	2-sided	2-sided
Usual			2.5%	10 or 20%	95%
Non-inferiority	$\delta \geq \varepsilon$ Inferiority	$\delta < \varepsilon$ Non-inferiority	1-sided	1-sided	1-sided
Usual			2.5%	10 or 20%	97.5%

Figure 9.2 Comparison of hypotheses tested in two group trials of superiority, bioequivalence, equivalence and non-inferiority comparing a test (T) with a standard (S), $\delta = \theta_{Test} - \theta_{Standard}$.

will usually be randomised equally between the two sequences TR and RT, that is, m subjects per sequence.

Food and Drug Administration (FDA) recommendations

In the context of bioequivalence, β, which is the probability of erroneously concluding bio-inequivalence, is often called the 'producer risk', while α, which is the probability of erroneously accepting bioequivalence, is termed the 'consumer risk'. Because small trials, which are in routine use in bioequivalence studies, have a low power to detect differences, large and perhaps clinically important differences would not be statistically significant following an appropriate hypothesis test. This difficulty has led regulatory bodies to specify rules for the conduct of bioequivalence studies (CPMP 1998; FDA 2000, 2001). For example, the 80/20 rule was introduced. This rule specifies that a test of bioequivalence must have at least 80% power of detecting a 20% difference between the parameters of interest. It was also suggested that 90% CIs are used in such circumstances (**Figure 9.2**).

Comparing (paired) means
Difference

If μ_{Test} and $\mu_{Reference}$ are the anticipated mean values of the Test and Reference formulations respectively, then, bioequivalence may be assessed by the difference between the two means, $\mu_{Test} - \mu_{Reference}$. In this case, lower and upper bounds of bioequivalence are set above and below zero, which represents the *true* equality of the means. If the bounds are θ_L and θ_U, then $\theta_L < 0 < \theta_U$. On this difference scale, commonly used and FDA recommended values are, $\theta_L = -0.2\mu_{Reference}$ and $\theta_U = 0.2\mu_{Reference}$. Bioequivalence is generally conceded if the two-sided $100(1 - \alpha)$% CI for the difference $\mu_{Test} - \mu_{Reference}$ is completely contained within the interval (θ_L, θ_U).

Ratio

The logarithms of many measures of drug absorption have an approximate Normal distribution form and so studies may focus on the ratio of the two means, $\mu_{\text{Test}}/\mu_{\text{Reference}}$, rather than their difference. In this situation, the lower and upper bounds of bioequivalence θ_L and θ_U are expressed as above and below the null hypothesis value of unity so that $\theta_L < 1 < \theta_U$. On the ratio scale, commonly used values are $\theta_L = 0.8$ and $\theta_U = 1.25$. These are equidistant from unity on a logarithmic scale, since $\log 1.25 = -\log 0.8 = 0.22$ and $\log 1 = 0$. Bioequivalence is conceded if the two-sided $100(1 - \alpha)\%$ CI for the ratio $\mu_{\text{Test}}/\mu_{\text{Reference}}$, is included within the interval $(\theta_L = 0.80, \theta_U = 1.25)$. In practice, by using a logarithmic transformation one can use the same equations as for the difference of two means; but we then compare $\log \mu_{\text{Test}}$ and $\log \mu_{\text{Reference}}$ for this situation.

Paired *t*-test

Sample size

Since bioequivalence studies are usually small, the sample-size equations use Student's t-distribution rather than the Normal distribution. Further since they are small, rounding upwards but only to the nearest integer following the sample-size calculations is generally advised.

Adapting Equation 7.10 for the *superiority* of one of two paired means in larger sample sizes, then the number of subjects required, half to receive the sequence TR and half RT, in a bioequivalence study in which it is assumed $\mu_{\text{Reference}} = \mu_{\text{Test}} = \mu$ is

$$N = \frac{2\sigma^2(t_{df,1-\alpha} + t_{df,1-\beta/2})^2}{\varepsilon^2}.$$ (9.3)

Essentially, to obtain Equation 9.3 we are merely replacing the ordinate z of the Normal distribution in Equation 7.10 by that of the t-distribution and ignoring the final term of that equation. Further α replaces $\alpha/2$ and $\beta/2$ replaces β.

If we define $\Omega = \varepsilon/\mu$, then the FDA (1992a) recommendations suggest that $\Omega \leq 0.2$ or 20%. In this case Equation 9.3 can be expressed in terms of the coefficient of variation, $CV (= \sigma/\mu)$, and Ω as

$$N = \frac{2CV^2(t_{df,1-\alpha} + t_{df,1-\beta/2})^2}{\Omega^2}.$$ (9.4)

These equations are applicable to calculations of sample size made on both the difference or ratio scales. However, since the way in which bioequivalence is defined on the two scales are not mathematically equivalent, there will be differences in the sample size resulting from these equations depending on the approach.

If the ratio of the means is used

$$CV = \sqrt{\exp(\sigma^2) - 1}.$$ (9.5)

Further, if σ is small,

$$CV \approx \sigma.$$ (9.6)

Degrees of freedom (df)

Besides depending on α, $t_{df,1-\alpha}$ of Equations 9.3 and 9.4 also depends on the number of degrees of freedom, *df*, utilised to estimate the standard deviation, σ, in the final analysis. For a two-period cross-over design, if analysis is by means of a paired *t*-test of the *N* differences, there are $df = 2m - 1 = N - 1$ degrees of freedom. This form of analysis assumes the absence of a period effect. If this cannot be assumed then an analysis of variance approach is required, in which case the number of degrees of freedom will depend on the model specification as pointed out by Senn (2002).

Iteration

The values of $t_{df,1-\alpha}$ and $t_{df,1-\beta/2}$ of Equations 9.3 and 9.4 depend on the sample size *N* whereas $z_{1-\alpha}$ and $z_{1-\beta/2}$ do not. As a consequence, to obtain the sample size using either expression, we require an iterative procedure. This would usually start by assuming infinite degrees of freedom, that is, using *z*'s in place of *t*'s and obtain a starting value for the sample size as N_∞. This is then used to obtain a provisional figure for the degrees of freedom, $df = N_\infty - 1$. The value of $t_{df,1-\alpha}$ and $t_{df,1-\beta/2}$ can then be determined by reference to **Table 2.4** of the *t*-distribution. This, in turn, provides a second estimate of the sample size, N_2. The whole process is then repeated as often as necessary until convergence.

9.4 Non-inferiority

Bioequivalence is a special case of the more general problem of equivalence which can be applied to other situations. In many cases the corresponding sample sizes are somewhat larger so that the Normal distribution *z* rather than the *t*-distribution can be used for sample-size estimation purposes. Thus, for example, a paired comparison for the equivalence situation utilises Equation 9.3 with $z_{1-\alpha}$ and $z_{1-\beta/2}$ replacing the *t*-distribution terms. However in the case of a trial investigating non-inferiority, $\beta/2$ reverts to β as in the superiority situation.

For bioequivalence, one may want the drug to be *neither* less than the Standard *nor* more than a Standard by the specified amount, ε, whereas for 'non-inferiority', if the Test turns out to be more efficacious than the Standard this would be regarded as a bonus. In this context, and most situations in practice, the concept of non-inferiority replaces that of therapeutic equivalence. In these circumstances the $-\varepsilon$ of **Figure 9.1** is replaced by $-\infty$ thereby implying that we are only concerned that the Test treatment should not be worse than the Standard. As a consequence, the two-sided confidence intervals of **Figure 9.1** would be replaced by one-sided intervals. In this case the confidence limits are no longer (even in large studies) symmetric about the estimated difference. If we imagine, that these confidence intervals have an upper limit corresponding to the right hand arrows in **Figure 9.1**, while the lower limits stretch to the left beyond the figure margin then all except *CI* : A and B would be supportive of non-inferiority.

The corresponding $100(1 - \alpha)\%$ *CI* for δ, in circumstances equivalent to a one-sided test situation, is

$$LL \text{ to } d + z_{1-\alpha}SE(d). \tag{9.7}$$

This extends from the lower limit (*LL*) of the possible difference δ which only depends on the *type* of data being considered, not their actual values, to the upper limit (*UL*) which would depend on the observations made.

In general, in testing for non-inferiority, we are trying to show that the Test treatment is the same or not significantly worse than the Standard treatment. Consequently we will be considering *one-sided* tests of the null hypothesis, since we are not trying to prove that the Test is better than the Standard. It is also necessary to specify a probability (power), $1 - \beta$, that the upper confidence limit (*UL*) for δ, calculated once the study is completed, will not exceed this pre-specified value ε.

Difference of means

When two means are compared, the lower limit for the *CI* of Equation 9.3 is $LL = -\infty$. Thus if a comparison of two means were being made, then the *LL* of all the corresponding confidence intervals of **Figure 9.1** would be negative infinity. This is due to the fact that, in repeated sampling, we wish the interval to fail to cover the population mean difference only when this is *greater* than the upper limit of the *CI*. To ensure that the lower limit of the CI is never greater than the population value we take it to be $-\infty$.

Sample size—paired differences

This situation has been described earlier by Equation 9.3 in the context of bioequivalence studies. However, for studies at the later stage of the drug development process much larger studies are the norm. Thus the large sample situation merely replaces the components from the *t*-distribution with those of *z* from the Normal distribution.

Sample size—independent groups

The sample size required for the Standard treatment, with patients randomised in the ratio 1 to φ to the treatments, for a comparison of two means $\mu_{Standard}$ and μ_{Test} from two Normal distributions with the same standard deviation, σ, is given by

$$m_{Standard} = \left(\frac{1+\varphi}{\varphi}\right)\frac{\sigma^2(z_{1-\alpha} + z_{1-\beta})^2}{[(\mu_{Standard} - \mu_{Test}) - \varepsilon]^2}, \mu_{Standard} > \mu_{Test}. \tag{9.8}$$

Thus, the total number of subjects to be recruited is $N = m(1 + \varphi)$. This is an adaptation of Equation 9.3.

For the situation in which it is assumed $\mu_{Standard} = \mu_{Test}$ Equation 9.8 simplifies to

$$m = \left(\frac{1+\varphi}{\varphi}\right)\frac{\sigma^2(z_{1-\alpha} + z_{1-\beta})^2}{\varepsilon^2}. \tag{9.9}$$

These are similar in form to Equation 5.2 for comparing two means although that includes an additional correction factor for small sample size situations. Consequently, the component of ^SS_S within that chapter can be used to evaluate Equations 9.8 or 9.9 by setting the effect size $\Delta = (\mu_{Standard} - \mu_{Test} - \varepsilon)/\sigma$ and using a one-sided test size α and power $1 - \beta$.

Two proportions

We assume that the outcome of the trial can be measured by one of two possibilities, for example, 'cured' or 'not-cured', and the true probability of success under Standard treatment is π_{Standard} and under Test is π_{Test}. However, for notational simplicity in the following we term these π_1 and π_2 respectively. After testing for equivalence of treatments we would wish to assume that, for all practical purposes $\pi_1 = \pi_2$ although we might have evidence that they, in fact, differ by a small amount. For the comparison of two proportions, the LL of Equation 9.7 is determined by the maximum possible difference between the two treatments; this occurs when $\pi_1 = 0$ and $\pi_2 = 1$ so that $LL = \pi_1 - \pi_2 = -1$.

Sample size—independent groups

The sample size required for Treatment 1 with patients randomised to the treatments in the ratio $1 : \varphi$, for anticipated proportions π_1 and π_2, maximal difference ε, one-sided test size α and power $1 - \beta$ is

$$m = \frac{\left\{ z_{1-\alpha}\sqrt{[\varphi\overline{\pi}_{1D}(1 - \overline{\pi}_{1D}) + \overline{\pi}_{2D}(1 - \overline{\pi}_{2D})]} + z_{1-\beta}\sqrt{[\varphi\pi_1(1 - \pi_1) + \pi_2(1 - \pi_2)]} \right\}^2}{\varphi[|\pi_2 - \pi_1| - \varepsilon]^2}. \tag{9.10}$$

In Equation 9.10 $\overline{\pi}_{1D}$ and $\overline{\pi}_{2D}$ are the maximum likelihood estimates of the true values of π_1 and π_2 under the hypothesis that they differ by ε. The total number of patients required to test for equivalence of the two treatments is $N = m + n = m(1 + \varphi)$.

Technical note

In Equation 9.10 $\overline{\pi}_{1D}$ is the solution of $ax^3 + bx^2 + cx + d = 0$ where $a = (1 + \varphi)/\varphi$, $b = -[1 + \varphi + \varphi\pi_1 + \pi_2 + \varepsilon(1 + 2\varphi)]/\varphi$, $c = [\varphi\varepsilon^2 + \varepsilon(2\varphi\pi_1 + 1 + \varphi) + \varphi\pi_1 + \pi_2]/\varphi$ and $d = -\pi_1\varepsilon(1 + \varepsilon)$. It can be shown that $\overline{\pi}_{1D} = 2u\cos(w) - (b/3a)$, $\overline{\pi}_{2D} = \overline{\pi}_{1D} - \varepsilon$, where $w = [\pi + \arccos(v/u^3)]/3$, and π is the irrational number $3.14159\ldots$ and not a Binomial proportion. Further, $v = b^3/(3a)^3 - bc/(6a^2) + d/(2a)$ and $u = \text{sgn}(v)\sqrt{[b^2/(3a)^2 - c/(3a)]}$.

An alternative approach to sample-size calculation is to replace $\overline{\pi}_{1D}$ and $\overline{\pi}_{2D}$ in Equation 9.10 by π_1 and π_2 respectively and this leads to

$$m = \frac{(z_{1-\alpha} + z_{1-\beta})^2[\varphi\pi_1(1 - \pi_1) + \pi_2(1 - \pi_2)]}{\varphi[|\pi_2 - \pi_1| - \varepsilon]^2}. \tag{9.11}$$

For the special case when we can assume the two treatments are likely to be equally effective (not just equivalent as defined here) then $\pi_1 = \pi_2 = \pi$ and Equation 9.11 simplifies to

$$m = \left(\frac{1 + \varphi}{\varphi}\right)\frac{(z_{1-\alpha} + z_{1-\beta})^2[\pi(1 - \pi)]}{\varepsilon^2}. \tag{9.12}$$

This is similar to Equation 5.2 for comparing two means, with $\Delta = \dfrac{\varepsilon}{\sqrt{\pi(1 - \pi)}}$ as the measure similar to effect size, although that includes an additional correction factor for small sample-size situations.

Although we use Equation 9.10 for **Table 9.1** and $\boxed{SS}$, it is clear that Equations 9.11 and 9.12 can be more readily evaluated and so provide a quick check on these calculations.

Hazard ratio

Sample size—independent groups

Although earlier in this chapter we expressed the null hypothesis for a trial with a survival time endpoint as a difference between two rates $H_{\text{Null}} : \delta = \lambda_1 - \lambda_2 = 0$ it is more usual to describe it in terms of their ratio so that non-inferiority is expressed through the Hazard Ratio (*HR*) defined by

$$\theta = \frac{\lambda_2}{\lambda_1}. \tag{9.13}$$

In which case a value $\theta_\varepsilon (> 1)$ is set as the limit of non-inferiority in *HR* that we wish to rule out within the hypothesis framework; $H_{\text{Null}} : \theta \geq \theta_\varepsilon$ against $H_{\text{Alt}} : \theta < \theta_\varepsilon$. We then wish to determine the sample size such that the null hypothesis is rejected at a one-sided test α with power $1 - \beta$ for a specified alternative $\theta < \theta_\varepsilon$ against $\theta \geq \theta_\varepsilon$. For patients randomised to the two groups in the ratio $1 : \varphi$ the required sample size for the first group is given by

$$m = \frac{(z_{1-\alpha} + z_{1-\beta})^2}{\varphi(\log\theta_0 - \log\theta_1)^2}\left[\frac{f(\theta_1\lambda_1,\eta)}{\theta_1^2\lambda_1^2} + \frac{f(\lambda_1,\eta)}{\lambda_1^2}\right]. \tag{9.14}$$

The sample size for the second group is $n = \varphi m$.

Here $f(.,.)$ is defined below but depends on the anticipated duration of patient entry to the trial, D, and the follow-up period beyond recruitment closure, F, while η is the anticipated loss to follow-up or censoring rate. The median survival time of group 1, M_1, is used as the unit of time in calculating D and F. Since, for the Exponential distribution, the relationships of Equation 9.15 below hold, M_1 and M_2 can be used to provide values for λ_1 and λ_2 for Equation 9.14.

Note

In the situation where the survival can be assumed to follow an Exponential distribution, the relationships between the hazard rate, λ, the proportion alive, π, at a fixed point of time, T, and the median survival time, M, can be summarised by

$$\lambda = \frac{-\log\pi_T}{T} = \frac{-\log 0.5}{M}. \tag{9.15}$$

If there is a constant recruitment rate over D, and the censoring follows an Exponential distribution, then $f(\lambda, \eta)$ of Equation 9.14 is

$$f(\lambda,\eta) = \lambda\left\{\frac{1}{\eta + \lambda}\left[1 - \frac{\exp[-F(\eta + \lambda)] - \exp[-(D + F)(\eta + \lambda)]}{D(\eta + \lambda)}\right]\right\}^{-1}. \tag{9.16}$$

To evaluate this, it is necessary for the design team to specify D, F and η, then calculate this for each group separately by setting $\lambda = \lambda_1$ and $\lambda = \lambda_1\theta_1$ respectively.

Equivalence

If the less common situation arises and equivalence rather than non-inferiority is appropriate, then the sample-size formulae of this section would still apply but α is replaced by $\alpha/2$ in all the respective formulae. Consequently, with all other conditions held the same, the corresponding sample sizes would therefore all be larger.

9.5 Bibliography

Roebruck and Kühn (1995) recommend the Farrington and Manning (1990) approach of Equation 9.4 in determining equivalence rather than that of Makuch and Simon (1978) and Blackwelder (1982) who use Equation 9.11.

ICH E10 (2000) E10 have issued general guidance on non-inferiority studies and CPMP (2000) discuss issues with moving from superiority to non-inferiority designs and CHMP (2005, 2006) the choice of the non-inferiority margin. Both FDA (1992b) and CPMP (2004) discuss non-inferiority in the context of bacterial infections. Guidance on some of the more technical issues is given by Julious (2004) who also details many of the appropriate regulatory guidelines.

Philips (1990) discusses bioequivalence for the measure of equivalence expressed as a difference. Julious (2004) and Diletti, Hauschke and Steinijans (1991) extend this to when bioequivalence is defined in terms of ratio, and provide sample-size tables for both situations. Sample sizes for bioequivalence studies are also discussed by Metzler (1991). Chow and Liu (1992) and Lin (1995) point out that in certain situations a two-sided value for β is appropriate. FDA (2000, 2001) and CPMP (1998) have issued guidance on bioequivalence studies

As we have already noted, for bioequivalence studies the sample size is likely to be relatively small, and so t-functions are used in Equations 9.10, 9.11 and 9.12. We also note, however, that Kupper and Hafner (1989) state that the commonly used Normal approximations '. . . perform amazingly well even for very small sample sizes . . .'.

The case of survival or time-to-event data is described by Crisp and Curtis (2007) who give Equations 9.14 and 9.16. They also discuss the situation when the recruitment is assumed to follow a truncated exponential distribution rather than occurring at a uniform rate and give an illustrative example of this situation. This requires a further parameter to be provided at the design stage.

Piaggio, Elbourne, Altman *et al.* (2006) set standards for the reporting of non-inferiority and equivalence trials while the issue of determining the equivalence limit is discussed in the CHMP (2006) guidelines.

9.6 Examples and the use of tables

Table 9.1 and Equation 9.4

Example 9.1—bioequivalence—difference between two means
Wooding (1994) gives an example of data on C_{max} obtained from a two-period cross-over trial of 12 patients. The mean C_{max} was 30.89 for one drug and 39.17 for the other and the pooled within-subject variation had standard deviation 14.7327. Assuming the study is to be repeated, how large should it be?

> For a 10% one-sided test size, $\alpha = 0.1$, the value from **Table 2.2** is $z_{0.90} = 1.2816$ and for a two-sided power with $\beta = 0.2$, $z_{0.90} = 1.2816$.

Here, the combined mean is $\mu = (30.89 + 39.17)/2 = 35.03$ and standard deviation $\sigma = 14.7327$ so that the $CV = \sigma/\mu = 14.7327/35.03 = 0.42$ or approximately 40%.

The FDA (1992a) recommendations suggest $\Omega = 0.2$, a two-sided power of 80% and a one-sided test size of 10%, then first assuming that a large sample size will result so that z can be used in place of t, Equation 9.4 suggests initially that $N_\infty = \dfrac{2 \times 0.4^2 \times (1.2816 + 1.2816)^2}{0.2^2} = 52.6$

or 53 subjects. Since this is relatively large, z and t are almost equal so that more exact calculations of **Table 9.1**, suggests that $N = 54$ subjects would need to be recruited. This is confirmed by the use of $^S S_S$ with the corresponding input values.

Table 9.1 and Equation 9.4

Example 9.2—bioequivalence—ratio of two means
Wooding (1994) gives the mean of log C_{max} for one drug as 3.36 and that for the other 3.54 while the pooled within-subject standard deviation is 0.40. Assuming the study is to be repeated, how large should it be?

> For a 10% one-sided test size, $\alpha = 0.1$, the value from **Table 2.2** is $z_{0.90} = 1.2816$ and for a two-sided power with $\beta = 0.80$, $z_{0.90} = 1.2816$.

Here, the combined mean is $\mu = (3.36 + 3.54)/2 = 3.45$ and $\sigma = 0.40$ so that $CV = 0.40/3.45 = 0.115$ or 12%. Then with $\Omega = 0.2$, two-sided power set as 80% and the one-sided test size at 10%, and first assuming that a large sample size will result so that z can be used in place of t, Equation 9.4 suggests initially that $N_\infty = \dfrac{2 \times 0.12^2 \times (1.2816 + 1.2816)^2}{0.2^2} = 4.73$ or 5 subjects.

Since this is very small, z (= 1.2816) and t will be very different. From **Table 2.4** of Student's t-distribution $df = 5 - 1 = 4$ degrees of freedom $t_{4, 0.9} = 2.132$. Now using these values in Equation 9.4 we obtain $N_2 = \dfrac{2 \times 0.12^2 \times (2.132 + 2.132)^2}{0.2^2} = 13.1$ or 14. Repeating this process

with $df = 13$, gives $N_3 = \dfrac{2 \times 0.12^2 \times (1.771 + 1.771)^2}{0.2^2} = 9.03$ or 10. This process eventually

converges and gives $N_{Final} = 6$ subjects that would need to be recruited, as does $^S S_S$ or Table 9.1 which also gives $N_{Final} = 6$ subjects, with $CV = 10\%$, the nearest tabular entry.

This is in marked contrast to the sample size of 54 in *Example 9.1* where bioequivalence was being assessed on a difference as opposed to a ratio scale.

Examples 9.4 and 9.5 make it clear that it is very important to utilise the most appropriate scale for the definition of bioequivalence. An examination of the data provided by Wooding (1994) would suggest that the ratio approach is the correct one for these particular data.

Table 9.2, Equations 9.8 and 9.9

Example 9.3—equivalence of two means

It is anticipated that patients on a particular drug have a mean diastolic BP of 96 mmHg, as against 94 mmHg on an alternative. It is also anticipated that the standard deviation of diastolic BP was approximately 8 mm. If one wishes to confirm that the difference is likely to be less than 5 mmHg, that is, one wishes to show equivalence, how many patients are required? We assume 80% power and a test size of 5%.

> For a 5% one-sided test size, $\alpha = 0.05$, the value from **Table 2.2** is $z_{0.95} = 1.6449$ and for a two-sided $\beta = 0.2$, $z_{0.90} = 1.2816$.

Here $\mu_1 = 94$, $\mu_2 = 96$, $\varepsilon = 5$ and $\sigma = 8$ and Equation 9.8 with $\varphi = 1$ gives $m = \left(\dfrac{1+1}{1}\right)\dfrac{8^2 \times (1.6449 + 1.2816)^2}{[|96 - 94| - 5]^2} = 121.8$ or approximately $N = 2 \times 125 = 250$ in total. ^SS_S or Table 9.2 give $N = 244$ subjects.

If it can be assumed that $\mu_1 = \mu_2$, then from Equation 9.9 we require only $m = 43.8$ or 44 per group giving a total of $N = 88$ in all.

Note that, under the assumption of equal population means, the calculations result in very similar values to those obtained from Equation 5.2 or **Table 5.1** which are used for the comparison of two means, although the specifications of the null hypothesis are different.

Table 9.3, Equations 9.9 and 9.11

Example 9.4—equivalence of two proportions

Bennett, Dismukes, Duma *et al.* (1979) designed a clinical trial to test whether combination chemotherapy for a shorter period would be at least as good as conventional therapy for patients with cryptococcal meningitis. They recruited 39 patients to each treatment arm and wished to conclude that a difference of less than 20% in response rate between the treatments would indicate equivalence. Assuming a one-sided test size of 10%, a power of 80% and an overall response rate of 50%, what would be a realistic sample size if the trial were to be repeated?

> For a 10% one-sided test size, $\alpha = 0.1$, the value from **Table 2.2** is $z_{0.90} = 1.2816$ and for a two-sided $\beta = 0.2$, $z_{0.90} = 1.2816$ also.

Here the maximum allowable difference $\varepsilon = 0.2$, $\varphi = 1$, $\pi_1 = \pi_2 = 0.5$, one-sided $\alpha = 0.1$ and $1 - \beta = 0.8$. Direct entry into **Table 9.3** or ^SS_S both give $m = 81$ so the total sample size would be $N = 162$.

A rough check on this calculation is provided by utilising Equation 9.12 to give $m = \left(\dfrac{1+1}{1}\right) \times \dfrac{(1.2816 + 1.2816)^2 \times 0.5 \times 0.5}{0.2^2} = 82.1$ or a total sample size $N = 164$.

Equations 9.11 and 9.13

Example 9.5—non-inferiority of hazards

Consider a clinical trial to compare two treatments for Stage I breast cancer. The treatments are either total mastectomy or simple removal of the lump, but leaving the remainder of the breast intact. We would like to show that, at worst, lump removal is only 10% inferior to mastectomy. Assuming the 5-year survival rate of Stage I breast cancer after mastectomy (M) is 60% how large a trial would be needed to show that the 5-year survival rate for lump (L) removal was not less than 50%?

For a 5% one-sided test size, $\alpha = 0.05$ and from **Table 2.2** $z_{0.95} = 1.6449$ while for one-sided $\beta = 0.2$, $z_{0.80} = 0.8416$.

These design characteristics with survival rates at 5-years of $\pi_M = 0.6$ and $\pi_L = 0.5$ give $\lambda_M = -\log 0.6/5 = 0.1022$ and $\lambda_L = -\log 0.5/5 = 0.1386$. From which $\theta_0 = 0.1386/0.1022 = 1.36$ (equivalently $\log \pi_L/\log \pi_M = \log 0.5/\log 0.6 = 1.36$). The value set for the alternative hypothesis is $\theta_1 = 1$. The 5-year survival rate of those receiving mastectomy is 0.6 so that, based on the expression used in Equation 9.12, their median survival time is $M_M = -\log 0.5/0.1022 = 6.78$ or approximately 7 years. If we set $D = 1$ then this implies the duration of recruitment to the trial will be 7 years and, and with $F = 0.5$ this implies $7 \times 0.5 = 3.5$ more years of follow-up once trial entry is closed. The design team further estimate the censoring rate as $\eta = 0.01$.

With these values Equation 9.16 gives $f(0.1022, 0.01) = 0.1085$ for Group M and exactly the same for Group L as $\theta_1 = 1$. From these, and an allocation ratio $\varphi = 1$, Equation 9.11 gives $m = \dfrac{(1.6449 + 0.8416)^2}{1 \times (\log 1.36 - \log 1)^2} \left[\dfrac{0.1085}{0.1022^2} + \dfrac{0.1085}{0.1022^2} \right] = 1358.6$ or approximately 1400. The total planned trial size is therefore approximately $N = 2800$ women. Direct input into $\boxed{^S S_S}$ gives $m = 1380$ or approximately $N = 2800$ also.

It should be emphasised that the resulting sample size may be very sensitive to the planning assumptions made, for example, reducing the *HR* from 1.36 to $\theta_0 = 1.3$ increases the sample size to $N = 3537$ or 3600 women.

9.7 References

Bennett JE, Dismukes WE, Duma RJ, Medoff G, Sande MA, Gallis H, Leonard J, Fields BT, Bradshaw M, Haywood H, McGee Z, Cate TR, Cobbs CG, Warner JF and Alling DW (1979). A comparison of amphotericin B alone and combined with flucytosine in the treatment of cryptococcal meningitis. *New England Journal of Medicine*, **301**, 126–131.

Blackwelder WC (1982). 'Proving the null hypothesis' in clinical trials. *Controlled Clinical Trials*, **3**, 345–353.

CHMP (2005). Guideline on the choice of the non-inferiority margin. Doc EMEA/CPMP/EWP/2158/99. Available at URL: http://www.emea.europa.eu/pdfs/human/ewp/215899en.pdf.

CHMP (2006). Guideline on the choice of the non-inferiority margin. *Statistics in Medicine*, 25, 1628–1638.

Chow S-C and Liu J-P (1992). *Design and Analysis of Bioavailability and Bioequivalence Studies*. Marcel Dekker, New York.

CPMP (1998). Notes for guidance on the investigation of bioavailability and bioequivalence. Doc. CPMP/EWP/QWP1401/98. Available at URL: http://www.emea.eu.int/pdfs/human/ewp/140198en.pdf.

CPMP (2000). Points to consider on switching between superiority and non-inferiority. Doc CPMP/EWP/482/99. Available at URL: http://www.emea.eu.int/pdfs/human/ewp/048299en.pdf.

CPMP (2004). Notes for guidance on the evaluation of medicinal products indicated for the treatment of bacterial infections. Doc CPMP/EWP/558/95. Available at URL: http://www.emea.eu.int/pdfs/human/ewp/055895en.pdf.

Crisp A and Curtis P (2007). Sample size estimation for non-inferiority trials of time-to-event data. *Pharmaceutical Statistics*, in press.

Diletti E, Hauschke D and Steinijans VW (1991). Sample size determination for bioequivalence assessment by means of confidence intervals. *International Journal of Clinical Pharmacology, Therapy and Toxicology*, 29, 1–8.

Farrington CP and Manning G (1990). Test statistics and sample size formulae for comparative binomial trials with null hypothesis of non-zero risk difference or non-unity relative risk. *Statistics in Medicine*, 9, 1447–1454.

FDA (1992a). Statistical procedures for bioequivalence studies using a standard two-treatment crossover design. US Department of Health and Human Services, Public Health Service, Food and Drug Administration, Washington D.C.

FDA (1992b). Points to consider. Clinical evaluation of anti-infective drug products. Available at URL: http://www.fda.gov/cder/guidance/old043fn.pdf.

FDA (2000). Guidance for industry. Bioavailability and bioequivalence studies for orally administered drug products—general considerations. Available at URL: http://www.fda.gov/cder/guidance/3615fnl.pdf.

FDA (2001). Statistical approaches to establishing bioequivalence. Available at URL: http://www.fda.gov/cder/guidance/3616fnl.pdf.

ICH E10 (2000). Choice of control group in clinical trials. Available at URL: http://www.ifpma.org/ich5e.html.

Jones B, Jarvis P, Lewis JA and Ebbutt AF (1996). Trials to assess equivalence: the importance of rigorous methods. *British Medical Journal*, 313, 36–39.

Julious SA (2004). Sample size for clinical studies with Normal data. *Statistics in Medicine*, 23, 1921–1986.

Kupper LL and Hafner KB (1989). How appropriate are popular sample size formulas? *American Statistician*, 43, 101–105.

Lin SC (1995). Sample size for therapeutic equivalence based on confidence intervals. *Drug Information Journal*, 29, 45–50.

Machin D and Campbell MJ (2005). *Design of Studies for Medical Research*, John Wiley & Sons, Chichester.

Makuch R and Simon R (1978). Sample size requirements for evaluating a conservative therapy. *Cancer Treatment Reports*, **62**, 1037–1040.

Metzler CM (1991). Sample sizes for bioequivalence studies (with discussion). *Statistics in Medicine*, **10**, 961–970.

Piaggio G, Elbourne DR, Altman DG, Pocock SJ and Evans SJW (2006). Reporting of non-inferiority and equivalence randomized trials: An extension of the CONSORT statement. *Journal of the American Medical Association*, **295**, 1152–1172.

Philips KE (1990). Power of the two one-sided tests procedure in bioequivalence. *Journal of Pharmacokinetics and Biopharmaceutics*, **18**, 137–143.

Roebruck P and Kühn A (1995). Comparison of tests and sample size formulae for proving therapeutic equivalence based on the difference of binomial probabilities. *Statistics in Medicine*, **14**, 1583–1594.

Senn S (2002). *Cross-over Trials in Clinical Research*, 2nd edn. John Wiley & Sons, Chichester.

Wooding WM (1994). *Planning Pharmaceutical Clinical Trials*. John Wiley & Sons, New York.

Table 9.1 Sample sizes for bioequivalence studies—difference between two means or ratio of two means. Each cell gives the total number of patients, N, that should be entered into study.

One-sided α	Two-sided β	CV	Ω 0.1	0.15	0.2	0.25
0.05	0.1	0.05	8	6	20	–
		0.1	24	12	8	6
		0.15	52	24	14	10
		0.2	90	42	24	16
		0.25	138	62	36	24
		0.3	198	90	52	34
		0.35	268	120	70	46
		0.4	350	156	90	58
		0.45	442	198	112	72
		0.5	544	244	138	90
	0.2	0.05	6	6	12	–
		0.1	20	10	6	6
		0.15	42	20	12	8
		0.2	72	34	20	14
		0.25	110	50	30	20
		0.3	156	72	42	28
		0.35	212	96	56	36
		0.4	276	124	72	46
		0.45	350	156	90	58
		0.5	430	192	110	72
0.1	0.1	0.05	6	6	12	–
		0.1	20	10	6	6
		0.15	42	20	12	8
		0.2	72	34	20	14
		0.25	110	50	30	20
		0.3	156	72	42	28
		0.35	212	96	56	36
		0.4	276	124	72	46
		0.45	350	156	90	58
		0.5	430	192	110	72
	0.2	0.05	6	10	–	–
		0.1	16	8	6	4
		0.15	32	16	10	6
		0.2	54	26	16	10
		0.25	84	38	22	16
		0.3	120	54	32	22
		0.35	164	74	42	28
		0.4	212	96	54	36
		0.45	268	120	68	44
		0.5	330	148	84	54

Table 9.2 Sample sizes for testing the equivalence of two means. Each cell gives the number of subjects for each group, m. Hence, the total sample size for the study is $N = 2m$.

One-sided α	μ_{Diff}	σ	$\beta = 0.1$ Maximal difference, ε 1	3	5	$\beta = 0.2$ Maximal difference, ε 1	3	5
0.05	2	2	87	87	10	69	69	8
		4	347	347	39	275	275	31
		6	780	780	87	617	617	69
		8	1386	1386	154	1097	1097	122
	4	2	10	87	87	8	69	69
		4	39	347	347	31	275	275
		6	87	780	780	69	617	617
		8	154	1386	1386	122	1097	1097
	6	2	4	10	87	3	8	69
		4	14	39	347	11	31	275
		6	32	87	780	25	69	617
		8	56	154	1386	44	122	1097
	8	2	2	4	10	2	3	8
		4	8	14	39	6	11	31
		6	16	32	87	13	25	69
		8	29	56	154	23	44	122
	10	2	2	2	4	1	2	3
		4	5	8	14	4	6	11
		6	10	16	32	8	13	25
		8	18	29	56	14	23	44
	15	2	1	1	1	1	1	1
		4	2	3	4	2	2	3
		6	4	6	8	4	5	7
		8	8	10	14	6	8	11
	20	2	1	1	1	1	1	1
		4	1	2	2	1	1	2
		6	3	3	4	2	3	3
		8	4	5	7	4	4	5

Table 9.2 (*continued*): Sample sizes for testing the equivalence of two means. Each cell gives the number of subjects for each group, *m*. Hence, the total sample size for the study is $N = 2m$.

One-sided α	μ_{Diff}	σ	Two-sided Type II error, β					
			$\beta = 0.1$			$\beta = 0.2$		
			Maximal difference, ε			Maximal difference, ε		
			1	3	5	1	3	5
0.1	2	2	69	69	8	53	53	6
		4	275	275	31	211	211	24
		6	617	617	69	474	474	53
		8	1097	1097	122	841	841	94
	4	2	8	69	69	6	53	53
		4	31	275	275	24	211	211
		6	69	617	617	53	474	474
		8	122	1097	1097	94	841	841
	6	2	3	8	69	3	6	53
		4	11	31	275	9	24	211
		6	25	69	617	19	53	474
		8	44	122	1097	34	94	841
	8	2	2	3	8	2	3	6
		4	6	11	31	5	9	24
		6	13	25	69	10	19	53
		8	23	44	122	18	34	94
	10	2	1	2	3	1	2	3
		4	4	6	11	3	5	9
		6	8	13	25	6	10	19
		8	14	23	44	11	18	34
	15	2	1	1	1	1	1	1
		4	2	2	3	2	2	3
		6	4	5	7	3	4	5
		8	6	8	11	5	6	9
	20	2	1	1	1	1	1	1
		4	1	1	2	1	1	1
		6	2	3	3	2	2	3
		8	4	4	5	3	3	4

Table 9.3 Sample sizes for testing the equivalence of two proportions. Each cell gives the number of subjects for each group, m. Hence, the total sample size for the study is $N = 2m$.

One-sided α	π_1	π_2	Two-sided Type II error, β							
			$\beta = 0.1$				$\beta = 0.2$			
			Maximal difference, ε				Maximal difference, ε			
			0.05	0.1	0.15	0.2	0.05	0.1	0.15	0.2
0.05	0.1	0.1	795	208	97	58	631	166	78	46
		0.2	1119	–	1180	302	889	–	943	242
		0.3	152	348	1410	–	121	278	1127	–
		0.4	62	98	175	395	50	78	140	316
		0.5	34	47	67	104	28	38	54	84
		0.6	21	27	35	47	17	22	28	38
		0.7	14	17	21	26	12	14	17	21
		0.8	10	11	13	16	8	9	11	13
		0.9	7	8	9	10	6	6	7	8
	0.2	0.2	1389	350	157	89	1100	277	125	71
		0.3	1621	–	1634	410	1284	–	1297	325
		0.4	198	447	1787	–	158	355	1419	–
		0.5	76	118	208	466	60	94	166	371
		0.6	39	53	76	118	32	43	61	94
		0.7	23	29	38	51	19	24	31	41
		0.8	15	18	22	27	12	15	18	22
		0.9	10	11	13	16	8	9	11	13
	0.3	0.3	1818	454	202	113	1439	360	160	90
		0.4	1960	–	1949	485	1552	–	1543	383
		0.5	226	508	2019	–	180	403	1600	–
		0.6	82	128	225	502	66	102	179	399
		0.7	41	55	79	122	33	44	63	98
		0.8	23	29	38	51	19	24	31	41
		0.9	14	17	21	26	12	14	17	21
	0.4	0.4	2076	518	229	128	1643	410	181	101
		0.5	2130	–	2110	523	1687	–	1668	413
		0.6	236	528	2097	–	187	419	1662	–
		0.7	82	128	225	502	66	102	179	399
		0.8	39	53	76	118	32	43	61	94
		0.9	21	27	35	47	17	22	28	38
	0.5	0.5	2162	539	238	133	1711	426	188	105
		0.6	2130	–	2110	523	1687	–	1668	413
		0.7	226	508	2019	–	180	403	1600	–
		0.8	76	118	208	466	60	94	166	371
		0.9	34	47	67	104	28	38	54	84

Table 9.3 (*continued*): Sample sizes for testing the equivalence of two proportions. Each cell gives the number of subjects for each group, *m*. Hence, the total sample size for the study is $N = 2m$.

One-sided α	π_1	π_2	\multicolumn{8}{c}{Two-sided Type II error, β}

One-sided α	π_1	π_2	\multicolumn{4}{c}{$\beta = 0.1$ Maximal difference, ε}				\multicolumn{4}{c}{$\beta = 0.2$ Maximal difference, ε}			
			0.05	0.1	0.15	0.2	0.05	0.1	0.15	0.2
0.1	0.1	0.1	628	164	76	45	483	127	59	35
		0.2	882	–	924	236	680	–	716	183
		0.3	120	273	1105	–	93	211	856	–
		0.4	49	77	137	309	38	60	106	240
		0.5	27	37	52	82	21	29	41	64
		0.6	17	21	27	37	13	17	21	29
		0.7	11	13	16	20	9	11	13	16
		0.8	8	9	10	12	6	7	8	10
		0.9	5	6	7	7	4	5	5	6
	0.2	0.2	1099	277	124	71	843	213	96	54
		0.3	1281	–	1290	323	984	–	992	249
		0.4	157	352	1408	–	121	271	1085	–
		0.5	59	93	164	366	46	72	127	283
		0.6	31	42	60	92	24	33	46	72
		0.7	18	23	30	40	14	18	23	31
		0.8	12	14	17	21	9	11	13	17
		0.9	8	9	10	12	6	7	8	10
	0.3	0.3	1439	360	160	90	1104	276	123	69
		0.4	1550	–	1543	384	1190	–	1184	295
		0.5	179	401	1595	–	138	308	1226	–
		0.6	65	101	178	396	50	78	137	305
		0.7	32	44	62	96	25	34	48	74
		0.8	18	23	30	40	14	18	23	31
		0.9	11	13	16	20	9	11	13	16
	0.4	0.4	1643	410	182	102	1260	314	139	78
		0.5	1685	–	1671	415	1293	–	1281	318
		0.6	186	417	1658	–	143	321	1273	–
		0.7	65	101	178	396	50	78	137	305
		0.8	31	42	60	92	24	33	46	72
		0.9	17	21	27	37	13	17	21	29
	0.5	0.5	1711	427	189	106	1313	327	145	81
		0.6	1685	–	1671	415	1293	–	1281	318
		0.7	179	401	1595	–	138	308	1226	–
		0.8	59	93	164	366	46	72	127	283
		0.9	27	37	52	82	21	29	41	64

Confidence intervals

10

SUMMARY

This chapter describes how sample sizes may be derived by pre-specifying the width or relative width of the confidence interval the investigator wishes to obtain at the end of the study. Formulae are given when a single estimate is required and also for the comparison of two groups for both binary and continuous outcome measures in two independent groups and paired or matched groups.

10.1 Introduction

A sample-size calculation is required for all clinical investigations. However, often a preliminary or pilot investigation is conducted with the objective of estimating any possible clinical effect with a view to doing a later definitive study. In such exploratory pilot or *learning* studies, what is proposed in this chapter is that the sample size be selected in order to provide a given level of precision, and not to power in the traditional fashion for a desirable and pre-specified difference of interest.

For precision-based studies, rather than testing a formal hypothesis, an estimation approach through the provision of confidence intervals for the true difference δ, is more appropriate.

A similar situation occurs where the sample size is determined primarily by practical considerations and the trial is not powered to detect any pre-specified effect. In such circumstances the estimation approach may be adopted to give the precision for the fixed sample size in the study.

Another instance where precision calculations can be useful is where one wishes to power on a primary endpoint overall, but also to have sufficient precision on some secondary endpoint(s) or within given subgroups which will not be formally statistically assessed.

It is not just in clinical trials where precision based sample size estimation is important. For example in an epidemiological survey the objective may be to estimate the prevalence of a particular disease in a population, for example, the prevalence of asthma in young children in a particular locality. An unbiased estimate of the prevalence can be provided by a sample if the sample is selected from the population by simple random sampling. In designing such a survey the epidemiologist is likely to ask: 'How many subjects do I need to examine in order to assess prevalence with a reasonable degree of accuracy?'

The sample size chosen is determined by a number of factors. Firstly, how precise should the estimate be? If the investigator can allow only a small margin of uncertainty, then he will

Sample Size Tables for Clinical Studies, 3rd edition. By David Machin, Michael J. Campbell, Say Beng Tan, and Sze Huey Tan. Published 2009 by Blackwell Publishing, ISBN: 978-1-4051-4650-0

need a large sample. This uncertainty can be expressed as the width of the corresponding confidence interval (*CI*), with a wider confidence interval corresponding to greater uncertainty.

The second factor is the required probability that the estimate is close to the population parameter we are trying to estimate. Although it is possible that the confidence interval obtained from a sample does not contain the actual prevalence. This means that, if we conducted a large number of surveys all of the same size, we could claim that 95% of the 95% *CIs* then calculated would contain the true prevalence.

Power implications

There is a relationship between conventional significance testing and confidence intervals. Thus, for example, if zero lies outside the 95% *CI* for the difference of two means, a significance test would yield a result significant at 5%. Hence, one might question the disappearance of $z_{1-\beta}$ from the sample-size equations below.

The calculations themselves are equivalent to assuming a power 50% or $1 - \beta = 0.5$, that is, setting $z_{1-\beta} = 0$. However, there is no formal power-based calculation as neither a null or alternative hypothesis has been declared. Thus one cannot declare the null to be rejected if *a priori* it was not set. The studies as stated are exploratory only and so although the range of plausible values may exclude zero a definitive formally powered study may be required to get the necessary level of proof.

Nevertheless conventional equations or tables for power calculations of significance tests can be used to estimate the equivalent sample size for confidence intervals simply by setting the power to be 50%.

10.2 Single proportion

Samples from large populations

Suppose we are designing a study for which the underlying population prevalence of the disease of interest is π_{Pop}. If N subjects are involved, then $p = r/N$, where r is the number of individuals observed to have the disease and p is the estimate of π_{Pop}. Provided that both Np and $N(1 - p)$ are not too small (a good guide is that they are both greater than 10) then we can use the Normal approximation to the Binomial distribution and obtain from these data a $100(1 - \alpha)\%$ *CI* for π_{Pop} as

$$p - z_{1-\alpha/2}\sqrt{\frac{p(1 - p)}{N}} \text{ to } p + z_{1-\alpha/2}\sqrt{\frac{p(1 - p)}{N}}. \tag{10.1}$$

With some change in notation this is the same expression as Equation 2.15.

At the design stage of the prevalence study, we have not yet observed p, and so we replace it by its anticipated value π_{Plan} in Equation 10.1. This then represents the target *CI* for the study we have in mind. The width of this *CI*, for a specific choice of α, will depend on π_{Plan} and critically on the ultimate sample size, N chosen.

For a pre-specified width $\omega = 2z_{1-\alpha/2}\sqrt{\dfrac{\pi_{\text{Plan}}(1 - \pi_{\text{Plan}})}{N}}$ from Equation 10.1 the corresponding sample size is given by

$$N = 4 \left[\frac{\pi_{\text{Plan}}(1 - \pi_{\text{Plan}})}{\omega^2} \right] z_{1-\alpha/2}^2. \tag{10.2}$$

Alternatively, instead of pre-specifying the width ω we might wish to estimate π_{Pop} to within a certain percentage of its anticipated value, say $100\varepsilon\%$, that is from $-\pi\varepsilon$ to $+\pi\varepsilon$. This is equivalent to specifying that the CI should be no wider than $\omega = 2\pi\varepsilon$. To obtain the sample size we substitute this value for ω in Equation 10.2 to obtain:

$$N = \frac{(1 - \pi_{\text{Plan}})z_{1-\alpha/2}^2}{\pi_{\text{Plan}}\varepsilon^2}. \tag{10.3}$$

Expressions 10.2 and 10.3 will clearly not be useful if the anticipated value of π is either 0 or 1. In either case, Equation 10.5 below would be used in their place. Indeed prudence suggests that this latter equation should always be used and this forms the basis of **Table 10.1**.

High or low anticipated response

As we have noted above and in **Chapter 2**, if the sample size is not large or π close to 0 or 1, then the 'traditional' method, which is a large sample approximation of Equation 10.1, for calculating a confidence interval should not be used. Further we should note that although Equation 10.1 is symmetric about the estimate p, strictly this is only the case if $p = 0.5$, otherwise the confidence interval is not symmetric. Despite this we can still plan a study on the basis of the width of the interval, ω, even though the centre of the interval may not be p. In so doing we use the 'recommended' method of Equation 2.14 described by Altman and Newcombe (2000, pp. 46–47) and which we reproduce here with some small notational changes, including replacing r by $N\pi_{\text{Plan}}$, as we are now at the planning (rather than the analysis) stage.

First defining $A = 2N\pi_{\text{Plan}} + z_{1-\alpha/2}^2$; $B = z_{1-\alpha/2}\sqrt{z_{1-\alpha/2}^2 + 4N\pi_{\text{Plan}}(1 - \pi_{\text{Plan}})}$; and $C = 2(N + z_{1-\alpha/2}^2)$ then the corresponding confidence interval is given by

$$(A - B)/C \text{ to } (A + B)/C. \tag{10.4}$$

From this the width of the confidence interval is $\omega = \dfrac{2B}{C}$ which, after some algebra, leads to a planning sample size

$$N = -z_{1-\alpha/2}^2(1 - 2\Omega) + z_{1-\alpha/2}^2\sqrt{\frac{1}{\omega^2} - 4\Omega + 4\Omega^2}, \tag{10.5}$$

where $\Omega = \dfrac{\pi_{\text{Plan}}(1 - \pi_{\text{Plan}})}{\omega^2}$. This latter term appears as part of Equation 10.2.

Samples from finite populations

In some cases, the size of the population from which the researcher is sampling is known precisely and may be of limited size. For example, the researcher may wish to assess the prevalence of impotence amongst patients on a diabetic register. The researcher could investigate everyone on the register and get an answer for the 'truth'. However, instead of investigating everyone the researcher may take a sample from the register and use this sample (with corresponding confidence interval) to estimate the truth.

It is clear that if one sampled 60 out of a total register of 100 subjects one would have a more accurate assessment of the prevalence than if one took a sample of 60 from a register of size 1000. In these circumstances, if p is estimated by the ratio of r cases from a sample of N diabetic patients from a register population of size $N_{\text{Population}}$ then Equation 10.1 is modified somewhat to give an approximate $100(1 - \alpha)\%$ CI for the true prevalence π_{Pop} of

$$p - z_{1-\alpha/2}\sqrt{\left[\frac{p(1 - p)}{N} \cdot \frac{N_{\text{Population}} - N}{N_{\text{Population}}}\right]} \text{ to } p + z_{1-\alpha/2}\sqrt{\left[\frac{p(1 - p)}{N} \cdot \frac{N_{\text{Population}} - N}{N_{\text{Population}}}\right]}. \quad (10.6)$$

Given that N is the sample size given by Equation 10.2 or 10.3 for an (effectively) *infinite* population then the sample size required for population that is *finite* is:

$$N_{\text{Finite}} = FN, \quad (10.7)$$

where

$$F = \frac{N_{\text{Population}}}{N + N_{\text{Population}}}. \quad (10.8)$$

The purpose of sampling is to reduce the number of observations to be made by the investigator. However, if the required sample size is a major proportion of the total population, say 80% or more, then it may be sensible to examine the whole population rather than a sample of it.

10.3 Proportions in two groups

Independent groups
Difference in proportions
At the design stage of a study, it may be difficult to specify planning values of π_1 and π_2. Instead investigators may find it easier to specify the difference that they expect to be able to detect.

The $100(1 - \alpha)\%$ CI for a true difference in proportions, $\delta = \pi_1 - \pi_2$, takes form similar to Equation 10.1 but now concerns $p_1 - p_2$ and the corresponding $SE(p_1 - p_2)$. It is estimated by

$$(p_1 - p_2) - z_{1-\alpha/2}\sqrt{\frac{p_1(1 - p_1)}{m} + \frac{p_2(1 - p_2)}{n}} \text{ to } (p_1 - p_2) + z_{1-\alpha/2}\sqrt{\frac{p_1(1 - p_1)}{m} + \frac{p_2(1 - p_2)}{n}},$$

$$(10.9)$$

where p_1 and p_2 are the corresponding observed proportions in each of the two groups of size m and n respectively.

Thus, one may wish to calculate the number of patients required to be able to obtain a confidence interval of a specified width,

$$\omega = 2z_{1-\alpha/2}\sqrt{\frac{\pi_1(1 - \pi_1)}{m} + \frac{\pi_2(1 - \pi_2)}{n}},$$

where π_1 and π_2 are the anticipated proportions provided by the design team. In which case, and first specifying $n = \varphi m$, the corresponding sample size is given by

$$m = \frac{4[\varphi\pi_1(1 - \pi_1) + \pi_2(1 - \pi_2)]z^2_{1-\alpha/2}}{\varphi\omega^2}. \tag{10.10}$$

As a consequence, a total of $N = m(1 + \varphi)$ subjects are required for the corresponding study.

However, in the case of $\varphi = 1$, instead of $SE(p_1 - p_2) = \sqrt{\dfrac{\pi_1(1 - \pi_1)}{m} + \dfrac{\pi_2(1 - \pi_2)}{m}}$ in

Equation 10.10 the following approximation can be used $SE(p_1 - p_2) \approx \sqrt{\dfrac{2\bar{\pi}(1 - \bar{\pi})}{m}}$. Here

$\bar{\pi} = (\pi_1 + \pi_2)/2$ which is the mean proportion anticipated across both the groups. This approximate standard error (SE) holds for response proportions whose magnitudes do not differ by more than 0.3, that is $|\pi_1 - \pi_2| < 0.3$, and thus covers many practical situations.

Using this approximation to the SE the sample size per group is

$$m = 8\left[\frac{\bar{\pi}(1 - \bar{\pi})}{\omega^2}\right]z^2_{1-\alpha/2}. \tag{10.11}$$

This expression also gives a convenient check of the more complex calculations of Equation 10.12.

In the case of equal numbers of subjects in each group Bristol (1989) suggested a more accurate approximation to the required study size, is given by

$$m = \frac{\left\{z_{1-\alpha/2}\sqrt{\pi_1(1 - \pi_1) + \pi_2(1 - \pi_2)} + \sqrt{z^2_{1-\alpha/2}[\pi_1(1 - \pi_1) + \pi_2(1 - \pi_2)] + 2\omega}\right\}^2}{\omega^2}. \tag{10.12}$$

However, *Example 10.5* suggests this may not be the case if π_1 or π_2 are close to 0 or 1.

Recommended method

Newcombe and Altman (2000, p. 49) provide a recommended method of calculating a confidence interval for the difference between two proportions. It is an extension of the methodology of Equation 10.4 for calculating the confidence interval for a single proportion. This leads to the following expression for the width of the $100(1 - \alpha)\%$ CI

$$\omega = \sqrt{(\pi_1 - L_1)^2 + (U_2 - \pi_2)^2} + \sqrt{(\pi_2 - L_2)^2 + (U_1 - \pi_1)^2}. \tag{10.13}$$

Here $L_1 = (A_1 - B_1)/C_1$ and $U_1 = (A_1 + B_1)/C_1$ with similar expressions for L_2 and U_2. Further $A_1 = 2m\pi_1 + z^2_{1-\alpha/2}$; $B_1 = z_{1-\alpha/2}\sqrt{z^2_{1-\alpha/2} + 4m\pi_1(1 - \pi_1)}$; $C_1 = 2(m + z^2_{1-\alpha/2})$ with similar expressions for A_2, B_2 and C_2 and with m replaced by $n = \varphi m$. For given planning values for π_1 and π_2, Equation 10.13 can be solved for m using an iterative procedure.

Since Equation 10.13 can be used for all resulting sample sizes, whether small or large, this procedure is used in $^S\!S_S$ rather than Equations 10.10, 10.11 or 10.12 above.

Odds ratio

The difference between two proportions can also be expressed through the odds ratio (OR) where

$$OR = \frac{p_2(1 - p_1)}{p_1(1 - p_2)}.$$ (10.14)

The estimated $100(1 - \alpha)\%$ CI for OR_{Pop} is given by

$$\exp[\log OR - z_{1-\alpha/2}SE(\log OR)] \text{ to } \exp[\log OR + z_{1-\alpha/2}SE(\log OR)],$$ (10.15)

where

$$SE(\log OR) = \left[\frac{1}{m\pi_1(1 - \pi_1)} + \frac{1}{n\pi_2(1 - \pi_2)} \right]^{1/2}.$$ (10.16)

The confidence interval given by Equation 10.15 is not symmetric about the estimate of the odds ratio and so for sample size purposes one can more easily specify the requirement as a proportion of the odds ratio itself, that is, εOR, rather than by the width of the interval. In which case, to estimate an OR to within $100\varepsilon\%$ of the true value, the sample size required for one group is

$$m = \frac{\left[\frac{1}{\pi_1(1 - \pi_1)} + \frac{1}{\varphi\pi_2(1 - \pi_2)} \right] z_{1-\alpha/2}^2}{[\log(1 - \varepsilon)]^2}.$$ (10.17)

Thus, the total sample size required is $N = m + n = m(1 + \varphi)$.

An alterative approximation to the SE of $\log OR$ is

$$SE(\log OR) = \left[\frac{4}{m\bar{\pi}(1 - \bar{\pi})} \right]^{1/2},$$ (10.18)

where $\bar{\pi} = \dfrac{\pi_1 + \varphi\pi_2}{1 + \varphi}$. This leads to a sample size given by

$$m = \frac{2z_{1-\alpha/2}^2}{\bar{\pi}(1 - \bar{\pi})[\log(1 - \varepsilon)]^2}$$ (10.19)

Equations 10.17 and 10.19 tend to give similar sample size answers provided $|\pi_1 - \pi_2| < 0.2$.

Paired groups
Difference in proportions
Newcombe and Altman (2000, p. 52) provide a recommended method of calculating a confidence interval for the difference between two proportions when the data are matched or paired. In the paired sample situation the estimates of the two population pair means are correlated and this leads to the following rather complex expression for the width of the $100(1 - \alpha)\%$ CI

$$\omega = \sqrt{(\pi_1 - L_1)^2 - 2\rho(\pi_1 - L_1)(U_2 - \pi_2) + (U_2 - \pi_2)^2}$$

$$+ \sqrt{(\pi_2 - L_2)^2 - 2\rho(\pi_2 - L_2)(U_1 - \pi_1) + (U_1 - \pi_1)^2},$$ (10.20)

where $L_1 = (A_1 - B_1)/C_1$ and $U_1 = (A_1 - B_1)/C_1$ with similar expressions for L_2 and U_2. Further $A_1 = 2N_{\mathrm{Pairs}}\pi_1 + z_{1-\alpha/2}^2$; $B_1 = z_{1-\alpha/2}\sqrt{z_{1-\alpha/2}^2 + 4N_{\mathrm{Pairs}}\pi_1(1 - \pi_1)}$; $C_1 = 2(N_{\mathrm{Pairs}} + z_{1-\alpha/2}^2)$ and also for A_2, B_2 and C_2. Finally ρ corrects for the fact that p_1 and p_2 are not independent. For given planning values for π_1, π_2 and ρ, Equation 10.20 can be solved for N_{Pairs} using an iterative procedure.

10.4 Single mean

For a single mean μ_{Pop} estimated from continuous data assumed to have a Normal distribution, the estimate of the corresponding $100(1 - \alpha)\%$ CI is

$$\bar{x} - z_{1-\alpha/2}\frac{s}{\sqrt{N}} \text{ to } \bar{x} + z_{1-\alpha/2}\frac{s}{\sqrt{N}}. \tag{10.21}$$

With some change in notation this is the same expression as Equation 2.13.

In the same way as Equation 10.2 is derived, to estimate μ_{Pop} for a pre-specified confidence interval width ω, and a planning value for the standard deviation, s, as σ_{Plan}, the corresponding sample size is given by

$$N = 4\left[\frac{\sigma_{\text{Plan}}^2}{\omega^2}\right]z_{1-\alpha/2}^2 = 4\frac{z_{1-\alpha/2}^2}{\Lambda_{\text{Plan}}^2}. \tag{10.22}$$

where $\Lambda_{\text{Plan}} = \omega / \sigma_{\text{Plan}}$. Note that this has a similar structure to Equations 10.26 and 10.28 for the difference between two means for independent and paired groups respectively. As a consequence **Table 10.5** is used for the three situations but for the single mean situation the entries in the table should be divided by two and the *total* sample size N results.

For a confidence interval no wider than $\varepsilon\mu$, the corresponding expression is:

$$N = \frac{\sigma_{\text{Plan}}^2 z_{1-\alpha/2}^2}{\mu^2 \varepsilon^2}. \tag{10.23}$$

It is important to note that, to calculate N from Equations 10.22 or 10.23, an anticipated value of the population standard deviation is required—we denote this σ_{Plan}. In the absence of any data on the standard deviation, a rough estimate of σ_{Plan} is provided by the anticipated range, that is, the largest anticipated minus the smallest anticipated value, divided by 4.

10.5 Difference between two means

Independent groups

If the standard deviation can be assumed to be the same for both groups, then the confidence interval for the difference between two independent group means is

$$(\bar{x}_1 - \bar{x}_2) - z_{1-\alpha/2}s_{\text{Pool}}\sqrt{\left[\frac{1}{m} + \frac{1}{n}\right]} \text{ to } (\bar{x}_1 - \bar{x}_2) + z_{1-\alpha/2}s_{\text{Pool}}\sqrt{\left[\frac{1}{m} + \frac{1}{n}\right]}, \tag{10.24}$$

where s_{Pool} is a combined estimate of σ_{Pop} obtained from the two samples.

Denoting $n = \varphi m$, this leads to the total width of the anticipated confidence interval as

$$\omega = 2z_{1-\alpha/2}\sigma_{\text{Plan}}\sqrt{\left[\frac{1}{m} + \frac{1}{\varphi m}\right]}. \tag{10.25}$$

Thus, an estimate for the sample size for one of the groups for a confidence interval of width ω is given by

$$m = 4\left(\frac{1+\varphi}{\varphi}\right)\left[\frac{\sigma_{\text{Plan}}^2}{\omega^2}\right]z_{1-\alpha/2}^2 = 4\left(\frac{1+\varphi}{\varphi}\right)\frac{z_{1-\alpha/2}^2}{\Lambda_{\text{Plan}}^2}, \tag{10.26}$$

where $\Lambda_{\text{Plan}} = \omega / \sigma_{\text{Plan}}$. The total sample size is therefore $N = m + n = m(1 + \varphi)$.

Note that this has a similar structure to Equations 10.22 and 10.28 for the case of a single mean and for the difference of two means in paired groups. As a consequence **Table 10.5** is used for the three situations.

Paired or matched groups

When the units of observation are paired or matched, essentially the endpoint observations from the two members of each unit are linked and the difference between them is used as the endpoint for analysis. For example, if cases with a particular disease are matched perhaps, by age and gender to healthy controls, then the endpoint for pair i becomes $d_i = (x_i - y_i)$ where x_i is the observation from the case and y_i that from the control and there are N_{Pairs} pairs. The corresponding large sample confidence interval for a continuous variable is

$$\bar{d} - z_{1-\alpha/2}\frac{\sigma_{\text{Pairs}}}{\sqrt{N_{\text{Pairs}}}} \text{ to } \bar{d} + z_{1-\alpha/2}\frac{\sigma_{\text{Pairs}}}{\sqrt{N_{\text{Pairs}}}}. \tag{10.27}$$

By analogy with previous situations discussed in this chapter, an appropriate sample size for a given confidence interval width ω is

$$N_{\text{Pairs}} = 4\left[\frac{\sigma_{\text{Pairs}}^2}{\omega^2}\right]z_{1-\alpha/2}^2 = 4\frac{z_{1-\alpha/2}^2}{\Lambda_{\text{Pairs}}^2}. \tag{10.28}$$

where $\Lambda_{\text{Pairs}} = \omega / \sigma_{\text{Pairs}}$. However, in this case an anticipated value of σ_{Pairs} is required.

Note that this has a similar structure to Equations 10.22 and 10.26 for the case of a single mean and for the difference of two means in independent groups. As a consequence **Table 10.5** is used for the three situations.

10.6 Practicalities

When estimating a single mean based on a sample of size N the corresponding confidence interval is given by Equation 10.21 provided the sample size is sufficiently large. If it is small then the confidence interval should use Student's t-distribution and will take the form of Equation 2.14. This implies replacing $z_{1-\alpha/2}$ by $t_{df,1-\alpha/2}$ in Equation 10.21 where df are the degrees of freedom or $N - 1$ in this case.

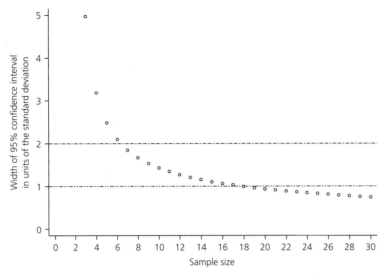

Figure 10.1 Reduction in the width of a 95% confidence interval for a mean with increasing sample size, for standard deviation, $\sigma = 1$.

However as df gets larger and larger $t_{df,1-\alpha/2}$ gets closer and closer to $z_{1-\alpha/2}$. For example using **Table 2.4**, $t_{8,0.975} = 2.306$, $t_{12,0.975} = 2.179$, $t_{16,0.975} = 2.120$ while $t_{\infty,0.975} = z_{0.975} = 1.960$. This is indicating that the estimate of the standard deviation, denoted s, is getting more and more reliable as we have more and more data. Further, in the same way as the value of $t_{df,1-\alpha/2}$ decreases with increasing N, so does the standard error (as it depends on $1/\sqrt{N}$). Combining these two aspects results in the width of the confidence interval rapidly declining as (small) sample sizes increase and then more slowly for larger values. This decline is illustrated in **Figure 10.1** with the standard deviation set as unity.

Thus to have a 95% CI of less than 2 SDs requires more than 6 subjects and for less than 1 SD about 20 or more subjects. We would be reluctant to recommend any study with less than 12 observations.

So a 'rule-of-thumb' in this context would suggest a minimum of 12 per group (12 pairs in a matched design) or for a two-group comparative study a sample size of 24. This does not mean a smaller study should never be envisaged but this rather alerts one to the probable consequences. It also provides a rough guide in other situations such as the comparison of two proportions, although in that case it specifies the number of events or non-events (whichever the less likely) that should be observed rather than the actual sample size.

10.7 Bibliography

Problems related to confidence intervals for proportions and their differences are discussed by Newcombe and Altman (2000). Day (1988) gives the approximate sample-size Equation 10.10 and Bristol (1989) Equation 10.12, used for a given width of the confidence interval for the difference in two proportions. The sample-size formula (Equation 10.17), for use when differences are expressed by the odds ratio, is given by Lemeshow, Hosmer and Klar (1988).

10.8 Examples and use of the tables

For a 95% CI, $\alpha = 0.05$ and the value from **Table 2.2** is $z_{0.975} = 1.96$ and that for a 99% CI, $\alpha = 0.01$ and $z_{0.995} = 2.5758$.

Table 10.1, Equations 10.2 and 10.5

Example 10.1—single binomial proportion—large population

The prevalence rate of a disease among children in a particular area is believed to be about 30%. How many subjects are required if we wish to determine this prevalence with 95% *CI* of width 10%?

It is anticipated that this will be a rather large study, so that Equation 10.2 may be used. This gives, with $\pi_{\mathrm{Plan}} = 0.30$ and $\omega = 0.1$, $N = \dfrac{4 \times 0.3 \times (1 - 0.3) \times 1.96^2}{0.1^2} = 322.7$ or approximately 330 children. However, if we use the more accurate expression of Equation 10.5, which is applicable whatever the sample size, then from **Table 10.1** the number of children to be surveyed is $N = 323$.

If the investigator decides that he would prefer to be 99%, rather than 95%, confident that the width of the *CI* will be 10% then SS evaluates Equation 10.5 to give $N = 558$ or approximately 560 children to be surveyed.

Table 10.1 and Equation 10.5

Example 10.2—single binomial proportion

Suppose all that is known about the prevalence of the disease is that it is anticipated to be somewhere between 10 and 40%. How does this effect the sample size calculated in *Example 10.1*?

If the prevalence was 10%, then for a 95% *CI* using the recommended confidence interval method from **Table 10.1** or SS with $\omega = 0.1$ and $\pi_{\mathrm{Plan}} = 0.1$ the investigator would require about $N = 139$ children. On the other hand, if $\pi_{\mathrm{Plan}} = 0.4$, $N = 369$ children. Thus if he decides to stick with the original estimate of 320 children from the first part of *Example 10.1*, then he will have a more precise estimate if the prevalence turns out to be near 10% than if turns out to be near 40%.

Equation 10.3

Example 10.3—single binomial proportion—large population

In the same situation as Example 10.1, how many subjects are required if we wish to determine the prevalence to within about 3%, that is have a confidence interval of width 6%, with 95% confidence that this is true?

Here $\pi_{Plan} = 0.3$, so $\varepsilon = 0.03/0.3 = 0.1$ which is equivalent to determining the prevalence to within 10% of its true value. Thus $\omega = 2\pi_{Plan}\varepsilon = 0.06$. From Equation 10.3 with $\pi_{Plan} = 0.3$ and $\varepsilon = 0.1$ we obtain $N = \dfrac{(1 - 0.3)1.96^2}{0.3 \times 0.1^2} = 896.4$ or approximately 900 children.

Alternatively using the recommended method, $\boxed{SS_S}$ gives $N = 897$ which agrees with the previous approximate calculation.

Equations 10.3 and 10.8

Example 10.4—single binomial proportion—finite population

Suppose that a register contains 1000 male patients with diabetes but no clinical details are included with respect to whether they are impotent or not. If the estimated prevalence of impotence amongst these diabetics is assumed to be 20%, how many patients do we require in a survey to determine the prevalence of impotence if we are willing to allow a 95% *CI* of 4 percentage points either side of the true prevalence?

Here $\pi_{Plan} = 0.2$ and 4 percentage points of this prevalence implies that $\pi_{Plan}\varepsilon = 0.04$, so that $\varepsilon = 0.04/0.20 = 0.2$. From Equation 10.3 we would require about $N = 390$ subjects for a 95% *CI* of the specified width. However, the population is of a finite size, $N_{Population} = 1000$, and therefore this sample comprises $N/N_{Population} = 0.39$ or approximately 40% of the diabetics on the register. To adjust for a finite population, the correction factor is

$$F = \frac{1000}{390 + 1000} = 0.7194.$$

Thus the actual number of subjects required to be sampled is reduced to $N_{Finite} = 0.7194 \times 390 = 280.6$ or approximately 300. This is a considerable reduction in the anticipated study size.

Alternatively using $\boxed{SS_S}$ with $\omega = 2\pi_{Plan}\varepsilon = 2 \times 0.2 \times 0.2 = 0.08$ gives $N = 385$ or $N_{Finite} = 0.7194 \times 385 = 277.0$ which agrees closely with the previous calculation.

Table 10.2, Equations 10.10 and 10.11

Example 10.5—difference between two proportions—independent groups

In a study of nausea after anaesthesia described by Day (1988), the anticipated nausea rates with two types of anaesthetics are 10% and 20%. How many patients are required if a width of −5% to +5% is set for the estimate of the difference with a 95% *CI*?

The anticipated values are $\pi_1 = 0.1$ and $\pi_2 = 0.2$, and $\omega = 2 \times 0.05 = 0.10$. Then use of Equation 10.10 with $\varphi = 1$ gives $m = \dfrac{4 \times [1 \times 0.1(1 - 0.1) + 0.2(1 - 0.2)] \times 1.96^2}{1 \times 0.10^2} = 384.2$.

Using the less precise method of Equation 10.11 with $\bar{\pi} = (0.1 + 0.2)/2 = 0.15$ gives $m = \dfrac{8 \times 0.15(1 - 0.15) \times 1.96^2}{0.10^2} = 391.8$.

However, since the allocation ratio $\varphi = 1$ in this case, Equation 10.12 gives $m = \dfrac{\left\{1.96\sqrt{0.1(1 - 0.1) + 0.2(1 - 0.2)} + \sqrt{1.96^2[0.1(1 - 0.1) + 0.2(1 - 0.2)] + 2 \times 0.10}\right\}^2}{0.10^2} = 423.2$.

This is somewhat different from the earlier estimates and also differs from that computed by $\boxed{^SS_S}$ which always defaults to the recommended method of Equation 10.13. This gives, as does **Table 10.2**, $m = 388$ or $N = 2m \approx 800$ patients.

Table 10.3, Equations 10.17 and 10.19

Example 10.6—odds ratio

In the study of nausea after anaesthesia of *Example 10.5* what sample size would be required if the odds ratio were to be determined to within 20% of its own value.

Here the planning $OR_{\text{Plan}} = \dfrac{\pi_2(1 - \pi_1)}{\pi_1(1 - \pi_2)} = \dfrac{0.2 \times 0.9}{0.1 \times 0.8} = 2.25$ and $\varepsilon = 0.2$. Use of Equation 10.17

with $\varphi = 1$ gives $m = \dfrac{\left[\dfrac{1}{0.1 \times 0.9} + \dfrac{1}{1 \times 0.2 \times 0.8}\right] \times 1.96^2}{[\log(1 - 0.2)]^2} = 1339.4$ or $N = 2m \approx 2700$ patients.

Using the less precise method of Equation 10.19 gives $m = \dfrac{2 \times 1.96^2}{0.15 \times 0.85 \times [\log 0.8]^2} = 1210.2$

or $N = 2m \approx 2500$ patients. The nearest tabular entries in **Table 10.3** are $\pi_1 = 0.1$, $OR = 2$ and $\pi_1 = 0.1$, $OR = 2.5$ with corresponding $m = 1376$ and 1311, the average of which is 1344. This is quite close to 1339 obtained above.

Table 10.4 and Equation 10.20

Example 10.7—difference between two proportions—paired groups

Bidwell, Sahu, Edwards *et al.* (2005) describe a study involving surveying patients attending a hospital clinic on their awareness and fear of blindness due to smoking, in comparison to stroke and other smoking-related diseases. 358 patients responded to the survey, with only 9.5% believing that smoking caused blindness, as compared to 70.6% for stroke.

The authors did not report any formal sample-size calculations carried out before the start of the study. But suppose they had wished to do this and had anticipated that 20% of patients believed smoking caused blindness while 60% believed smoking caused stroke. Moreover, they had planned to obtain a confidence interval on the difference in the proportions of width 0.1, with correlation coefficient 0.6.

Since Equation 10.20 must be solved iteratively for N, we use **Table 10.4** with $\pi_1 = 0.2$, $\pi_2 = 0.6$, $\omega = 0.1$ and $\rho = 0.6$ to obtain $N = 252$ patients for the study. However, the final study size is quite sensitive to the presumed value of ρ so that if it takes the values 0.5 and 0.7, the corresponding sample sizes of 312 and 192 are obtained from $\boxed{^SS_S}$.

Table 10.5 and Equation 10.24

Example 10.8—difference between two means—independent groups

In a clinical trial described by Day (1988) which involved comparing the diastolic blood pressure (BP) in two groups of patients, it was anticipated that the mean BP might be 100 and 90 mmHg respectively and past experience suggested that the standard deviation is likely to be 10 mmHg. In the event, however, the observed difference turned out to be 1 mmHg which is much less than the anticipated 10 mmHg. The corresponding 95% *CI* was −5 to +7 mmHg. Nevertheless, if the difference was truly as large as 7 mmHg, this might be medically worthwhile. As a consequence, a new study is planned, but with the anticipated difference set a 5 mmHg, rather than at 7 mmHg, which is towards the upper end of the above *CI*, as this is taken to be the smallest medically relevant difference. What sample size is required for obtaining a 95% *CI* of width 10 mmHg?

Here $\delta_{Plan} = 5$, although this is not needed for the sample-size calculation, $\sigma_{Plan} = 10$ and $\omega = 10$ is required, hence $\Lambda_{Plan} = 10/10 = 1.0$. Equation 10.26 with $\varphi = 1$ is used, to obtain

$$m = 4 \left[\frac{1+1}{1} \right] \frac{1.96^2}{1.0^2} = 30.7 \text{ or 31 patients per group or a total of } N = 62 \text{ in all. Direct entry with}$$

$\Lambda_{Plan} = 1$ in **Table 10.5** or use of $\boxed{{}^SS_S}$ lead to $N = 62$.

Table 10.5 and Equation 10.22

Example 10.9—single mean—enzymealanine aminopeptidase

Jung, Perganda, Schimke *et al.* (1988) give the mean and standard deviation of the tabular enzymealanine aminopeptidase (AAP) in 30 healthy male hospital staff members as 1.05 and 0.32 respectively. A repeat of the study is planned in a random sample of males in the neighbourhood. How large should the study be to ensure that the width of the corresponding 95% *CI* is 0.1?

Here the anticipated value of $\mu_{Plan} = 1.05$, the anticipated standard deviation is $\sigma_{Plan} = 0.32$ and $\omega = 0.1$, hence $\Lambda_{Plan} = 0.1/0.32 = 0.3125$. For a 95% *CI*, Equation 10.22 gives $N = 4 \times 1.96^2 / 0.3125^2 = 157.35$ or approximately 160 men. Direct entry with $\Lambda_{Plan} = 0.3$ in **Table 10.5** gives $m = 342$ and so, as we have a single mean situation, $N = m/2 = 171$. Use of $\boxed{{}^SS_S}$ with $\Lambda_{Plan} = 0.3125$ gives $N = 158$.

Table 10.5 and Equation 10.26

Example 10.10—difference between two means—paired groups—small samples

Suppose the study reported by Altman and Gardner (2000) in which systolic blood pressure levels in 16 middle-aged men before and after a standard exercise were to be repeated. In that study the mean 'After minus Before exercise' difference was 6.6 mmHg, the standard deviation of this difference was 6.0 mmHg and the corresponding 95% *CI* was from 3.4 to 9.8 mmHg. The new investigators would like to reduce the width of the resulting confidence interval to about 80% of that of the previous one.

The planning values are therefore $\omega = 0.8 \times (9.8 - 3.4) = 5.12$ and $\sigma_{Plan} = 6.0$, hence $\Lambda_{Plan} = 5.12/6.0 = 0.8533$. Using these values in Equation 10.28 for a 95% *CI* gives a sample

size of $N = \dfrac{4 \times 1.96^2}{0.8533^2} = 21.1$ or 22 middle-aged men, which agrees with $\boxed{{}^SS_S}$. **Table 10.5**

with Λ_{Plan} set to 0.85 gives $m = 43$, hence $N = 43/2 = 21.5$ or 22 once more.

In view of the modest sample size, the investigator may feel that a confidence interval should use Student's *t*-distribution in the calculations rather than the Normal distribution. This implies replacing $z_{1-\alpha/2}$ by $t_{df,1-\alpha/2}$ in Equation 10.28 where *df* are the degrees of freedom or $N - 1$ in this case. With $N = 22$, $df = 21$ and we have $t_{21,0.975} = 2.079$.

To obtain the sample size, we assume the sample size $N_0 = 22$ is that obtained from Equation 10.28 from which we have shown $t_{21,0.975} = 2.079$. This is then used to replace the 1.96 in the above calculations to give $N_2 = (4 \times 2.079^2)/0.8533^2 = 23.74$ or 24. This results in a second iteration with $t_{23,0.975} = 2.069$ and $N_1 = (4 \times 2.069^2)/0.8533^2 = 23.51$ or 24. As this gives the same result as the previous calculation the iteration stops and $N = 24$ middle-aged men are recruited to the study.

10.9 References

Altman DG and Gardner MJ (2000). Means and their differences. In Altman DG, Machin D, Bryant TN and Gardner MJ (eds). *Statistics with Confidence*, 2nd edn. British Medical Journal Books, London, 31–32.

Bidwell G, Sahu A, Edwards R, Harrison RA, Thornton J and Kelly SP (2005). Perceptions of blindness related to smoking: a hospital-based cross-sectional study. *Eye*, **19**, 945–948.

Bristol DR (1989). Sample sizes for constructing confidence intervals and testing hypotheses. *Statistics in Medicine*, **8**, 803–811.

Day SJ (1988). Clinical trial numbers and confidence intervals of a pre-specified size. *Lancet*, **ii**, 1427.

Jung K, Perganda M, Schimke E, Ratzmann KP and Ilius A (1988). Urinary enzymes and low-molecular-mass proteins as indicators of diabetic nephropathy. *Clinical Chemistry*, **34**, 544–547.

Lemeshow S, Hosmer DW and Klar J (1988). Sample size requirements for studies estimating odds ratios or relative risks. *Statistics in Medicine*, **7**, 759–764.

Newcombe RG and Altman DG (2000). Proportions and their differences. In Altman DG, Machin D, Bryant TN and Gardner MJ (eds). *Statistics with Confidence*, 2nd edn. British Medical Journal Books, London, 45–56.

Table 10.1 Sample sizes required to observe a given confidence interval width for a given proportion in a sample from a large population.

	Confidence interval (CI)							
	90%				95%			
	Width of CI, ω				Width of CI, ω			
π_{Plan}	0.05	0.1	0.15	0.2	0.05	0.1	0.15	0.2
0.01	43	11	5	3	61	16	7	4
0.02	85	22	10	6	121	31	14	8
0.03	126	32	14	8	179	45	20	12
0.04	167	42	19	11	237	60	27	15
0.05	206	52	23	13	292	73	33	19
0.06	245	62	28	16	347	87	39	22
0.07	282	71	32	18	401	101	45	26
0.08	319	80	36	20	453	114	51	29
0.09	355	89	40	23	504	126	56	32
0.10	390	98	44	25	554	139	62	35
0.11	424	106	48	27	602	151	67	38
0.12	458	115	51	29	650	163	73	41
0.13	490	123	55	31	696	174	78	44
0.14	522	131	58	33	741	186	83	47
0.15	552	138	62	35	784	196	88	49
0.16	582	146	65	37	827	207	92	52
0.17	611	153	68	39	868	217	97	55
0.18	639	160	71	40	908	227	101	57
0.19	667	167	75	42	946	237	106	60
0.20	693	174	77	44	984	246	110	62
0.25	812	203	91	51	1153	289	129	73
0.30	910	228	102	57	1291	323	144	81
0.35	985	247	110	62	1399	350	156	88
0.40	1039	260	116	65	1476	369	164	93
0.45	1072	268	120	67	1522	381	170	96
0.50	1083	271	121	68	1537	385	171	97

Table 10.2 Sample sizes required to observe a given confidence interval width for the difference between two proportions—independent groups. Each cell gives the number of subjects for each group, m. Hence, the total sample size for the study is $N = 2m$.

		Confidence intervals (CI)							
		90%				95%			
		Width of CI, ω				Width of CI, ω			
π_1	π_2	0.05	0.1	0.15	0.2	0.05	0.1	0.15	0.2
0.1	0.2	1085	274	123	70	1541	388	175	100
	0.3	1300	326	146	82	1846	463	207	117
	0.4	1429	358	159	90	2029	507	226	127
	0.5	1472	368	164	92	2090	522	232	130
	0.6	1428	357	159	89	2028	507	225	126
	0.7	1299	325	144	81	1844	461	205	115
	0.8	1083	271	121	68	1537	385	171	97
	0.9	782	197	89	51	1110	280	126	72
0.2	0.3	1601	400	178	100	2273	568	252	141
	0.4	1731	432	191	107	2457	613	272	152
	0.5	1774	442	196	110	2518	628	278	156
	0.6	1730	432	191	107	2456	613	271	152
	0.7	1600	399	177	99	2272	567	251	140
	0.8	1385	346	153	86	1966	491	217	122
	0.9	1083	271	121	68	1537	385	171	97
0.3	0.4	1946	485	215	120	2763	689	305	170
	0.5	1989	496	219	123	2824	704	311	174
	0.6	1946	485	215	120	2763	689	304	170
	0.7	1816	453	200	112	2579	643	284	159
	0.8	1600	399	177	99	2272	567	251	140
	0.9	1299	325	144	81	1844	461	205	115
0.4	0.5	2119	528	234	130	3008	750	331	185
	0.6	2076	517	229	128	2947	734	325	181
	0.7	1946	485	215	120	2763	689	304	170
	0.8	1730	432	191	107	2456	613	271	152
	0.9	1428	357	159	89	2028	507	225	126
0.5	0.6	2119	528	234	130	3008	750	331	185
	0.7	1989	496	219	123	2824	704	311	174
	0.8	1774	442	196	110	2518	628	278	156
	0.9	1472	368	164	92	2090	522	232	130

Table 10.3 Sample sizes required to observe a proportionate confidence interval width for the difference between two groups expressed via the odds ratio (OR). Each cell gives the number of subjects for each group, m. Hence, the total sample size for the study is $N = 2m$.

		90% CI				95% CI			
		Proportion of the odds ratio, ε				Proportion of the odds ratio, ε			
π_1	OR	0.1	0.15	0.2	0.25	0.1	0.15	0.2	0.25
0.1	1.25	4985	2095	1112	669	7077	2975	1578	950
	1.50	4699	1975	1048	631	6672	2804	1488	895
	1.75	4497	1890	1003	604	6385	2684	1424	857
	2.00	4347	1827	969	583	6172	2594	1376	828
	2.50	4141	1741	924	556	5880	2471	1311	789
0.2	1.25	2867	1205	640	385	4071	1711	908	546
	1.50	2753	1157	614	370	3908	1643	872	525
	1.75	2675	1125	597	359	3798	1596	847	510
	2.00	2621	1102	585	352	3721	1564	830	499
	2.50	2554	1074	570	343	3625	1524	809	487
0.3	1.25	2234	939	498	300	3172	1333	708	426
	1.50	2184	918	487	293	3101	1304	692	416
	1.75	2156	907	481	290	3061	1287	683	411
	2.00	2142	900	478	288	3041	1278	678	408
	2.50	2137	899	477	287	3034	1276	677	407
0.4	1.25	1999	840	446	269	2838	1193	633	381
	1.50	1991	837	444	267	2827	1188	631	380
	1.75	1997	839	446	268	2835	1192	632	381
	2.00	2011	846	449	270	2855	1200	637	383
	2.50	2056	864	459	276	2919	1227	651	392
0.5	1.25	1962	825	438	264	2786	1171	622	374
	1.50	1991	837	444	267	2827	1188	631	380
	1.75	2029	853	453	273	2880	1211	642	387
	2.00	2072	871	462	278	2942	1237	656	395
	2.50	2170	912	484	291	3080	1295	687	414
0.6	1.25	2090	879	466	281	2968	1248	662	399
	1.50	2160	908	482	290	3067	1289	684	412
	1.75	2236	940	499	300	3175	1335	708	426
	2.00	2316	974	517	311	3288	1382	733	441
	2.50	2482	1044	554	333	3524	1482	786	473
0.7	1.25	2443	1027	545	328	3468	1458	774	466
	1.50	2571	1081	574	345	3651	1535	814	490
	1.75	2703	1137	603	363	3838	1613	856	515
	2.00	2838	1193	633	381	4030	1694	899	541
	2.50	3112	1308	694	418	4418	1857	985	593
0.8	1.25	3279	1378	731	440	4655	1957	1038	625
	1.50	3514	1477	784	472	4989	2097	1113	670
	1.75	3752	1577	837	504	5327	2239	1188	715
	2.00	3991	1678	890	536	5667	2382	1264	761
	2.50	4473	1880	998	600	6351	2669	1416	852

Table 10.4 Sample sizes required to observe a given confidence interval width for the difference between two proportions from paired or matched groups. Each cell gives the number of pairs, N_{pairs}, required for the study.

ρ	π_1	π_2	Width of 90% CI, ω				Width of 95% CI, ω			
			0.05	0.1	0.15	0.2	0.05	0.1	0.15	0.2
0.2	0.1	0.3	1063	267	120	68	1508	379	170	96
		0.4	1175	294	131	74	1668	418	186	105
		0.5	1212	303	135	76	1721	430	191	107
		0.6	1174	293	130	73	1667	416	185	104
	0.2	0.4	1392	347	154	86	1976	493	218	122
		0.5	1427	356	158	88	2026	505	224	125
		0.6	1391	347	153	86	1975	492	218	122
		0.7	1283	320	142	79	1822	454	201	112
	0.3	0.5	1593	397	175	98	2261	563	249	139
		0.6	1557	388	171	96	2211	551	243	136
		0.7	1453	362	160	89	2063	514	227	126
		0.8	1283	320	142	79	1822	454	201	112
	0.4	0.6	1660	413	183	102	2357	587	259	144
		0.7	1557	388	171	96	2211	551	243	136
		0.8	1391	347	153	86	1975	492	218	122
		0.9	1174	293	130	73	1667	416	185	104
	0.5	0.7	1593	397	175	98	2261	563	249	139
		0.8	1427	356	158	88	2026	505	224	125
		0.9	1212	303	135	76	1721	430	191	107
0.4	0.1	0.3	825	208	94	54	1172	296	133	76
		0.4	921	231	103	58	1307	328	146	83
		0.5	953	238	106	60	1352	338	150	85
		0.6	920	230	102	57	1305	326	145	81
	0.2	0.4	1053	263	117	65	1494	373	165	93
		0.5	1081	270	119	67	1535	383	169	95
		0.6	1052	262	116	65	1493	372	164	92
		0.7	966	241	106	59	1371	341	151	84
	0.3	0.6	1169	291	128	71	1659	413	182	101
		0.7	1089	271	120	66	1546	385	169	94
		0.8	966	241	106	59	1371	341	151	84
	0.4	0.6	1245	310	136	76	1767	439	194	107
		0.7	1169	291	128	71	1659	413	182	101
		0.8	1052	262	116	65	1493	372	164	92
		0.9	920	230	102	57	1305	326	145	81
	0.5	0.7	1196	298	131	73	1698	423	186	104
		0.8	1081	270	119	67	1535	383	169	95
		0.9	953	238	106	60	1352	338	150	85

Table 10.4 (*continued*): Sample sizes required to observe a given confidence interval width for the difference between two proportions from paired or matched groups. Each cell gives the number of pairs, N_{pairs}, required for the study.

ρ	π_1	π_2	Width of 90% CI, ω				Width of 95% CI, ω			
			0.05	0.1	0.15	0.2	0.05	0.1	0.15	0.2
0.6	0.1	0.3	589	150	69	40	836	213	97	57
		0.4	667	168	75	43	946	238	107	61
		0.5	693	174	77	44	984	246	110	62
		0.6	665	166	74	41	944	236	105	59
	0.2	0.4	714	179	80	45	1014	254	113	64
		0.5	735	183	81	45	1044	260	115	64
		0.6	713	177	78	44	1012	252	111	62
		0.7	648	161	71	39	920	229	101	56
	0.3	0.5	800	199	88	49	1135	282	124	69
		0.6	780	194	85	47	1107	275	121	67
		0.7	726	180	79	44	1030	256	112	62
		0.8	648	161	71	39	920	229	101	56
	0.4	0.6	829	206	90	50	1177	292	128	71
		0.7	780	194	85	47	1107	275	121	67
		0.8	713	177	78	44	1012	252	111	62
		0.9	665	166	74	41	944	236	105	59
	0.5	0.7	800	199	88	49	1135	282	124	69
		0.8	735	183	81	45	1044	260	115	64
		0.9	693	174	77	44	984	246	110	62
0.8	0.1	0.3	353	93	44	27	500	131	62	38
		0.4	413	105	48	28	586	149	68	39
		0.5	433	109	48	27	615	154	69	39
		0.6	410	102	45	25	582	145	64	36
	0.2	0.4	377	96	44	25	535	136	62	36
		0.5	390	98	44	25	554	139	62	35
		0.6	374	93	41	23	530	132	58	32
		0.7	331	82	36	20	470	116	51	28
	0.3	0.5	403	100	44	24	572	142	62	34
		0.6	391	97	42	23	556	137	59	32
		0.7	362	89	39	21	514	126	55	30
		0.8	331	82	36	20	470	116	51	28
	0.4	0.6	413	102	44	24	587	144	62	34
		0.7	391	97	42	23	556	137	59	32
		0.8	374	93	41	23	530	132	58	32
		0.9	410	102	45	25	582	145	64	36
	0.5	0.7	403	100	44	24	572	142	62	34
		0.8	390	98	44	25	554	139	62	35
		0.9	433	109	48	27	615	154	69	39

Table 10.5 Sample sizes required to observe a given confidence interval width to estimate a single mean or the difference between two means for independent or matched groups. We denote the tabular value m, for the single mean $N = m/2$; for two independent groups $N = 2m$; whereas for a paired or matched design $N_{Pairs} = m/2$.

	Confidence intervals (CI)	
Λ	90%	95%
0.20	542	769
0.25	347	492
0.30	241	342
0.35	177	251
0.40	136	193
0.45	107	152
0.50	87	123
0.55	72	102
0.60	61	86
0.65	52	73
0.70	45	63
0.75	39	55
0.80	34	49
0.85	30	43
0.90	27	38
0.95	24	35
1.0	22	31
1.1	18	26
1.2	16	22
1.3	13	19
1.4	12	16
1.5	10	14
1.6	9	13
1.7	8	11
1.8	7	10
1.9	6	9
2.0	6	8

Post-marketing surveillance

11

SUMMARY

Once a drug or medical device has been approved for use in patients by the regulatory authorities, it will then usually go into routine clinical use and may be followed by studies involving their post-marketing surveillance. These will usually cover a wider pool of patient types than those recruited to the clinical trial(s) demonstrating their efficacy. There may be concerns about the short and longer term consequences of this wider use. This chapter describes sample-size calculations for some single or two-group designs, which are often referred to as post-marketing studies.

11.1 Introduction

After a drug or medical device has been accepted for general use it may be prudent to survey the corresponding treated patients to identify the type, and quantify the scale, of any adverse effects. In some circumstances it is possible that only one adverse reaction, such as a drug-related death, would be necessary for the drug to be considered unacceptable and withdrawn from a prescription list. In other situations a single adverse occurrence of a particular event would be put down to chance and two or three occurrences are required to confirm suspicion about the drug. In most situations the observed adverse reactions may occur in patients not receiving the drug in question; for example, in an elderly population deaths are likely to occur in any event. Many common adverse reactions such as nausea, drowsiness and headache are prevalent in the population, and we need to know whether the drug has provoked an increase in prevalence of such adverse reactions over this background rate. If the background incidence is known, then the sample-size calculations are relatively straightforward. If, as is more usual, the incidence is not known, then a control population might also be monitored for comparison purposes.

An alternative to a prospective study is to conduct a case-control study in which patients who have experienced the adverse event of particular interest are matched to individuals who have not experienced such a reaction. Cases and controls are then checked to see if they have taken the drug under study.

Sample Size Tables for Clinical Studies, 3rd edition. By David Machin, Michael J. Campbell, Say Beng Tan, and Sze Huey Tan. Published 2009 by Blackwell Publishing, ISBN: 978-1-4051-4650-0

11.2 Cohort studies

No background incidence

Sample size

Suppose the expected incidence of adverse reactions is λ, the number of occurrences of a particular adverse reaction is a and the number of patients required to be monitored is N. If the incidence of adverse reactions is reasonably low then one might assume that they follow a Poisson distribution. With these assumptions and defining β to be the probability that, for given incidence λ, we will not find a reactions in a sample of N patients on the particular drug under study, then N satisfies

$$\sum_{x=0}^{a-1} \frac{(N\lambda)^x e^{-N\lambda}}{x!} = \beta. \tag{11.1}$$

For $a > 1$ there is no simple expression for the solution to Equation 11.1 but the equation can be solved using numerical methods.

For the special case $a = 1$, that is, when the particular adverse reaction need occur in only one patient, (Equation 11.1) simplifies to

$$N = \frac{-\log \beta}{\lambda}. \tag{11.2}$$

Quick formula

In certain circumstances, it may be that the experience to date with a new drug had not yet resulted in the occurrence of a side-effect which is of particular interest. For example, the event of a post-operative death may be of particular concern if a new type of anaesthesia has been introduced. If none of N patients showed the event of interest, then the upper 95% confidence limit of a $0/N$ (or 0%) rate is approximately $3/N$. Thus, in planning a study, for an anticipated incidence λ, this suggests a sample size of

$$N = 3 / \lambda. \tag{11.3}$$

Known background incidence

Sample size

If λ_0 is the known background incidence of the adverse reaction, and δ the additional incidence caused by use of the particular drug under study, then a one-sided test is appropriate. The sample size, for given significance level α and power $1 - \beta$ is

$$N = \frac{\left[z_{1-\alpha}\sqrt{\lambda_0} + z_{1-\beta}\sqrt{(\lambda_0 + \delta)} \right]^2}{\delta^2}. \tag{11.4}$$

This is an equivalent expression to Equation 3.7 with $\pi_{\text{Known}} = \lambda_0$ and $\pi_2 = \lambda_0 + \delta$ when both λ_0 and δ are very small as we would anticipate in this context.

Unknown background incidence

Sample size

If the background incidence is unknown then a control group is needed for comparison purposes. In this situation also, a one-sided test is likely to be the most appropriate. However, in order to estimate the number of subjects required in the study we would still need to anticipate the background incidence λ_0. We note that, in contrast to the randomised clinical trials described in **Chapter 3**, it is more usual in post-marketing surveillance studies to have more untreated controls, m, than subjects receiving the drug to be monitored, n, as they are usually more numerous in number so can improve the statistical efficiency of the design when numbers taking the drug are perhaps limited. We recognise this by specifying the sample size in terms of n and setting $m = Cn$. Thus, if the control group is indeed C times as large as the treated group then following Equation 3.2, the number of patients in the treated group, is

$$n = \frac{\left\{z_{1-\alpha}\sqrt{[(C+1)\bar{\lambda}(1-\bar{\lambda})]} + z_{1-\beta}\sqrt{[\lambda_0(1-\lambda_0) + C(\lambda_0+\delta)(1-\lambda_0-\delta)]}\right\}^2}{C\delta^2}, \tag{11.5}$$

where $\bar{\lambda} = [C\lambda_0 + (\lambda_0 + \delta)] / (1 + C)$. The total number of subjects recruited is $N = m + n = n(C + 1)$.

If the control group is the same size as the treated group, then $C = 1$ and Equation 11.5 can be approximated by

$$n = m = \frac{(z_{1-\alpha} + z_{1-\beta})^2[\lambda_0(1-\lambda_0) + (\lambda_0+\delta)(1-\lambda_0-\delta)]}{\delta^2}, \tag{11.6}$$

Moreover, if δ and λ_0 are small, this in turn, can be approximated by

$$n = m = \frac{(z_{1-\alpha} + z_{1-\beta})^2(2\lambda_0 + \delta)}{\delta^2}. \tag{11.7}$$

Several independent reactions

In practice, several adverse reactions to a particular drug are often monitored simultaneously. For planning purposes these are often assumed all to have approximately the same incidence and to act independently of each other. If s reactions are being monitored simultaneously, then to avoid getting many false positive results the significance level is changed from α to α/s. Thus the only change required is to replace $z_{1-\alpha}$ by $z_{1-\alpha/s}$ in these equations. However, this approach can result in very large studies.

11.3 Case-control studies

An alternative to the cohort studies approach to post-marketing surveillance is first to identify those patients experiencing the adverse event, perhaps over a pre-defined period, then obtain matched controls who have not experienced the event and finally to ascertain in each group how many have been exposed to the particular substance (drug) under scrutiny.

Sample size

The number of cases required, or equivalently the number of units of one case to C matched controls, is

$$n = \frac{1}{(\lambda_0 - \Omega)^2} \left\{ z_{1-\alpha} \sqrt{\left(1 + \frac{1}{C} \right) \Pi(1 - \Pi)} + z_{1-\beta} \sqrt{\frac{\lambda_0(1 - \lambda_0)}{C} + \Omega(1 - \Omega)} \right\}^2, \qquad (11.8)$$

where $\Pi = \dfrac{\lambda_0}{1 + C} \left[C + \dfrac{\Omega}{\lambda_0} \right]$, and $\Omega = \dfrac{\lambda_0 + \delta}{(1 + \delta)}$.

The corresponding number of controls is $m = Cn$. Thus, the total number of subjects recruited to such a study is $N = m + n = n(C + 1)$.

11.4 Bibliography

Post-marketing surveillance has been discussed by Lewis (1981, 1983) and Tubert-Bitter, Begaud, Moride and Abenhaim (1994) from the statistical point of view, and also by Skegg and Doll (1977) and Wilson (1977). The approximation of Equation 11.3 follows from the suggestion of Hanley and Lippman-Hand (1983) and is described by Eypasch, Lefering, Kum and Troidl (1995). Sample-size issues are also discussed by Strom (2005) who gives the formulae for a case-control design. A number of alternative approaches have also been proposed including those by Dupont (1988) and Edwardes (2001).

11.5 Examples and use of the tables

Table 11.1 and Equation 11.1

Example 11.1—cohort design—no background incidence

In a previous survey, a hypertensive drug produced cardiac arrhythmias in about one in 10 000 people. A researcher decides that if a new hypertensive drug produces three such arrhythmias then the drug will have to be withdrawn pending further research. He wishes to detect three events with a 99% probability of success.

Table 11.1 with $1 - \beta = 0.99$, incidence $\lambda = 1/10\ 000 = 0.0001$ and $a = 3$, gives $m = 84\ 060$ subjects as does $^S\!S_S$. Thus approximately $N = 85\ 000$ subjects are required.

If, on the other hand, the maximum number of subjects was restricted to 30 000 then one can see by scanning **Table 11.1** that he could detect one adverse reaction with a probability of success of 0.95, since with $\lambda = 0.0001$, $a = 1$ then $1 - \beta = 0.95$; or two reactions with probability of 0.80, since with $\lambda = 0.0001$, $a = 2$ then $1 - \beta = 0.80$. The corresponding calculations using $^S\!S_S$ confirm the actual sample sizes as 29 958 and 29 944 respectively.

Equation 11.3

Example 11.2—cohort design—quick formula

The incidence of a particular adverse event is thought to be of less than one per 10 000. How many patients would need to be observed for the researcher to be reasonably confident that the upper 95% confidence interval is less than one in 10 000?

Here, $\lambda = 1/10\,000 = 0.0001$ and use of Equation 11.3 suggests that $N = 3/0.0001 = 30\,000$ patients would need to be observed amongst which not a single adverse reaction is to be anticipated.

Table 11.2 and Equation 11.4

Example 11.3—cohort design—known background incidence

Suppose that a possible side-effect of a drug is an increased incidence of gastric cancer. In an elderly population, suppose that the annual incidence of gastric cancer is 1%, and the drug will be deemed unacceptable if this increases to 1.5%. What size of study is required? Further suppose there was also concern with respect to possible cardiovascular events of much the same magnitude. How would this affect the sample size?

> For a 5% one-sided test size, $\alpha = 0.05$, **Table 2.2** gives $z_{0.95} = 1.6449$ and for a power of 90% with one-sided $1 - \beta = 0.90$, $z_{0.90} = 1.2816$. For $s = 2$, $\alpha/s = 0.025$ and for a one-sided test $z_{0.975} = 1.96$.

If an experimenter is prepared to discount any result that states that the drug actually prevents gastric cancer, then this is a one-sided test, at say $\alpha = 0.05$. Furthermore, if he requires a power $1 - \beta = 0.9$ to detect this increase, then with $\lambda_0 = 0.01$ and $\delta = 0.005$ Equation 11.4 gives

$$N = \frac{\left[1.6449 \times \sqrt{0.01} + 1.2816 \times \sqrt{(0.01 + 0.005)}\right]^2}{0.005^2} = 4133.3$$ so that he would be required to

study $N = 4200$ subjects receiving the drug. The calculations using ^SS_S give $N = 4134$ as does **Table 11.2**.

If cardiovascular events were also to be monitored, then the study team may set α/s, where $s = 2$, in place of α in the above calculations. Thus, for example, calculation using ^SS_S then gives $N = 4984$ which is an increase of 850 subjects so clearly a larger study is suggested.

Table 11.3 and Equation 11.5

Example 11.4—cohort design—unknown background incidence

If the experimenter of *Example 11.3* did not know the annual incidence of gastric cancer, but was prepared to monitor a comparable population of equal size, how many subjects should be monitored in each group?

> For a 5% one-sided test size, $\alpha = 0.05$, **Table 2.2** gives $z_{0.95} = 1.6449$ and for a power of 90% with one-sided $1 - \beta = 0.90$, $z_{0.90} = 1.2816$.

For one-sided $\alpha = 0.05$, $1 - \beta = 0.90$, $\lambda_0 = 0.01$, $\delta = 0.005$ and $C = 1$,

$$\bar{\lambda} = \frac{0.01 + 1 \times (0.01 + 0.005)}{1 + 1} = 0.0125$$ and from Equation 11.5 $n = m =$

$$\frac{\left\{1.6449 \times \sqrt{2 \times 0.0125 \times 0.9875} + 1.2816\sqrt{(0.01 \times 0.99) + (0.015 \times 0.985)}\right\}^2}{0.005^2} = 8455.5 \quad \text{or}$$

approximately the 8500, implying a total of $N = 17\,000$ subjects. The calculations using either **Table 11.3** or ^SS_S give $n = 8455$.

It should be emphasised that, although he does not know the actual incidence for the control group, he has to provide its anticipated value in order to estimate the required number of patients. Patient numbers are quite sensitive to the anticipated value of the incidence λ_0. Thus, in this example, if $\lambda_0 = 0.005$ rather than 0.01 then the number of subjects in each group, for the same test size and power, would be $n = m = 5100$ or approximately $N = 10\ 000$ subjects.

Table 11.3 and Equation 11.5

Example 11.5—cohort design—unknown background incidence—multiple controls
Suppose that an investigator planning the study described in *Example 11.3* has access to a cancer registry as a source for controls, and this enables him to monitor many more patient controls than patients receiving the drug of interest. What effect does this have on the number of patients to be monitored?

As in *Example 11.4*, assuming one-sided $\alpha = 0.05$, $1 - \beta = 0.90$, $\lambda_0 = 0.01$, $\delta = 0.005$, and that $C = 5$ then **Table 11.3** or $^S S_S$ suggest recruiting $n = 4968$ or 5000 patients to receive the drug and $m = 5 \times 5000 = 25\ 000$ controls. This suggests a study of $N = 5000 + 25\ 000 = 30\ 000$ subjects.

Equations 11.4 and 11.5

Example 11.6—randomised trial—unknown background incidence
In a randomised trial conducted by Silverstein, Faich, Goldstein *et al.* (2000) celecoxib was compared with non-steroidal anti-inflammatory drugs (NSAIDs) for osteoarthritis and rheumatoid arthritis. The annualized incidence rates of upper GI ulcer complications alone and combined with symptomatic ulcers were 0.76% with celecoxib and 1.45% with NSAIDs. Were this to be repeated, but with a concern that the level reported for celecoxib was perhaps less than what might be anticipated, what size of study might be contemplated?

Assuming one-sided $\alpha = 0.05$, and power $1 - \beta = 0.8$, then if we further assume the celecoxib rate is in fact nearer 0.95%, this suggests we set $\lambda_0 = 0.0095$ and $\delta = 0.005$. Equation 11.5 and $^S S_S$ then give $n = 5863$ or a post-marketing trial size of approximately 12 000 patients. Were we to assume that the background incidence for NSAIDs is known, Equation 11.4 and $^S S_S$ gives $n = 2739$ or a post-marketing study of approximately 3000 patients all receiving celecoxib.

Table 11.4 and Equation 11.9

Example 11.7—case-control design
It is postulated that a relatively new analgesic may be associated with a particular type of adverse reaction. To investigate if indeed this is so, a case-control study is planned in which it is important to detect a possible relative risk of 1.2 by use of the new analgesic as compared to those that have been in current use. It is anticipated that the adverse event has a prevalence of 0.05 amongst users of standard analgesics. How many cases experiencing the adverse reaction ought the investigators to recruit?

For a 5% one-sided test size, $\alpha = 0.05$, **Table 2.2** gives $z_{0.95} = 1.6449$ and for a power of 80% with one-sided $1 - \beta = 0.80$, $z_{0.80} = 0.8416$.

Here $\lambda_0 = 0.05$ and the relative risk, $RR_{Plan} = \lambda_1/\lambda_0 = 1.2$, where $\lambda_1 = 1.2 \times 0.05 = 0.06$ is the anticipated prevalence in the new analgesic users. From this we have $\delta = \lambda_1 - \lambda_0 = 0.01$, and assuming $C = 1$, $\Omega = (0.05 + 0.01)/(1 + 0.01) = 0.0594$, $\Pi = \dfrac{0.05}{1+1}\left[1 + \dfrac{0.0594}{0.05}\right] = 0.0547$, then with one-sided test size $\alpha = 0.05$ and power $1 - \beta = 0.8$, Equation 11.8 gives $n =$

$$\frac{1}{(0.05 - 0.0594)^2}\left\{1.6449\sqrt{\left(1 + \frac{1}{1}\right) \times 0.0547 \times 0.9453} + 0.8416\sqrt{\frac{0.05 \times 0.95}{1} + (0.0594 \times 0.9406)}\right\}^2$$

$= 7235.1$. **Table 11.4** and ^SS_S with $C = 1$, give $n = 7227$ or approximately 7500. This implies a total study size of $N = 15\,000$ subjects. On the other hand, if $C = 5$, then ^SS_S gives 4257 or approximately $n = 4500$. This gives a total study size of $N = m + n = 5 \times 4500 + 4500 = 27\,000$.

11.6 References

Dupont WD (1988). Power calculations for matched case-control studies. *Biometrics*, **44**, 1157–1168.

Edwardes MD (2001). Sample size requirements for case-control study designs. *BMC Medical Research Methodology*, **1**, 11.

Eypasch E, Lefering R, Kum CK and Troidl H (1995) Probabiliy of adverse events that have not yet occurred: a statistical reminder. *British Medical Journal*, **311**, 619–620.

Hanley JA and Lippman-Hand A (1983). If nothing goes wrong, is everything alright? *Journal of the American Medical Association*, **259**, 1743–1745.

Lewis JA (1981). Post-marketing surveillance: how many patients? *Trends in Pharmacological Sciences*, **2**, 93–94.

Lewis JA (1983). Clinical trials: statistical developments of practical benefit to the pharmaceutical industry. *Journal of the Royal Statistical Society (A)*, **146**, 362–393.

Silverstein FE, Faich G, Goldstein JL and 13 others (2000). Gastrointestinal toxicity with celecoxib vs nonsteroidal anti-inflammatory drugs for osteoarthritis and rheumatoid arthritis. *Journal of the American Medical Association*, **284**, 1247–1255.

Skegg DCG and Doll R (1977). The case for recording events in clinical trials. *British Medical Journal*, **2**, 1523–1524.

Strom BL (2005) Sample size considerations for pharmacoepidemiology studies. In Strom BL (ed.) *Pharmacoepidemiology*, 4th edn. John Wiley & Sons, Chichester, pp. 29–56.

Tubert-Bitter P, Begaud B, Moride Y and Abenhaim L (1994). Sample size calculations for single group post-marketing cohort studies. *Journal of Clinical Epidemiology*, **47**, 435–439.

Wilson AB (1977). Post-marketing surveillance of adverse reactions to new medicines. *British Medical Journal*, **2**, 1001–1003.

Table 11.1 Sample sizes required to observe a total of *a* adverse reactions with a given probability $1 - \beta$ and anticipated incidence λ.

λ	*a*	Probability $1 - \beta$				
		0.5	0.8	0.9	0.95	0.99
0.0001	1	6932	16 095	23 026	29 958	46 052
	2	16 784	29 944	38 898	47 439	66 384
	3	26 741	42 791	53 224	62 958	84 060
	4	36 721	55 151	66 808	77 537	100 452
	5	46 710	67 210	79 936	91 536	116 047
0.0005	1	1387	3219	4606	5992	9211
	2	3357	5989	7780	9488	13 277
	3	5349	8559	10 645	12 592	16 812
	4	7345	11 031	13 362	15 508	20 091
	5	9342	13 442	15 988	18 308	23 210
0.001	1	694	1610	2303	2996	4606
	2	1679	2995	3890	4744	6639
	3	2675	4280	5323	6296	8406
	4	3673	5516	6681	7754	10 046
	5	4671	6721	7994	9154	11 605
0.005	1	139	322	461	600	922
	2	336	599	778	949	1328
	3	535	856	1065	1260	1682
	4	735	1104	1337	1551	2010
	5	935	1345	1599	1831	2321
0.01	1	70	161	231	300	461
	2	168	300	389	475	664
	3	268	428	533	630	841
	4	368	552	669	776	1005
	5	468	673	800	916	1161

Table 11.2 Sample sizes required for detection of a specific adverse reaction with background incidence, λ_0, known.

λ_0	One-sided $\alpha = 0.05$; Power $1 - \beta = 0.8$					
	Additional incidence, δ					
	0.001	0.005	0.01	0.05	0.1	0.15
0.005	32 943	1608	–	–	–	
0.01	63 886	2864	804	–	–	
0.05	311 214	12 778	3295	161	–	
0.1	620 345	25 146	6389	287	81	
0.15	929 474	37 512	9481	411	112	54

λ_0	One-sided $\alpha = 0.05$; Power $1 - \beta = 0.9$					
	Additional incidence, δ					
	0.001	0.005	0.01	0.05	0.1	0.15
0.005	46 474	2391	–	–	–	
0.01	89 339	4134	1196	–	–	
0.05	431 933	17 868	4648	240	–	
0.1	860 130	35 001	8934	414	120	
0.15	1 288 324	52 130	13 218	586	164	80

Table 11.3 Sample sizes required for detection of a specific adverse reaction with background incidence unknown. Each cell gives the number of cases, n. Hence, the total sample size for the study is $N = (C + 1)n$.

λ_0	δ	One-sided $\alpha = 0.05$; Power $1 - \beta = 0.8$				
		Controls per case, C				
		1	2	3	4	5
0.005	0.001	67 634	50 221	44 410	41 502	39 757
0.01	0.001	128 470	95 858	84 984	79 546	76 282
	0.005	6105	4477	3931	3657	3492
0.05	0.005	24 603	18 362	16 281	15 240	14 615
	0.01	6426	4774	4223	3947	3781
0.1	0.005	45 500	34 045	30 227	28 317	27 171
	0.01	11 620	8675	7693	7202	6907
	0.05	540	398	350	325	311
0.15	0.005	63 924	47 873	42 523	39 848	38 242
	0.01	16 195	12 111	10 750	10 069	9661
	0.05	714	528	467	436	417
	0.1	197	145	127	118	113

λ_0	δ	One-sided $\alpha = 0.05$; Power $1 - \beta = 0.9$				
		Controls per case, C				
		1	2	3	4	5
0.005	0.001	93 683	69 983	62 073	58 115	55 738
0.01	0.001	177 951	133 195	118 271	110 807	106 328
	0.005	8455	6283	5554	5188	4968
0.05	0.005	34 078	25 510	22 652	21 224	20 366
	0.01	8901	6651	5899	5524	5298
0.1	0.005	63 024	47 225	41 958	39 325	37 745
	0.01	16 094	12 049	10 700	10 026	9621
	0.05	748	556	492	460	441
0.15	0.005	88 545	66 371	58 980	55 284	53 066
	0.01	22 432	16 805	14 929	13 991	13 428
	0.05	988	737	653	611	586
	0.1	273	203	179	167	160

Table 11.4 Number of cases to be observed in a case-control study. Each cell gives the number of cases, n. Hence, the total sample size for the study is $N = (C + 1)n$.

| λ_0 | δ | \multicolumn{5}{c}{One-sided $\alpha = 0.05$; Power $1 - \beta = 0.8$} | | | | |
| | | \multicolumn{5}{c}{Controls per case, C} | | | | |
		1	2	3	4	5
0.005	0.001	68 415	50 804	44 927	41 986	40 220
0.01	0.001	131 273	97 955	86 845	81 289	77 955
	0.005	6273	4601	4041	3760	3591
0.05	0.005	27 466	20 504	18 183	17 022	16 325
	0.01	7227	5372	4753	4443	4257
0.1	0.005	56 608	42 367	37 619	35 246	33 821
	0.01	14 567	10 880	9651	9036	8667
	0.05	718	529	466	434	415
0.15	0.005	89 178	66 801	59 342	55 612	53 374
	0.01	22 770	17 036	15 125	14 169	13 595
	0.05	1066	791	699	653	625
	0.1	316	233	205	191	183

| λ_0 | δ | \multicolumn{5}{c}{One-sided $\alpha = 0.05$; Power $1 - \beta = 0.9$} | | | | |
| | | \multicolumn{5}{c}{Controls per case, C} | | | | |
		1	2	3	4	5
0.005	0.001	94 765	70 793	62 792	58 788	56 385
0.01	0.001	181 833	136 104	120 855	113 229	108 653
	0.005	8688	6457	5708	5332	5106
0.05	0.005	38 045	28 482	25 293	23 698	22 741
	0.01	10 010	7481	6637	6214	5961
0.1	0.005	78 411	58 760	52 209	48 934	46 968
	0.01	20 176	15 108	13 418	12 573	12 066
	0.05	993	740	655	612	587
0.15	0.005	123 525	92 600	82 291	77 136	74 044
	0.01	31 540	23 632	20 996	19 678	18 887
	0.05	1475	1102	977	915	877
	0.1	438	326	288	269	258

12 The correlation coefficient

SUMMARY

The strength of the linear association between two continuous or ranked variables is estimated by the correlation coefficient. Recommendations as to what may be considered 'small', 'medium' and 'large' associations are given and the formulae for sample sizes to detect such are included, as well as for the situation where lack of association is required to be demonstrated.

12.1 Introduction

An investigator may wish to show that two measurements are associated. Note that this is not the same as showing that two measurements are in agreement with each other. For example, in patients with a particular disease, the number of monocytes in the blood may be correlated with the estrone-to-estradiol conversion rate in that the ratio between the two measurements remains approximately constant, even though the values themselves may not be similar to each other. One method of measuring association is to compute Pearson's product-moment correlation coefficient r. This measures the degree of linear relationship between two variables but is inappropriate in the case of non-linear relationships. Thus a correlation of $r = 0$ indicates that there is no linear relation between the two variables, while $r = +1$ or -1 indicates perfect positive or negative linear correlation respectively. A hypothesis test could also be conducted, the corresponding null hypothesis being that the true correlation coefficient $\rho_{Pop} = 0$. A small p-value will then indicate evidence *against* that true correlation coefficient being zero. However this does not then imply that ρ_{Pop} is necessarily close to $+1$ or -1. Given that the number of monocytes in the blood and the estrone-to-estradiol conversion rates differ between patients, one can calculate the requisite number of patients to be observed by specifying the magnitude of the correlation coefficient to be detected. Specifying the correlation coefficient avoids the problem of defining the ranges (largest to smallest values) of the two variables under consideration; however, the wider their ranges, the more sensitive the study.

12.2 Theory and formulae

Effect size

The correlation coefficient is a dimensionless quantity and so can (itself) act as an effect-size index. Before the study, we need to specify the anticipated size of the correlation coefficient ρ

Sample Size Tables for Clinical Studies, 3rd edition. By David Machin, Michael J. Campbell, Say Beng Tan, and Sze Huey Tan. Published 2009 by Blackwell Publishing, ISBN: 978-1-4051-4650-0

that we think might represent the true correlation between the two variables. Clearly the smaller the true correlation coefficient the larger the study has to be to detect it. To get a feel for the correlation coefficient between the two variables, we note that ρ^2 is the proportion of variance in either of the variables which may be accounted for by the other, using a linear relationship. Cohen (1988) suggested values of ρ of 0.1, 0.3 and 0.5 as 'small', 'medium' and 'large' effects.

Usually the direction of the relationship will be specified in advance. For example, systolic and diastolic blood pressures are certain to be positively associated and so one would use a one-sided test. However, if one is looking for an association with no sign specified, then a two-sided test is warranted.

Sample size

To calculate appropriate sample sizes, we assume that we are investigating the association between two Normally distributed variables with correlation coefficient ρ. It can be shown that:

$$u_p = \frac{1}{2}\log\frac{1+\rho}{1-\rho} + \frac{\rho}{2(N-1)}, \tag{12.1}$$

is approximately Normally distributed with standard deviation $\sqrt{[1/(N-3)]}$, where N is the sample size. This leads to the appropriate sample size to detect a correlation ρ for significance level α and power of $1 - \beta$ as:

$$N = \frac{(z_{1-\alpha} + z_{1-\beta})^2}{u_\rho^2} + 3. \tag{12.2}$$

Note that we have used $z_{1-\alpha}$ rather than $z_{1-\alpha/2}$ as one-sided comparisons are more usual in this situation. However, it should be emphasized that to calculate u_ρ for Equation 12.2 we require some value for N (the number we are trying to estimate!) to substitute in Equation 12.1. To circumvent this problem an initial value for u_ρ, labelled u_ρ^0, is calculated where:

$$u_\rho^0 = \frac{1}{2}\log\left[\frac{1+\rho}{1-\rho}\right]. \tag{12.3}$$

Equation 12.3 is the first term on the right-hand side of Equation 12.1. The value obtained is then used in Equation 12.2 to give an initial value for N labelled N_0. This N_0 is then used in Equation 12.1 to obtain a new value for u_ρ, say u_ρ^1 which is now used in Equation 12.2 to obtain a new value N, and the whole process is repeated again.. To calculate the entries for **Table 12.1** the iteration was repeated until two consecutive values of N within unity of each other were found.

Lack of association

Cohen (1988) cites an example of a social psychologist planning an experiment in which college students would be subjected to two questionnaires, one on personality, $y_{\text{Personality}}$, and one on social desirability, y_{Social}. He wishes to show that $y_{\text{Personality}}$ and y_{Social} are *not* associated. This is a similar situation to that described in **Chapter 9**, where we are trying to do the impossible and prove the null hypothesis. We circumvent this problem by attempting to demonstrate that ρ is small, for example, no greater in absolute value than 0.10.

12.3 Bibliography

Cohen (1988) described sample sizes for tests of significance of the correlation coefficient while problems connected with their use and interpretation in medical studies are discussed by Campbell, Machin and Walters (2007).

12.4 Use of the table

Table 12.1 and Equation 12.2

Example 12.1—forced expiratory volume and forced vital capacity

In respiratory physiology, suppose the correlation between the forced expiratory volume in 1 second (FEV_1), and the forced vital capacity (FVC) in healthy subjects is thought to be about 0.6. Also, suppose that patients with a certain lung disease are available at a clinic and one wishes to test if there is a significant correlation between the FEV_1 and the FVC in these patients. We do not expect a negative correlation, and so the test is a one-sided one, say at the 5% level, and power 80%. How many subjects are required?

> Using **Table 2.2** with a 5% one-sided test size, $\alpha = 0.05$ gives $z_{0.95} = 1.6449$ and for a power of 80% a one-sided $1 - \beta = 0.80$ gives $z_{0.80} = 0.8416$.

Here, one-sided $\alpha = 0.05$, $1 - \beta = 0.8$ and $\rho = 0.6$. An initial value to start the iteration to find N in Equation 12.2 is $u_{0.6}^0 = \dfrac{1}{2}\log\left[\dfrac{1 + 0.6}{1 - 0.6}\right] = 0.6931$. Substituting this in Equation 12.2 gives

$$N_0 = \frac{(1.6449 + 0.8416)^2}{0.6931^2} + 3 = 15.9 \approx 16.$$ Following this $u_1 = \dfrac{1}{2}\log\dfrac{1 + 0.6}{1 - 0.6} + \dfrac{0.6}{2(16 - 1)} = 0.7131$

with $N_1 = \dfrac{6.1827}{0.7131^2} + 3 = 15.2$ or 16 once more. Thus the iteration process need go no further.

This is the same value as is obtained from **Table 12.1** or directly from $\boxed{{}^S S_S}$ so we require at least $N = 16$ subjects on which both FEV_1 and FVC are measured.

Table 12.1 and Equation 12.2

Example 12.2—blood pressure and viscosity

If subjects suffering from mild hypertension are given a certain dose of a drug, the subsequent fall in blood pressure is associated with a decrease in blood viscosity, with a correlation coefficient of about 0.3. Suppose we conduct the same experiment on patients with severe hypertension and observe their fall in blood pressure and decrease in viscosity following ingestion of the drug. How many patients do we need to recruit to obtain a significant correlation, given that its magnitude is anticipated to be 0.3?

> Using **Table 2.2** with a two-sided 5% test size, $\alpha = 0.05$ gives $z_{0.975} = 1.96$ and for a power of 90% a one-sided $1 - \beta = 0.90$ gives $z_{0.90} = 1.2816$.

In this case, suppose we do not know which way the correlation may go, that is, it may be positive or negative, so that we are using a two-sided test with significance level 5%, and power 90%. Thus, two-sided $\alpha = 0.05$, $1 - \beta = 0.90$, $\rho = 0.3$, and from **Table 12.1** or directly from ^SS_S, we would require $N = 112$ patients to be investigated.

Table 12.1 and Equation 12.2

Example 12.3—lack of association
A psychologist wishes to plan an experiment in which medical students are asked questions from which measures of personality and social desirability can be obtained. The investigator wishes to show that these two variables are not associated. How many students must he recruit to his study?

> Using **Table 2.2** with a 20% one-sided test size, $\alpha = 0.20$ gives $z_{0.80} = 0.8416$ and for a power of 95% a one-sided $1 - \beta = 0.95$ gives $z_{0.95} = 1.6449$.

It is first necessary to specify the size of the Type I error α. In such a situation, as described here, the investigator may be willing to be effectively assume that $\rho = 0$ when it is small and so choose a large Type I error, $\alpha = 0.2$. However, he will require a relatively small Type II error and perhaps choose $\beta = 0.05$. In addition he must set a value of ρ below which he would regard the association as effectively zero, he chooses $\rho = 0.1$. Using ^SS_S with one-sided $\alpha = 0.2$, $1 - \beta = 0.95$ and $\rho = 0.1$, gives the number of students to be recruited $N = 617$ or approximately 700.

12.5 References

Campbell MJ, Machin D and Walters SJ (2007). *Medical Statistics: A Textbook for the Health Sciences*, 4th edn. John Wiley & Sons, Chichester.

Cohen J (1988). *Statistical Power Analysis for Behavioral Sciences*, 2nd edn. Lawrence Earlbaum, New Jersey.

Table 12.1 Sample sizes for detecting a statistically significant correlation coefficient.

	α		Power $1 - \beta$	
ρ	One-sided	Two-sided	0.8	0.9
0.1	0.025	0.05	782	1046
	0.05	0.10	617	853
	0.10	0.20	450	655
0.2	0.025	0.05	193	258
	0.05	0.10	153	211
	0.10	0.20	112	162
0.3	0.025	0.05	84	112
	0.05	0.10	67	92
	0.10	0.20	50	71
0.4	0.025	0.05	46	61
	0.05	0.10	37	50
	0.10	0.20	28	39
0.5	0.025	0.05	29	37
	0.05	0.10	23	31
	0.10	0.20	18	24
0.6	0.025	0.05	19	25
	0.05	0.10	16	21
	0.10	0.20	12	16
0.7	0.025	0.05	13	17
	0.05	0.10	11	14
	0.10	0.20	9	12
0.8	0.025	0.05	10	12
	0.05	0.10	8	10
	0.10	0.20	7	8
0.9	0.025	0.05	7	8
	0.05	0.10	6	7
	0.10	0.20	5	6

Reference intervals and receiver operating curves

13

SUMMARY

An important part of the process of examining a patient is to check clinical measures taken from the patient against a 'normal' or 'reference' range of values. Evidence of the measure lying outside these values may be taken as indicative of the need for further investigation. In this chapter we describe sample sizes for establishing such reference intervals. The value of disease screening tests are often summarised by their sensitivity and specificity and so sample sizes for comparing a diagnostic test's sensitivity to that of a standard as well as for the comparison between two tests are given. We also describe sample-size calculations for determining receiver operating curves (ROC) which are utilised for distinguishing diseased from non-diseased subjects.

13.1 Introduction

When a physician is in the process of establishing a diagnosis in a patient who presents with particular symptoms, the patient may be subjected to a series of tests, the results from which may then suggest an appropriate course of action. For example, a patient complaining of not feeling well may be tested for the presence of a bacterium in their urine. On the basis of the reading obtained the patient may then be compared with the normal range of values expected from healthy individuals, if outside the range, then infection is suspected. It is this infection that is then presumed to be the cause of 'not feeling well'.

The objective of a study to establish a normal range or reference interval (RI) is to define the interval for a particular clinical measurement within which the majority of values, often 95%, of a defined population will lie.

Such an interval is then used as a screen in a clinical context to identify patients presenting with particular symptoms that are 'outside' this interval—the purpose being to give an indication of a possible pathology causing their symptoms. However, for truly diagnostic purposes merely being outside the RI is not sufficient as it is necessary to know the range of values of patients with the disease in question rather than the range for the general population at large. For example, in patients suspected of liver cancer it is routine to take blood samples from which their α-feta protein (AFP) levels are determined. A high level is indicative of liver cancer although further and more detailed examination will be required to confirm the eventual diagnosis. The judgement as to whether or not a particular patient has a high AFP is made by comparison with AFP measured in individuals who are known to be free of the disease in question. In most circumstances, the range of values of AFP in patients who do

Sample Size Tables for Clinical Studies, 3rd edition. By David Machin, Michael J. Campbell, Say Beng Tan, and Sze Huey Tan. Published 2009 by Blackwell Publishing, ISBN: 978-1-4051-4650-0

indeed have liver cancer will overlap with healthy subjects who are free of the disease. In view of this overlap, and to help distinguish the diseased from the non-diseased, receiver operating curves (ROC) are constructed to help determine the best cut-point value for diagnosis.

In clinical practice diagnostic tests are never used in healthy persons but only in groups for which the diagnostic test is indicated. These will include some patients without the disease in question and others with the disease present at various levels of severity. Consequently the best approach to evaluate the diagnostic accuracy of a new diagnostic test is to use a sample of consecutive patients for whom the test is indicated. A careful description of the eligibility characteristics of this group needs to be provided.

The patients in this group will undergo the new diagnostic test and also those for the reference test by which they will be categorised as non-diseased or diseased. The reference test is usually the currently accepted best available and feasible diagnostic tool to determine the presence or absence of the disease in question. Thus, for every patient, there is their test result and the ultimate clinical decision on their diagnosis.

13.2 Reference intervals

Choosing the subjects

Samples are taken from populations of individuals to provide estimates of the population parameters of which we are interested; in our situation the cut-off-point(s) of the RI indicating boundaries of high (and/or low) values. The purpose of summarising the behaviour of a particular group is usually to draw some inference about a wider population of which the group is a sample. Thus although a group of volunteers comprise the sample, and are duly investigated, the object is to represent the RI of the general population as a whole. The wider population will include the healthy as well as those who are not. As a consequence, it is clearly important that the 'volunteers' are chosen carefully so that they do indeed reflect the population as a whole and not a particular subset of that population. If the 'volunteers' are selected at random from the population of interest then the calculated RI will be an estimate of the true RI of the population. If they are not, then it is no longer clear what the interval obtained represents and at worst it may not even be appropriate for clinical use.

Normal distribution

If the variable that has been measured has a Normal distribution form, then the data x_1, x_2, $\ldots x_N$ from the N subjects can be summarised by the sample mean, $\bar{x}$, and sample SD, s. These provide estimates of the associated population mean μ and SD σ respectively.

In this situation, the $100(1 - \alpha)\%$ RI is estimated by

$$\bar{x} - z_{1-\alpha/2} s \text{ to } \bar{x} + z_{1-\alpha/2} s. \tag{13.1}$$

Often a 95% reference interval is required in which case $\alpha = 0.05$ and from **Table 2.1**, $z_{1-\alpha/2} = z_{0.975} = 1.9600$.

If we denote the cut-points of the lower and upper limits of this reference interval as R_{Lower} and R_{Upper}, then its width is

$$W_{\text{Reference}} = R_{\text{Upper}} - R_{\text{Lower}} = 2z_{1-\alpha/2} s. \tag{13.2}$$

Study size

A key property of any reference interval is the precision with which the cut-points are estimated. Thus of particular relevance to design, are the width of the confidence intervals for the estimated cut-points R_{Lower} and R_{Upper}. If the sample is large ($N > 100$) then the standard error (SE) of these cut-points is

$$SE(R_{\text{Lower}}) = SE(R_{\text{Upper}}) = \sigma\sqrt{(3/N)} = 1.7321\sigma/\sqrt{N}. \tag{13.3}$$

Thus the approximate $100(1-\gamma)\%$ CI for the true R_{Lower} is

$$R_{\text{Lower}} - z_{1-\gamma/2} \times \frac{1.7321s}{\sqrt{N}} \text{ to } R_{\text{Lower}} + z_{1-\gamma/2} \times \frac{1.7321s}{\sqrt{N}}, \tag{13.4}$$

and there is a similar expression for R_{Upper}. The width of these confidence intervals is

$$W_{\text{Cut}} = 2 \times z_{1-\gamma/2} \times \frac{1.7321s}{\sqrt{N}}. \tag{13.5}$$

One design criteria for determining an appropriate study size to establish a RI is to fix a value for the ratio of W_{Cut} to $W_{\text{Reference}}$. The design therefore sets $\rho = \dfrac{W_{\text{Cut}}}{W_{\text{Reference}}}$ to some pre-specified value. In this case it follows, from dividing Equation 13.5 by Equation 13.2 and rearranging, that the sample size is estimated by

$$N = 3\left[\frac{z_{1-\gamma/2}}{\rho z_{1-\alpha/2}}\right]^2. \tag{13.6}$$

For the particular case when we choose α and γ to have the same value, Equation 13.6 simplifies to

$$N = 3/\rho^2. \tag{13.7}$$

Practical values for ρ suggested by Linnet (1987) range from 0.1 to 0.3.

Non-Normal situation

Logarithmic transformation

If the data do not have a Normal distribution then, in some circumstances, a logarithmic transformation of the data may have to be made. In which case, the reference interval for $y = \log x$ will take the form of Equation 13.1 but with y replacing x in the calculation of the mean and SD. Further the sample size can still be estimated by Equations 13.6 and 13.7. However, the corresponding reference interval on the x-scale is then obtained from the antilogarithms of the lower and upper limits of this range. That is the reference range for x is

$$\exp(\bar{y} - z_{1-\alpha/2}s_y) \text{ to } \exp(\bar{y} + z_{1-\alpha/2}s_y). \tag{13.8}$$

Ranked data

If the data cannot be transformed to the Normal distribution form then a reference interval can still be calculated. In this case, the data $x_1, x_2, \ldots x_N$ are first ranked from largest to smallest. These are labelled $x_{(1)}, x_{(2)}, \ldots x_{(j)}, \ldots x_{(N)}$. The lower limit of the $100(1-\alpha)\%$ reference range is then $x_{(j)}$, where $j = N\alpha/2$ (interpolating between adjacent observations if $N\alpha/2$ is not an integer). Similarly the upper limit is the observation corresponding to $j = N(1 - \alpha/2)$. These limits provide what is often known as the *empirical* normal range.

The ranks of the lower and upper limits of a $100(1 - \gamma)\%$ CI for any quantile q, are

$$r_q = Nq - [z_{1-\gamma/2} \times \sqrt{Nq(1 - q)}]$$

and

$$s_q = 1 + Nq + [z_{1-\gamma/2} \times \sqrt{Nq(1 - q)}].$$

(13.9)

These values are then rounded to the nearest integer. These integers provide the r_qth and s_qth observations in this ranking and hence the relevant lower and upper confidence limits. To determine those for R_{Lower}, one sets $q = \alpha/2$ in Equation 13.9 and for R_{Upper}, $q = 1 - (\alpha/2)$ is used.

However, these are the *ranks* of the observed values corresponding to R_{Lower} and R_{Upper} not the values themselves and so there is no equivalent algebraic form to W_{Cut} of Equation 13.5 in this case. However, an approximate SE is provided by that which is appropriate for quantiles estimated using ranks *but* assuming these ranks had arisen from data having a Normal distribution form. This gives, in place of Equation 13.3,

$$SE(R_{Lower}) = SE(R_{Upper}) = \eta \frac{\sigma}{\sqrt{N}},$$

(13.10)

where

$$\eta = \sqrt{\frac{(\gamma/2)[1 - (\gamma/2)]}{\phi_{1-\gamma/2}^2}}$$

(13.11)

and $\phi_{1-\gamma/2} = \dfrac{1}{\sqrt{2\pi}} \exp\left(-\dfrac{1}{2}z_{1-\gamma/2}^2\right)$ is the height of the Normal distribution at $z_{1-\gamma/2}$.

Thus an approximation to the $100(1 - \gamma)\%$ CI for the true R_{Lower} of the $100(1 - \alpha)\%$ RI is

$$R_{Lower} - z_{1-\gamma/2} \times \eta \frac{\sigma}{\sqrt{N}} \text{ to } R_{Lower} + z_{1-\gamma/2} \times \eta \frac{\sigma}{\sqrt{N}}.$$

(13.12)

This confidence interval has width

$$W_{CI} = 2 \times \eta \times z_{1-\gamma/2} \times \frac{\sigma}{\sqrt{N}}.$$

(13.13)

Study size

Sample size is determined by first using Equation 13.6 to give $N_{Initial}$ and then inflate this to obtain

$$N_{Final} = \eta \, N_{Initial}/\sqrt{3}.$$

(13.14)

This will lead to a larger study size to establish a reference interval than those given by Equation 13.6. This is why, if at all possible, transforming the scale of measurement to one that is approximately Normal in distribution is very desirable.

13.3 Sensitivity and specificity

As we have indicated, diagnostic test results are often given in the form of a continuous variable, such as diastolic blood pressure or haemoglobin level. However, for the purposes of diagnosis of a particular disease or condition, a cut-off point along this scale is required. Thus, for every laboratory test or diagnostic procedure with the corresponding cut-point chosen, if the disease is present the probability that the test will be positive is required. The sensitivity of the test, Se, is the proportion of those with the disease who also have a positive test result. Conversely, if the disease is absent, the probability that the test result will be negative is required. Thus the specificity of the test, Sp, is the proportion of those without the disease who also have a negative test result.

In the following discussions on sample sizes, we only mention Se. However, the formulae will equally extend to Sp as well.

One sample design

Sample size

In this situation, we require the number of subjects, N, necessary to show that a given Se differs from a target value $Se = Se_{Known}$. Given a significance level α and a power $(1 - \beta)$ against the specified alternative Se_{Plan} then the required number of patients with the disease, is approximately

$$N_{Disease} = \frac{\left\{z_{1-\alpha/2}\sqrt{Se_{Known}(1 - Se_{Known})} + z_{1-\beta}\sqrt{Se_{Plan}(1 - Se_{Plan})}\right\}^2}{(Se_{Plan} - Se_{Known})^2}. \tag{13.15}$$

Values for $z_{1-\alpha/2}$ and $z_{1-\beta}$ can be obtained from **Table 2.2**.

This is the same as Equation 3.7 but with Se_{Known} and Se_{Plan} replacing π_{Known} and π_2.

However, to determine the number of subjects for the study, of whom $N_{Disease}$ are anticipated to ultimately have the disease in question, it is necessary to divide this by the prevalence of the disease, $\pi_{Disease}$ amongst the cohort of subjects to which the test will be applied. Thus

$$N = \frac{N_{Disease}}{\pi_{Disease}}. \tag{13.16}$$

Equation 13.15, and hence this affects Equation 13.16, is a large sample approximation and Li and Fine (2004) have indicated how the exact method using the binomial probabilities may be calculated. Their methodology is implemented in ^SS_S.

Two sample design

Independent groups

If two diagnostic tests are to be compared then the total number of diseased individuals required is given by

$$N_{Disease} = \frac{\left\{z_{1-\alpha/2}\sqrt{(Se_1 + Se_2)(2 - Se_1 - Se_2)} + z_{1-\beta}\sqrt{2[Se_1(1 - Se_1) + Se_2(1 - Se_2)]}\right\}^2}{(Se_2 - Se_1)^2}. \tag{13.17}$$

Values for $z_{1-\alpha/2}$ and $z_{1-\beta}$ can be obtained from **Table 2.2**.

This is the same expression as Equation 3.2 but with Se_1 and Se_2 replacing π_1 and π_2. Finally the number of subjects to recruit is given by Equation 13.16. It is important to stress that once the sample sizes to receive the two tests have been established then the subjects concerned should be randomly allocated to the two alternative tests.

Paired design

If two diagnostic tests are to be compared but both within the same subjects then this is a paired design as each subject provides a sample from both. Thus each subject also has two distinct diagnoses, one from one test—one from the other. These may or may not agree with each other. Given a significance level α and a power $(1 - \beta)$, the number of patients required who have the disease in question is

$$N_{\text{Disease}} = \frac{\left\{ z_{1-\alpha/2}\Lambda + z_{1-\beta}\sqrt{\Lambda^2 - \zeta^2(3 + \Lambda)/4} \right\}^2}{\Lambda\zeta^2}, \tag{13.18}$$

where $\Lambda = (1 - Se_1)Se_2 + (1 - Se_2)Se_1$ and $\zeta = (1 - Se_1)Se_2 - (1 - Se_2)Se_1$.

Once again the number of subjects to recruit is then given by using Equation 13.16. It is important to stress that once the sample size to receive both tests has been established then the order in which they are determined from the patient should be randomised half to have Test 1 before Test 2 and half the reverse. The details of how this may be achieved will vary with the clinical situation concerned.

13.4 Receiver operating curves (ROC)

When a diagnostic test produces a continuous measurement, then a diagnostic cut-point is selected. This is then used ultimately to divide future subjects into those who are suspected to have the disease and those who are not. This diagnostic cut-point is determined by first calculating the sensitivity and specificity at each potential cut-point along the measurement scale.

As we have indicated, the sensitivity, Se, of a diagnostic test is the proportion of those *with* the disease who also have a positive diagnostic result. It is also termed the true positive rate (TPR). On the other hand, the specificity is the proportion of those *without* the disease who also have a *negative* result, that is, they do not have the disease and their test is below the cut-point. Those who do not have the disease but have a test value above the cut-point are termed false positives. The corresponding false positive rate (FPR) = (1 − specificity) or $(1 - Sp)$.

Once a study is completed Se on the (vertical) y-axis is plotted against $(1 - Sp)$ on the (horizontal) x-axis for each possible cut-point to produce the ROC.

In order to divide the diseased from the non-diseased, the final (diagnostic) cut-point, C, chosen is usually made at a point that provides a sensible balance between the sensitivity and the specificity. For a particular test this requires an assessment of the relative medical consequences, and costs, of making a false diagnosis of disease (false positive, FP) or of not diagnosing disease that is present (false negative, FN).

A perfect diagnostic test would be one with no FP or FN outcomes and would be represented by a line that started at the origin and went up the y-axis to $Se = 1$, while keeping a false positive rate of $(1 - Sp) = 0$, and then horizontally across the x-axis until it reaches $(1 - Sp) = 1$. A test that produces FP results at the same rate as TP results would produce a ROC on the diagonal line $y = x$.

The sensitivity and specificity in the context of sample size determination for ROC are analogous to the test size and power of other chapters.

Study size

If the objective is to estimate the area, AUC, under an ROC, then sample size can be determined using an expression similar to Equation 10.20 and from which the width, ω, of this confidence interval can be calculated. The study size is then

$$m_{\text{Diseased}} = 4\left[\frac{\sigma^2}{\omega^2}\right]z^2_{1-\alpha/2}.$$ (13.19)

The right-hand side of this equation is identical in form to Equation 10.20 but because evaluation of a diagnostic test is determined through the ROC, this requires two subject groups, the diseased and non-diseased. Further, the method of estimating σ has to take this into account. In fact σ is a rather complex function of the anticipated ratio of non-diseased subjects to diseased patients, R, and the required sensitivity and specificity. It is given by,

$$\sigma = \frac{\exp(-\frac{1}{4}A^2)}{2\sqrt{\pi}}\sqrt{\left(1 + \frac{1}{R} + \frac{5A^2}{8} + \frac{A^2}{8R}\right)},$$ (13.20)

where $A = z_{1-\text{FPR}} - z_{1-\text{TPR}}$ which can be evaluated using **Table 2.1**.

This is used in Equation 13.19 to determine the required m_{Diseased}, after which $m_{\text{Non-diseased}} = R \times m_{\text{Diseased}}$ is calculated. The final estimated study size is $N = m_{\text{Diseased}} + m_{\text{Non-diseased}}$.

13.5 Bibliography

Harris and Boyd (1995) give the large sample estimate of the standard error of cut-points of Equation 13.3 while the ranks of the lower and upper limits of a $100(1 - \gamma)\%$ CI for any quantile are given by Campbell and Gardner (2000). Methods to calculate reference intervals and associated sample sizes are also discussed in Altman (1991). Li and Fine (2004) provide sample size formulae for determining sensitivity and specificity in a variety of situations. Obuchowski and McClish (1997), who refer to the AUC as the accuracy of the test, derive Equation 13.20.

13.6 Examples and use of tables

Table 13.1 and Equation 13.6
Example 13.1—myocardial iron deposition
Anderson, Holden, Davis *et al.* (2001) established normal ranges for T2-star (T2*) values in the heart. T2* is a magnetic resonance technique which can quantify myocardial iron

deposition, the levels of which indicate the need for ventricular dysfunction treatment. They quote a 95% normal range for T2* as 36−68 ms obtained from 15 healthy volunteers (9 males, 6 females, aged 26−39 years).

> For a 5% two-sided reference interval, $\alpha = 0.05$, **Table 2.2** gives $z_{0.975} = 1.96$ while for a confidence interval with $\gamma = 0.1$, $z_{0.90} = 1.6449$.

We presume that we are planning to estimate the 95% RI for myocardial T2* and we have the above study available. From that study, $W_{\text{Reference}} = 68 - 36 = 32$ ms and we intend to quote a 90% *CI* for the cut-point(s) so determined.

Use of Equation 13.6 with $\rho_{\text{Plan}} = 0.1$ gives $N = 3 \times [1.6449/(0.1 \times 1.96)]^2 \approx 215$. Direct entry into **Table 13.1** or use of $^{S}S_{S}$ with a 95% RI ($\alpha = 0.05$), a 90% CI ($\gamma = 0.10$) for the cut-point and $\rho_{\text{Plan}} = 0.1$ gives $N = 212$ subjects. Had $\rho_{\text{Plan}} = 0.2$ been specified then, $N \approx 53$ subjects are required.

These estimates of study size contrast markedly with the 15 volunteers used by Anderson, Holden, Davis *et al.* (2001). In terms of the design criteria we have introduced here their study corresponds to the use of $\rho_{\text{Plan}} \approx 0.4$, which is outside the range recommended by Linnet (1987).

Table 13.2 and Equations 13.11 and 13.14

Example 13.2—empirical normal range—cerebrospinal fluid opening pressure

Whiteley, Al-Shahi, Warlow *et al.* (2006) conducted a study involving the prospective recording of the cerebrospinal fluid (CSF) opening pressure in 242 adults who had lumbar puncture. Their objective was to obtain the 95% RI for lumbar CSF opening pressure and relate this to the body mass index.

In their report, the authors plotted the distribution of CSF opening pressures in the 242 subjects and used a Kolmogorov–Smirnov test to conclude that the data was not normally distributed. They then used a non-parametric approach to calculate the 95% reference interval. No mention was made on how they arrived at a sample size of 242.

> For a 5% two-sided reference interval, $\alpha = 0.05$, **Table 2.2** gives $z_{0.975} = 1.96$ while for a confidence interval with $\gamma = 0.1$, $z_{0.90} = 1.6449$.

Assuming that the authors had computed the sample size using the approach discussed, from Equation 13.6 with 95% RI and 90% *CI* ($\alpha = 0.05$, $\gamma = 0.10$) and $\rho_{\text{Plan}} = 0.1$, we have $N_{\text{Initial}} =$

$$3\left[\frac{1.6449}{0.1 \times 1.96}\right]^2 = 211.3 \text{ or } 212. \text{ Use of Equations 5.11 then gives } \phi_{0.95} = \frac{1}{\sqrt{2\pi}}\exp\left(-\frac{1.6449^2}{2}\right)$$

$$= 0.1031 \text{ and } \eta = \sqrt{\frac{(0.1/2)[1 - (0.1/2)]}{0.1031^2}} = \sqrt{\frac{0.05 \times 0.95}{0.1031^2}} = 2.1139 \text{ so that, from Equation 13.14,}$$

$N_{\text{Final}} = 2.1139 \times 212/\sqrt{3} = 258.7$ or approximately 260 individuals. Direct entry into **Table 13.2** or use of $^{S}S_{S}$ give $N = 259$ subjects. This is larger than the 242 actually recruited to the study.

The sample size of 242 utilised by Whiteley, Al-Shahi, Warlow *et al.* (2006) would correspond to setting $\alpha = 0.05$, $\gamma = 0.10$ and $\rho_{\text{Plan}} \approx 0.104$ in $^{S}S_{S}$.

Table 13.3 and Equations 13.15 and 13.16

Example 13.3—sensitivity—excessive daytime somnolence (EDS)

Hosselet, Ayappa, Norman *et al.* (2001) conducted a study to evaluate the utility of various measures of sleep-disordered breathing (SDB) to find that which best identifies excessive daytime somnolence (EDS). They concluded that a total respiratory disturbance index ($\text{RDI}_{\text{Total}}$ – sum of apnoea, hypopnoea, and flow limitation events) of 18 events per hour or more had the best discriminant ability. This was then tested prospectively in 103 subjects, of whom 68 had EDS and 35 did not, giving a disease prevalence of $\rho_{\text{Disease}} = 68/103 = 0.66$. The sensitivity of the test was reported to be 86%.

In a confirmatory study of the value of $\text{RDI}_{\text{Total}}$ as a screen for EDS, how many subjects need to be recruited?

> Using **Table 2.2** with a 5% one-sided test size, $\alpha = 0.05$ gives $z_{0.95} = 1.6449$ and for a power of 80% a one-sided $1 - \beta = 0.80$ gives $z_{0.80} = 0.8416$.

The investigators felt that the subject population in the confirmatory study may differ in several respects from the earlier study and so anticipated that the sensitivity of the test may be somewhat higher at $Se_{\text{Plan}} = 0.95$, with the disease prevalence also lower at $\pi_{\text{Disease}} = 0.55$. Then assuming a one-sided test of 5% and a power of 80%, with $Se_{\text{Known}} = 0.86$, Equation 13.15

$$\text{gives } N_{\text{Disease}} = \frac{\left\{1.6449 \times \sqrt{0.86(1 - 0.86)} + 0.8416 \times \sqrt{0.95(1 - 0.95)}\right\}^{2}}{(0.95 - 0.86)^{2}} = 70.2 \approx 75.$$

From Equation 13.17, the number of subjects to be tested is $N = N_{\text{Disease}} / \pi_{\text{Disease}} = 75/0.55 = 136.4$ or approximately 140 patients. Using the more accurate exact binomial approach implemented in $^{S}S_{S}$, gives $N = 133$. This approach is also used to generate the values given in **Table 13.3**, where supposing instead that $Se_{\text{Known}} = 0.8$, $Se_{\text{Plan}} = 0.9$ and $\pi_{\text{Disease}} = 0.5$, the required sample size would be $N = 164$.

Tables 13.4 and 13.5, Equations 13.16, 13.17 and 13.18

Example 13.4—comparative sensitivity of two tests—periodontal disease

Nomura, Tamaki, Tanaka, *et al.* (2006) conducted a study to evaluate the utility of various salivary enzyme tests for screening of periodontitis. Amongst the biochemical markers, salivary lactate dehydrogenase (LDH), with a cut at 371 IU/L appeared the best, and free haemoglobin (f-HB) with a cut at 0.5 IU/L the worst, with sensitivities: 0.66 and 0.27 respectively.

If a repeat study is planned, how many subjects per group are needed if only one test can be given to each individual? The anticipated proportion with periodontal disease is anticipated to be 1 in 4.

> Using **Table 2.2** with a 5% two-sided test size, $\alpha = 0.05$ gives $z_{0.975} = 1.96$ and for a power of 80% a one-sided $1 - \beta = 0.80$ gives $z_{0.80} = 0.8416$.

If the difference anticipated is the same as that observed by Nomura, Tamaki, Tanaka et al. (2006), then the planning difference is $Se_2 - Se_1 = 0.66 - 0.27 = 0.39$. Thus for a two-sided test of 5% and power 80% the total number with the disease to be recruited is

$$N_{\text{Disease}} = \frac{\left\{1.96 \times \sqrt{(0.27 + 0.66)(2 - 0.27 - 0.66)} + 0.8416\sqrt{2[0.27(1 - 0.27) + 0.66(1 - 0.66)]}\right\}^2}{(0.66 - 0.27)^2}$$

$= 48.9$ or approximately 50. To identify 50 subjects with the disease from Equation 13.17, the number of subjects to be tested is $N = N_{\text{Disease}} / \pi_{\text{Disease}} = 50/0.25 = 200$. Using the more accurate approach implemented in $\boxed{SS_S}$ gives $N = 196$. Alternatively **Table 13.4** could be used, although since the table does not have the particular input values tabulated, the nearest values of $Se_1 = 0.3$, $Se_2 = 0.7$ and $\pi_{\text{Disease}} = 0.3$ would need to be used, to give $N = 158$.

If on the other hand, it was possible to make both diagnostic tests in each individual, then a paired design using Equation 13.18 could be used for determining sample size. Thus in this situation $\Lambda = (1 - Se_1)Se_2 + (1 - Se_2)Se_1 = 0.5736$, $\zeta = (1 - Se_1)Se_2 - (1 - Se_2)Se_1 = 0.3900$ and

$$\text{so } N_{\text{Disease}} = \frac{\left\{1.96 \times 0.5736 + 0.8416\sqrt{0.5736^2 - 0.3900^2(3 + 0.5736)/4}\right\}}{0.5736 \times 0.3900^2} = 25.6 \text{ or } 26 \text{ diseased}$$

subjects. Thus the number of subjects to be tested is $N = N_{\text{Disease}} / \pi_{\text{Disease}} = 26/0.25 = 92$ or approximately 100. In this situation, the choice of a paired design reduces the size of the proposed study considerably. Using $\boxed{SS_S}$ directly gives $N = 80$, or **Table 13.5** with $Se_1 = 0.3$, $Se_2 = 0.7$ and $\pi_{\text{Disease}} = 0.3$ gives $N = 64$.

Table 13.6 and Equation 13.20

Example 13.5—ROC curves—cartilage abnormalities

Obuchowski and McClish (1997) consider the planning of a study to estimate the accuracy of magnetic resonance imaging (MRI) for detecting cartilage abnormalities in patients with symptomatic knees. Patients in the study were to undergo MRI for arthroscopy, which is considered the gold standard for determining the presence/absence of abnormalities. Following a five-point scoring, it was anticipated that 40% of patients will have a cartilage abnormality, so $R = 60/40 = 1.5$. They stipulated an anticipated specificity of 90% and sensitivity of 45%. The width of the 95% confidence interval was set as 0.1.

The anticipated specificity and sensitivity imply FPR = 0.1 and TPR = 0.45 respectively.

> A 10% FPR is equivalent to setting a one-sided, $\alpha = 0.1$ in **Table 2.2** hence $z_{0.9} = 1.2816$. A 45% TPR is equivalent to setting a one-sided, $\alpha = 0.45$ in **Table 2.2** hence, $z_{0.55} = 0.1257$.

From the values in the panel, $A = 1.2816 - 0.1257 = 1.1559$. Hence $\sigma =$

$$\frac{\exp(-\frac{1}{4} \times 1.1559^2)}{2\sqrt{\pi}} \sqrt{\left(1 + \frac{1}{1.5} + \frac{5 \times 1.1559^2}{8} + \frac{1.1559^2}{8 \times 1.5}\right)} = 0.3265. \text{ From which, for a 95% } CI,$$

$$m_{\text{Diseased}} = 4\left[\frac{0.3265^2}{0.1^2}\right] \times 1.96^2 = 163.8 \text{ or approximately 164. This differs marginally from}$$

$m_{\text{Diseased}} = 161$ given by Obuchowski and McClish (1997) due to rounding error. Finally $m_{\text{Non-diseased}} = R \times m_{\text{Diseased}} = 1.5 \times 164 = 246$ so that the final estimated study size is $N = m_{\text{Diseased}} + m_{\text{Non-diseased}} = 407$. Using $\boxed{SS_S}$ directly gives $N = 410$. **Table 13.6** does not have TPR = 0.45 tabulated, but using TPR = 0.40, the total sample size required would be $N = 2.5 \times 176 = 440$.

13.5 References

Altman DG (1991). *Practical Statistics for Medical Research*. Chapman & Hall/CRC, Boca Raton.

Anderson LJ, Holden S, Davis B, Prescott E, Charrier CC, Bunce NH, Firmin DN, Wonke B, Porter J, Walker JM and Pennell DJ (2001). Cardiovascular T2-star (T2*) magnetic resonance for the early diagnosis of myocardial iron overload. *European Heart Journal*, **22**, 2171–2179.

Campbell MJ and Gardner MJ (2000). Medians and their differences. In: Altman DG, Machin D, Bryant TN and Gardner MJ (eds) *Statistics with Confidence*, 2nd edn. British Medical Journal, London, pp. 171–190.

Harris EK and Boyd JC (1995). *Statistical Bases of Reference Values in Laboratory Medicine*. Marcel Dekker, New York.

Hosselet J-J, Ayappa I, Norman RG, Krieger AC and Rapoport DM (2001). Classification of sleep-disordered breathing. *American Journal of Respiratory Critical Care Medicine*, **163**, 398–405.

Li J and Fine J (2004). On sample size for sensitivity and specificity in prospective diagnostic accuracy studies. *Statistics in Medicine*, **23**, 2537–2550.

Linnet K (1987). Two-stage transformation systems for normalization of reference distributions evaluated. *Clinical Chemistry*, **33**, 381–386.

Nomura Y, Tamaki Y, Tanaka T, Arakawa H, Tsurumoto A, Kirimura K, Sato T, Hanada N and Kamoi K (2006). Screening of periodontitis with salivary enzyme tests. *Journal of Oral Science*, **48**, 177–183.

Obuchowski NA and McClish DN (1997). Sample size determination for diagnostic accuracy studies involving binormal ROC curve indices. *Statistics in Medicine*, **16**, 1529–1542.

Whiteley W, Al-Shahi R, Warlow CP, Zeideler M and Lueck CJ (2006). CSF opening pressure: Reference interval and the effect of body mass index. *Neurology*, **67**, 1690–1691.

Table 13.1 Sample sizes in order to obtain a required reference interval—Normal distribution. Each cell gives the total number of patients, N, that should be entered into study.

Reference interval (%)	ρ	Confidence interval of the estimated cutoff (%)		
		80	90	95
90	0.025	2914	4800	6816
	0.05	729	1200	1704
	0.075	324	534	758
	0.1	183	300	426
	0.125	117	192	273
	0.15	81	134	190
	0.175	60	98	140
	0.2	46	75	107
	0.3	21	34	48
	0.4	12	19	27
95	0.025	2053	3381	4800
	0.05	514	846	1200
	0.075	229	376	534
	0.1	129	212	300
	0.125	83	136	192
	0.15	58	94	134
	0.175	42	69	98
	0.2	33	53	75
	0.3	15	24	34
	0.4	9	14	19
99	0.025	1189	1958	2780
	0.05	298	490	695
	0.075	133	218	309
	0.1	75	123	174
	0.125	48	79	112
	0.15	34	55	78
	0.175	25	40	57
	0.2	19	31	44
	0.3	9	14	20
	0.4	5	8	11

Table 13.2 Sample sizes in order to obtain a required reference interval—non-Normal distribution. Each cell gives the total number of patients, N, that should be entered into study.

Reference interval (%)	ρ	Confidence interval of the estimated cutoff (%)		
		80	90	95
90	0.025	2876	5857	10 513
	0.05	720	1465	2629
	0.075	320	652	1170
	0.1	181	367	658
	0.125	116	235	422
	0.15	80	164	294
	0.175	60	120	216
	0.2	46	92	166
	0.3	21	42	75
	0.4	12	24	42
95	0.025	2027	4125	7403
	0.05	508	1033	1851
	0.075	227	459	824
	0.1	128	259	463
	0.125	82	166	297
	0.15	58	115	207
	0.175	42	85	152
	0.2	33	65	116
	0.3	15	30	53
	0.4	9	18	30
99	0.025	1174	2389	4288
	0.05	295	598	1072
	0.075	132	266	477
	0.1	75	151	269
	0.125	48	97	173
	0.15	34	68	121
	0.175	25	49	88
	0.2	19	38	68
	0.3	9	18	31
	0.4	5	10	17

Table 13.3 Sample sizes required to observe a given sensitivity or specificity in diagnostic accuracy studies—single sample. Each cell gives the number of subjects for the study, *N*.

| | | One-sided $\alpha = 0.05$; Power $1 - \beta = 0.8$ | | | | |
| | | Disease prevalence, $\pi_{Disease}$ | | | | |
Se_{Known}	Se_{Plan}	0.01	0.1	0.3	0.5	0.7
0.1	0.2	7800	780	260	156	112
	0.3	2500	250	84	50	36
	0.4	1300	130	44	26	19
	0.5	800	80	27	16	12
	0.6	600	60	20	12	9
	0.7	500	50	17	10	8
	0.8	300	30	10	6	5
	0.9	200	20	7	4	3
0.2	0.3	11 600	1160	387	232	166
	0.4	3500	350	117	70	50
	0.5	1700	170	57	34	25
	0.6	1000	100	34	20	15
	0.7	700	70	24	14	10
	0.8	400	40	14	8	6
	0.9	200	20	7	4	3
0.3	0.4	14 400	1440	480	288	206
	0.5	3900	390	130	78	56
	0.6	1700	170	57	34	25
	0.7	1000	100	34	20	15
	0.8	700	70	24	14	10
	0.9	500	50	17	10	8
0.4	0.5	15 800	1580	527	316	226
	0.6	4200	420	140	84	61
	0.7	1900	190	64	38	28
	0.8	1100	110	37	22	16
	0.9	600	60	20	12	9
0.5	0.6	15 800	1580	527	316	226
	0.7	3700	370	124	74	53
	0.8	1800	180	60	36	26
	0.9	800	80	27	16	12
0.6	0.7	14 300	1430	477	286	205
	0.8	3600	360	120	72	52
	0.9	1400	140	47	28	20
0.7	0.8	11 900	1190	397	238	170
	0.9	2800	280	94	56	40
0.8	0.9	8200	820	274	164	118

Table 13.3 (*continued*): Sample sizes required to observe a given sensitivity or specificity in diagnostic accuracy studies—single sample. Each cell gives the number of subjects for the study, *N*.

Se_{Known}	Se_{Plan}	Two-sided $\alpha = 0.05$; Power $1 - \beta = 0.9$				
		Disease prevalence, $\pi_{Disease}$				
		0.01	0.1	0.3	0.5	0.7
0.1	0.2	10 900	1090	364	218	156
	0.3	3300	330	110	66	48
	0.4	1800	180	60	36	26
	0.5	1200	120	40	24	18
	0.6	700	70	24	14	10
	0.7	600	60	20	12	9
	0.8	500	50	17	10	8
	0.9	300	30	10	6	5
0.2	0.3	16 000	1600	534	320	229
	0.4	4700	470	157	94	68
	0.5	2100	210	70	42	31
	0.6	1300	130	44	26	19
	0.7	900	90	30	18	13
	0.8	600	60	20	12	9
	0.9	400	40	14	8	6
0.3	0.4	19 300	1930	644	386	276
	0.5	5300	530	177	106	76
	0.6	2500	250	84	50	36
	0.7	1400	140	47	28	20
	0.8	900	90	30	18	13
	0.9	500	50	17	10	8
0.4	0.5	21 400	2140	714	428	306
	0.6	5600	560	187	112	80
	0.7	2500	250	84	50	36
	0.8	1300	130	44	26	19
	0.9	800	80	27	16	12
0.5	0.6	21 300	2130	710	426	305
	0.7	5300	530	177	106	76
	0.8	2300	230	77	46	33
	0.9	1100	110	37	22	16
0.6	0.7	19 700	1970	657	394	282
	0.8	4500	450	150	90	65
	0.9	1700	170	57	34	25
0.7	0.8	16 400	1640	547	328	235
	0.9	3700	370	124	74	53
0.8	0.9	11 200	1120	374	224	160

Table 13.4 Sample sizes required to observe a given sensitivity or specificity in diagnostic accuracy studies—two sample unpaired design. Each cell gives the total number of subjects for the study, N.

| Se_1 | Se_2 | Two-sided $\alpha = 0.05$; Power $1 - \beta = 0.8$ Disease prevalence, $\pi_{Disease}$ | | | | |
		0.01	0.1	0.3	0.5	0.7
0.1	0.2	39 800	3 980	1328	796	570
	0.3	12 400	1240	414	248	178
	0.4	6300	630	210	126	90
	0.5	3900	390	130	78	56
	0.6	2700	270	90	54	40
	0.7	1900	190	64	38	28
	0.8	1400	140	48	28	20
	0.9	1000	100	34	20	16
0.2	0.3	58 700	5870	1958	1174	840
	0.4	16 300	1630	544	326	234
	0.5	7700	770	258	154	110
	0.6	4500	450	150	90	66
	0.7	2900	290	98	58	42
	0.8	2000	200	68	40	30
	0.9	1400	140	48	28	20
0.3	0.4	71 200	7120	2374	1424	1018
	0.5	18 600	1860	620	372	266
	0.6	8400	840	280	168	122
	0.7	4700	470	158	94	68
	0.8	2900	290	98	58	42
	0.9	1900	190	64	38	28
0.4	0.5	77 500	7750	2584	1550	1108
	0.6	19 400	1940	648	388	278
	0.7	8400	840	280	168	122
	0.8	4500	450	150	90	66
	0.9	2700	270	90	54	40
0.5	0.6	77 500	7750	2584	1550	1108
	0.7	18 600	1860	620	372	266
	0.8	7700	770	258	154	110
	0.9	3900	390	130	78	56
0.6	0.7	71 200	7120	2374	1424	1018
	0.8	16 300	1630	544	326	234
	0.9	6300	630	210	126	90
0.7	0.8	58 700	5870	1958	1174	840
	0.9	12 400	1240	414	248	178
0.8	0.9	39 800	3980	1328	796	570

Table 13.4 (*continued*): Sample sizes required to observe a given sensitivity or specificity in diagnostic accuracy studies—two sample unpaired design. Each cell gives the total number of subjects for the study, *N*.

		Two-sided $\alpha = 0.05$; Power $1 - \beta = 0.9$				
		Disease prevalence, $\pi_{Disease}$				
Se_1	Se_2	0.01	0.1	0.3	0.5	0.7
0.1	0.2	53 200	5320	1774	1064	760
	0.3	16 400	1640	548	328	236
	0.4	8400	840	280	168	122
	0.5	5100	510	170	102	74
	0.6	3400	340	114	68	50
	0.7	2400	240	80	48	36
	0.8	1700	170	58	34	256
0.9		1200	120	40	24	18
0.2	0.3	78 400	7840	2614	1568	1120
	0.4	21 700	2170	724	434	310
	0.5	10 300	1030	344	206	148
	0.6	5900	590	198	118	86
	0.7	3800	380	127	76	56
	0.8	2500	250	84	50	36
	0.9	1700	170	58	34	26
0.3	0.4	95 300	9530	3177	1906	1362
	0.5	24 800	2480	828	496	356
	0.6	11 200	1120	374	224	160
	0.7	6200	620	208	124	90
	0.8	3800	380	128	76	56
	0.9	2400	240	80	48	36
0.4	0.5	103 700	10 370	3458	2074	1482
	0.6	25 900	2590	864	518	370
	0.7	11 200	1120	374	224	160
	0.8	5900	590	198	118	86
	0.9	3400	340	114	68	50
0.5	0.6	103 700	10 370	3458	2074	1482
	0.7	24 800	2480	828	496	356
	0.8	10 300	1030	344	206	148
	0.9	5100	510	170	102	74
0.6	0.7	95 300	9530	3178	1906	1362
	0.8	21 700	2170	724	434	310
	0.9	8400	840	280	168	122
0.7	0.8	78 400	7840	2614	1568	1120
	0.9	16 400	1640	548	328	236
0.8	0.9	53 200	5320	1774	1064	760

Table 13.5 Sample sizes required to observe a given sensitivity or specificity in diagnostic accuracy studies—two sample matched paired design. Each cell gives the total number of subjects for the study, N.

		Two-sided $\alpha = 0.05$; Power $1 - \beta = 0.8$				
		Disease prevalence, $\pi_{Disease}$				
Se_1	Se_2	0.01	0.1	0.3	0.5	0.7
0.1	0.2	15 401	1540	514	308	220
	0.3	4701	470	157	94	68
	0.4	2401	240	80	48	35
	0.5	1501	150	50	30	22
	0.6	1101	110	37	22	16
	0.7	801	80	27	16	12
	0.8	601	60	20	12	9
	0.9	501	50	17	10	8
0.2	0.3	23 001	2300	767	460	329
	0.4	6401	640	214	128	92
	0.5	3001	300	100	60	43
	0.6	1801	180	60	36	26
	0.7	1201	120	40	24	18
	0.8	801	80	27	16	12
	0.9	601	60	20	12	9
0.3	0.4	28 001	2800	934	560	400
	0.5	7401	740	247	148	106
	0.6	3301	330	110	66	48
	0.7	1901	190	64	38	28
	0.8	1201	120	40	24	18
	0.9	801	80	27	16	12
0.4	0.5	30 501	3050	1017	610	436
	0.6	7701	770	257	154	110
	0.7	3301	330	110	66	48
	0.8	1801	180	60	36	26
	0.9	1101	110	37	22	16
0.5	0.6	30 501	3050	1017	610	436
	0.7	7401	740	247	148	106
	0.8	3001	300	100	60	43
	0.9	1501	150	50	30	22
0.6	0.7	28 001	2800	934	560	400
	0.8	6401	640	214	128	92
	0.9	2401	240	80	48	35
0.7	0.8	23 001	2300	767	460	329
	0.9	4701	470	157	94	68
0.8	0.9	15 401	1540	514	308	220

Table 13.5 (*continued*): Sample sizes required to observe a given sensitivity or specificity in diagnostic accuracy studies—two sample matched paired design. Each cell gives the total number of subjects for the study, *N*.

| | | Two-sided $\alpha = 0.05$; Power $1 - \beta = 0.9$ | | | | |
| | | Disease prevalence, $\pi_{Disease}$ | | | | |
Se_1	Se_2	0.01	0.1	0.3	0.5	0.7
0.1	0.2	21 101	2110	704	422	302
	0.3	6301	630	210	126	90
	0.4	3201	320	107	64	46
	0.5	1901	190	64	38	28
	0.6	1301	130	44	26	19
	0.7	1001	100	34	20	15
	0.8	701	70	24	14	10
	0.9	501	50	17	10	8
0.2	0.3	31 701	3170	1057	634	453
	0.4	8701	870	290	174	125
	0.5	4101	410	137	82	59
	0.6	2401	240	80	48	35
	0.7	1501	150	50	30	22
	0.8	1001	100	34	20	15
	0.9	701	70	24	14	10
0.3	0.4	38 701	3870	1290	774	553
	0.5	10 001	1000	334	200	143
	0.6	4501	450	150	90	65
	0.7	2501	250	84	50	36
	0.8	1501	150	50	30	22
	0.9	1001	100	34	20	15
0.4	0.5	42 201	4220	1407	844	603
	0.6	10 501	1050	350	210	150
	0.7	4501	450	150	90	65
	0.8	2401	240	80	48	35
	0.9	1301	130	44	26	19
0.5	0.6	42 201	4220	1407	844	603
	0.7	10 001	1000	334	200	143
	0.8	4101	410	137	82	59
	0.9	1901	190	64	38	28
0.6	0.7	38 701	3870	1290	774	553
	0.8	8701	870	290	174	125
	0.9	3201	320	107	64	46
0.7	0.8	31 701	3170	1057	634	453
	0.9	6301	630	210	126	90
0.8	0.9	21 101	2110	704	422	302

Table 13.6 Sample sizes required to observe a given confidence interval width for receiver operating curves (ROC). Each cell gives the number of subjects for each group, *m*. Hence, the total sample size for the study is $N = (1 + R)m$.

			Confidence intervals (CI)							
			90%				95%			
			Width of CI, ω				Width of CI, ω			
R	**FPR**	**TPR**	**0.05**	**0.1**	**0.15**	**0.2**	**0.05**	**0.1**	**0.15**	**0.2**
1	0.1	0.4	568	142	64	36	806	202	90	51
		0.5	490	123	55	31	696	174	78	44
		0.6	400	100	45	25	568	142	64	36
		0.7	300	75	34	19	426	107	48	27
		0.8	195	49	22	13	277	70	31	18
		0.9	90	23	10	6	127	32	15	8
	0.2	0.4	655	164	73	41	930	233	104	59
		0.5	612	153	68	39	869	218	97	55
		0.6	549	138	61	35	779	195	87	49
		0.7	461	116	52	29	655	164	73	41
		0.8	345	87	39	22	490	123	55	31
		0.9	195	49	22	13	277	70	31	18
	0.3	0.4	683	171	76	43	969	243	108	61
		0.5	663	166	74	42	941	236	105	59
		0.6	625	157	70	40	887	222	99	56
		0.7	562	141	63	36	798	200	89	50
		0.8	461	116	52	29	655	164	73	41
		0.9	300	75	34	19	426	107	48	27
1.5	0.1	0.4	492	124	56	32	698	176	78	44
		0.5	430	108	48	28	610	154	68	40
		0.6	354	90	40	24	504	126	56	32
		0.7	270	68	30	18	382	96	44	24
		0.8	176	44	20	12	250	64	28	16
		0.9	82	22	10	6	116	30	14	8
	0.2	0.4	554	140	62	36	788	198	88	50
		0.5	526	132	60	34	746	188	84	48
		0.6	476	120	54	30	676	170	76	44
		0.7	406	102	46	26	576	144	64	36
		0.8	308	78	36	20	436	110	50	28
		0.9	176	44	20	12	250	64	28	16
	0.3	0.4	572	144	64	36	812	204	92	52
		0.5	560	140	64	36	794	200	90	50
		0.6	534	134	60	34	758	190	86	48
		0.7	488	122	56	32	692	174	78	44
		0.8	406	102	46	26	576	144	64	36
		0.9	270	68	30	18	382	96	44	24

Table 13.6 (*continued*): Sample sizes required to observe a given confidence interval width for receiver operating curves (ROC). Each cell gives the number of subjects for each group, *m*. Hence, the total sample size for the study is $N = (1 + R)m$.

			Confidence intervals (CI)							
			90%				95%			
			Width of CI, ω				Width of CI, ω			
R	*FPR*	*TPR*	0.05	0.1	0.15	0.2	0.05	0.1	0.15	0.2
2	0.1	0.4	453	114	51	29	642	161	72	41
		0.5	399	100	45	25	566	142	63	36
		0.6	331	83	37	21	470	118	53	30
		0.7	253	64	29	16	359	90	40	23
		0.8	167	42	19	11	237	60	27	15
		0.9	78	20	9	5	111	28	13	7
	0.2	0.4	504	126	56	32	715	179	80	45
		0.5	481	121	54	31	683	171	76	43
		0.6	440	110	49	28	625	157	70	40
		0.7	378	95	42	24	536	134	60	34
		0.8	289	73	33	19	409	103	46	26
		0.9	167	42	19	11	237	60	27	15
	0.3	0.4	515	129	58	33	732	183	82	46
		0.5	508	127	57	32	721	181	81	46
		0.6	488	122	55	31	693	174	77	44
		0.7	449	113	50	29	637	160	71	40
		0.8	378	95	42	24	536	134	60	34
		0.9	253	64	29	16	359	90	40	23
2.5	0.1	0.4	430	108	48	27	610	153	68	39
		0.5	381	96	43	24	540	135	60	34
		0.6	318	80	36	20	451	113	51	29
		0.7	243	61	27	16	345	87	39	22
		0.8	161	41	18	11	229	58	26	15
		0.9	76	19	9	5	107	27	12	7
	0.2	0.4	474	119	53	30	673	169	75	43
		0.5	455	114	51	29	645	162	72	41
		0.6	418	105	47	27	594	149	66	38
		0.7	361	91	41	23	512	128	57	32
		0.8	277	70	31	18	393	99	44	25
		0.9	161	41	18	11	229	58	26	15
	0.3	0.4	482	121	54	31	684	171	76	43
		0.5	477	120	53	30	676	169	76	43
		0.6	461	116	52	29	654	164	73	41
		0.7	426	107	48	27	605	152	68	38
		0.8	361	91	41	23	512	128	57	32
		0.9	243	61	27	16	345	87	39	22

14 Observer agreement studies

SUMMARY

In this chapter we describe sample-size calculations for observer agreement studies, with respect to the degree of lack of self-reproducibility of a single observer assessing the same material twice, or agreement between two observers both independently assessing the same specimens. In these situations, when binary decisions are to be made, sample sizes are then based on the pre-specified width of the confidence interval of either the estimated probability of lack of reproducibility (disagreement) or alternatively Cohen's κ statistic. For a study design comprising a combination of these two options, in which the two observers repeat their assessments on a proportion of the specimens but not on the remainder, the lack of reproducibility and disagreement are both estimated so sample size depends on pre-specified confidence interval widths of each of these components. When the measures taken by the reviewer(s) are continuous in nature then agreement is assessed using the intra-class correlation coefficient.

14.1 Introduction

Assessing the results of diagnostic procedures and the effects of therapies often involves some degree of subjective judgment. Observer agreement studies are conducted to investigate the reproducibility and level of consensus on such assessments. Typically, two observers make assessments on each of a series of specimens (assumed as one per subject or patient depending on the context) and these assessments are compared. For example, to examine the measurement of volume of intracranial gliomas from computed tomography, the two observers would evaluate scans from a series of patients and record their estimates of the tumour volume. In some circumstances, the assessments made are of binary form such as a decision on the presence or absence of metastases when examining liver scintigraphy charts.

An important consideration relevant to study design is the presence of both within-observer and between-observer variation. The apparent disagreement between observers may be due to either one of these components or both. It is important to distinguish between them, as any action taken to reduce disagreement will depend on which type of variation dominates. To do this, we require repeated observations of the same material by the same observer.

We consider observer agreement studies with binary assessments and designs; where each of two observers assesses all specimens once, where each observer assesses all specimens twice, and where each observer assesses a proportion of the specimenss once and the remainder twice. Also included are sample sizes for situations where Cohen's κ is used to assess binary decision agreement and those that have a continuous outcome and express agreement through the intra-class correlation coefficient.

Sample Size Tables for Clinical Studies, 3rd edition. By David Machin, Michael J. Campbell, Say Beng Tan, and Sze Huey Tan. Published 2009 by Blackwell Publishing, ISBN: 978-1-4051-4650-0

Observer-agreement studies are designed to estimate the level of observer agreement and so sample sizes are usually based on the achievement of sufficient precision of the estimate as expressed by the desired width of the relevant confidence interval (*CI*). Moreover, there are often no obvious hypotheses to test. The hypothesis of perfect agreement between observers is unrealistic as it can be refuted by a single case of disagreement and the hypothesis of agreement purely by chance is also unrealistic. Rejection of such a hypothesis does not provide useful information since the investigator needs to know more than the fact that the observed level of agreement is unlikely to be due to chance.

Nevertheless we describe a hypothesis testing approach to sample size for a continuous outcome in which a minimally acceptable inter-observer agreement (or reliability) and an anticipated level are set.

14.2 Theory and formulae

No replicate observations

Suppose two observers make a diagnostic decision after examining a patient (or perhaps a specimen taken from a patient), then how likely is it that the two observers draw the same diagnostic conclusion? If we assume the question is whether or not a particular disease is present or absent, then this review process generates, for each of the specimens reviewed, one of the four possible binary pairs $(0, 0)$, $(1, 0)$, $(0, 1)$ and $(1, 1)$ as indicated in **Figure 14.1**.

From **Figure 14.1**, it is clear that the estimates of the proportion of times the reviewer(s) agree or disagree are

$$p_{Agree} = \frac{d_{00} + d_{11}}{m_{Repeat}} \text{ and } p_{Dis} = \frac{d_{10} + d_{01}}{m_{Repeat}} \tag{14.1}$$

respectively.

Sample size

If the corresponding anticipated value for the probability of disagreement, π_{Dis}, is not too close to zero, and the sample size is anticipated to be reasonably large, then for a specified width W_{Dis} of the $100(1 - \alpha)\%$ *CI*, the sample size is

Second review(er)	First review(er)		
	Absent (0)	Present (1)	Total
Absent (0) Present (1)	d_{00} d_{10}	d_{01} d_{11}	
Total			m_{Repeat}

Figure 14.1 Possible outcomes for two observers each reviewing the same specimens but only once to determine the level of between observer disagreement (or a single observer reviewing the same material on two occasions to determine their own lack of reproducibility).

$$m_{\text{Two}} = \frac{4\pi_{\text{Dis}}(1 - \pi_{\text{Dis}})z^2_{1-\alpha/2}}{W^2_{\text{Dis}}}. \tag{14.2}$$

This equation has the same format as Equation 10.2 which was used for calculating the sample size to estimate a Binomial proportion for a given width of confidence interval.

As we have warned previously, it may not be reliable if π_{Dis} is close to 0 or 1 although the latter is very unlikely in this context. Typical values of π_{Dis} range from 0.05 to 0.4. In most situations high disagreement values would not be anticipated but low values may be quite common.

Replicate observations

If replicate observations on some specimens by the *same* observers are added to the design of the previous section, then observer disagreement can be factored into the two components of *between* and *within*-observer variation.

The statistical method assumes that for each specimen the observer, say A, has an unknown 'true' assessment, but owing to difficulties of assessment or other reasons, the observer sometimes makes an 'error' and records a result opposite to his own 'true' assessment. The probability of this is denoted, ξ_A. Further suppose the probability that the true assessment of observer A, for a particular specimen drawn at random, would be to diagnose the condition as present (denoted 1) and this is Θ_{A1}. The corresponding probability of diagnosing the condition as absent is Θ_{A0}. For a second observer B we have ξ_B, Θ_{B1} and Θ_{B0}.

These probabilities are combined into the four possible binary-pair outcomes, to give $\Theta_{00}(= \Theta_{A0} \times \Theta_{B0})$, Θ_{10}, Θ_{01} and Θ_{11} from which $\Theta_{\text{Dis}} = \Theta_{10} + \Theta_{01}$ is the probability they truly disagree. Thus Θ_{Dis} represents the true between-observer variation having extracted the contribution to the disagreement made by within-observer variation.

The aim of the study is to ascertain the level of *agreement* between two observers *and* to estimate the degree of *reproducibility* from each observer. As a consequence, each observer assesses the same set of N specimens independently. In addition, each observer assesses again a random sample of m_{Repeat} ($< N$) of these same specimens. Thus each observer makes $T = N + m_{\text{Repeat}}$ examinations.

Within-observer variation—reproducibility

For a single observer, the degree of reproducibility is quantified by the probability of making a chance error in diagnosis ξ. As indicated above, this is the probability of ascribing a 0 to a diagnosis when it should be 1, or a 1 to a diagnosis that should be 0. The estimate of this probability is

$$\xi = \{1 - \sqrt{2\pi_{\text{Dis}}}\}/2. \tag{14.3}$$

This has a $100(1 - \alpha)\%$ CI,

$$\xi - z_{1-\alpha/2} \times SE(\xi) \text{ to } \xi + z_{1-\alpha/2} \times SE(\xi) \tag{14.4}$$

where $SE(\xi) = \sqrt{\dfrac{\xi(1 - \xi)[1 - 2\xi(1 - \xi)]}{2(1 - 2\xi)^2 m_{\text{Repeat}}}}$.

Number of repeat observations

Sample-size calculations are based on the achievement of sufficient precision of the estimate of ξ which is governed primarily by the number of duplicate assessments, m_{Repeat}. For a given ξ, and desired width w_ξ, of the $100(1 - \alpha)\%$ CI, the number of repeats necessary is given by

$$m_{Repeat} = \frac{2\xi(1 - \xi)(1 - 2\xi + 2\xi^2)z_{1-\alpha/2}^2}{w_\xi^2(1 - 2\xi)^2}.$$ (14.5)

Between-observer variation—agreement

Each observer, say A and B, must make m_{Repeat} diagnoses and so we obtain measures of reproducibly for each, that is estimates of ξ_A and ξ_B respectively. The estimated probability of their disagreement is

$$\Theta_{Dis} = \frac{\theta_{01} + \theta_{10} - [(1 - \xi_A)\xi_B + \xi_A(1 - \xi_B)]}{(1 - 2\xi_A)(1 - 2\xi_B)},$$ (14.6)

where θ_{01} is the probability that on the first assessment observer A says 0 and observer B says 1, while θ_{10} is the same with the positions of A and B reversed.

Gold standard

If one of the observers, say B, can be regarded as defining the 'gold standard' for comparison then this is equivalent to specifying $\xi_B = 0$, so that Equation 14.6 becomes

$$\Theta_{Dis} = \frac{\theta_{01} + \theta_{10} - \xi_A}{(1 - 2\xi_A)}.$$ (14.7)

Equal error rates

At the design stage we will usually have no reason to expect one observer to have a greater error rate than the other, so we assume that $\xi_A = \xi_B = \xi$, and Equation 14.6 becomes

$$\Theta_{Dis} = \frac{\theta_{01} + \theta_{10} - 2\xi(1 - \xi)}{(1 - 2\xi)^2}.$$ (14.8)

We make this equal error rate assumption in the methods described below.

Sample size

As the design of the study has two objectives in mind, the final sample size chosen must be sufficient to meet both design objectives. In order to achieve this, the number of specimens, and the final number of repeats, required for the study is established based on the following considerations. First the number required to obtain a specified precision for Θ_{Dis} is established by setting the confidence interval width as w_Θ.

(i) If it is desired to minimize the number of subjects assessed twice by each observer, then for the width of the $100(1 - \alpha)\%$ CI set at w_Θ, the required sample size is

$$N = \frac{m_{Repeat}(E - Bm_{Repeat})}{Cm_{Repeat} - D},$$ (14.9)

where $B = \dfrac{G(1 - 2F)^2 w_\Theta^2}{4z_{1-\alpha/2}^2}$, $C = \dfrac{(H - G)(1 - 2F)^2 w_\Theta^2}{4z_{1-\alpha/2}^2}$, $D = (H - G)F(1 - F)(1 - 2\Theta_{Dis})^2/2$,

$E = H(H - G) + F(1 - 2\Theta_{Dis})^2[G(1 - F)/2 - H(1 - 2F)]$, $F = 2\xi(1 - \xi)$, $G = (2F - F^2)/4$ and $H = \Theta_{Dis}(1 - \Theta_{Dis}) + F(1 - F)(1 - 2\Theta_{Dis})^2$.

(ii) If it is desired to minimize the total number of subjects required to achieve the desired precision in Θ_{Dis}, when all subjects are assessed twice, then

$$N = \frac{[4\Theta_{Dis}(1 - \Theta_{Dis})(1 - 2F - 2F^2) + 3F^2]z_{1-\alpha/2}^2}{w_\Theta^2(1 - 2F)^2}. \tag{14.10}$$

It is useful to note that since $F = 2\xi(1 - \xi)$ this equation depends only on specified values for ξ, Θ_{Dis}, w_Θ and the confidence level required, $1 - \alpha$, and so is relatively easy to evaluate.

(iii) If it is desired to minimize the total number of assessments, $T = N + m_{Repeat}$. The value of the number of repeat assessments that achieves this minimum is given by

$$m_{Optimal} = \frac{D}{C}\left[1 + \sqrt{\left(\frac{CE - BD}{CD - BD}\right)}\right], \tag{14.11}$$

where B, C, D and E are defined as above. $N_{Optimal}$ is then determined from Equation 14.9 by replacing m_{Repeat} with $m_{Optimal}$.

Cohen's kappa, κ

Inter-observer agreement can also be assessed using Cohen's κ, which takes the form

$$\kappa = \frac{\pi_{Agree} - \pi_{Exp}}{1 - \pi_{Exp}} \tag{14.12}$$

where π_{Agree} is the proportion of observer pairs exhibiting perfect agreement and π_{Exp} the proportion expected to show agreement by chance alone. From **Figure 14.1**, as we have shown before, $p_{Agree} = (d_{00} + d_{11})/m_{Repeat}$. To get the expected agreement we use the row and column totals to estimate the expected numbers agreeing for each category. For negative agreement (Absent, Absent) the expected proportion is the product of $(d_{01} + d_{00})/m_{Repeat}$ and $(d_{10} + d_{00})/m_{Repeat}$, giving $(d_{00} + d_{01})(d_{00} + d_{10})/m_{Repeat}^2$. Likewise for positive agreement the expected proportion is $(d_{10} + d_{11})(d_{01} + d_{11})/m_{Repeat}^2$. The expected proportion of agreements for the whole table is the sum of these two terms, that is

$$p_{Exp} = \frac{(d_{00} + d_{01})(d_{00} + d_{10})}{m_{Repeat}^2} + \frac{(d_{10} + d_{11})(d_{01} + d_{11})}{m_{Repeat}^2}. \tag{14.13}$$

Study size

Suppose the same two observers each assess a sample from m_κ specimens independently then, if κ is not too close to zero and the study is reasonably large, for a specified width W_κ of the $100(1 - \alpha)\%$ CI, the sample size is

$$m_\kappa = 4 \times \frac{(1 - \kappa)}{W_\kappa^2}\left((1 - \kappa)(1 - 2\kappa) + \frac{\kappa(2 - \kappa)}{2\pi_{Dis}(1 - \pi_{Dis})}\right)z_{1-\alpha/2}^2. \tag{14.14}$$

Intra-class correlation coefficient

The intra-class correlation (ICC) is the equivalent to Cohen's κ when the observers are asked to record on a continuous rather than on a binary scale. Further, it allows more than two observers to be compared. It is defined by

$$\rho = \frac{\sigma^2_{\text{Between}}}{\sigma^2_{\text{Within}} + \sigma^2_{\text{Between}}}, \tag{14.15}$$

where σ_{Within} and σ_{Between} are the within and between observer standard deviations.

Study size—confidence interval approach

Suppose that k observers each assess $m_{\text{Specimens}}$ independently then, for a specified width W_ρ of the $100(1 - \alpha)\%$ CI, an approximate sample size is:

$$m_{\text{Specimens}} = 1 + \frac{8z^2_{1-\alpha/2}(1 - \rho_{\text{Plan}})^2[(1 + (k - 1)\rho_{\text{Plan}}]^2}{k(k - 1)W^2_\rho}. \tag{14.16}$$

The design choice is the combination $N_{\text{Observations}} = km_{\text{Specimens}}$.

Bonett (2002) points out that when there are only $k = 2$ raters and the anticipated intra-class correlation is $\rho_{\text{Plan}} > 0.7$, then the sample size required should be increased from $m_{\text{Specimens}}$ to $(m_{\text{Specimens}} + 5\rho_{\text{Plan}})$ or increasing the number of specimens by 4 or 5.

Study size—hypothesis testing approach

To estimate the study size, a minimally acceptable level of inter-observer reliability, say ρ_0, has to be specified. Further, ρ_{Plan} is then set as the value that we anticipate for our study. Once more, the design choice, is $N_{\text{Observations}} = km_{\text{Specimens}}$, that is the combination of numbers of observers available, k, and the associated numbers of specimens to examine, $m_{\text{Specimens}}$, which also depends on k. For this purpose the effect size is

$$C_0 = \frac{1 + k\left[\dfrac{\rho_0}{1 - \rho_0}\right]}{1 + k\left[\dfrac{\rho_{\text{Plan}}}{1 - \rho_{\text{Plan}}}\right]}. \tag{14.17}$$

The number of specimens, $m_{\text{Specimens}}$, then required for two-sided significance α and power $1 - \beta$ is given by

$$m_{\text{Specimens}} = 1 + \frac{2(z_{1-\alpha/2} + z_{1-\beta})^2 k}{(\log C_0)^2(k - 1)}. \tag{14.18}$$

This can be evaluated with the help of **Table 2.3** which gives $\theta = (z_{1-\alpha/2} + z_{1-\beta})^2$ for different values of α and β.

Cautionary note

Equation 14.18 is less robust to differing values of ρ than 14.16 of the confidence interval approach. For example, under a null hypothesis of $\rho_0 = 0.7$, with $\alpha = \beta = 0.05$ and $k = 3$, from Equation 14.18 for $\rho_{\text{Plan}} = 0.725$, 0.75 and 0.80, we require 3376, 786 and 167 specimens respectively. In comparison, the corresponding sample sizes required to estimate ρ with a

95% confidence interval of $W_\rho = 0.2$ from Equation 14.16 are 60, 52 and 37. This large reduction is caused by changing the value of ρ_{Plan} that, while resulting in large changes of the effect size C_0 of Equation 14.17 and hence the corresponding sample size, does not have such a big influence on the sample size obtained from Equation 14.16.

14.3 Bibliography

The early sections of this chapter are based on the work of Baker, Freedman and Parmar (1991) and Freedman, Parmar and Baker (1993) who include a derivation of the sample-size formulae referred to. For Cohen's κ, Donner and Eliasziw (1992) give the $SE(\kappa)$ from which Equation 14.14 is then derived. Although not included here, Cantor (1996) describe the situation in which π_{Dis} is different for each of the two raters. Cicchetti (2001) gives a general discussion of the problem of estimating a valid sample size in this area. He points out that clinically useful results can be obtained with relatively modest values of κ, and there is diminishing gain from increasing the sample size much above 100. Bonett (2002) proposed the confidence interval approach to sample size calculation for the intra-class correlation coefficient, while Walter, Eliasziw and Donner (1998) suggest a hypothesis testing approach and define the effect size, C_0, of Equation 14.17 for this purpose.

14.4 Examples and use of the tables

Table 14.1 or Table 10.1 and Equation 14.2

Example 14.1—two observers—no replicate observations—disagreement
It is anticipated that two observers will have a probability of disagreement of approximately 25% but it is desired to estimate this with a 95% *CI* of width 10%. How many observations should be made?

For a 95% two-sided confidence interval, $\alpha = 0.05$ and from **Table 2.2** $z_{0.975} = 1.96$.

Here, $\pi_{Dis} = 0.25$, $W_{Dis} = 0.1$ and $\alpha = 0.05$. Hence Equation 14.2 gives $m_{Two} = 4 \times \left(\dfrac{0.25(1 - 0.25)}{0.1^2} \right)$

$\times 1.96^2 = 288$. This agrees very closely with the more exact calculations of **Table 14.1** and SS which give $m_{Two} = 289$ or essentially 300. So for such a study, this implies that the two observers examine the same 300 specimens independently.

Table 14.2 and Equation 14.5

Example 14.2—single observer—repeat observations
An observer wishes to establish his own probability of error for making a particular diagnosis from patient specimens. He plans a study involving two assessments per specimen and judges his own probability of error as 5%. If he plans for a 95% confidence interval of width 0.1, how many repeat observations should be made?

For a 95% two-sided confidence interval, $\alpha = 0.05$ and from **Table 2.2** $z_{0.975} = 1.960$.

Here, $\xi = 0.05$, $w_\xi = 0.1$, and for $\alpha = 0.05$, Equation 14.5 gives

$$m_{Repeat} = \frac{2 \times 0.05 \times 0.95 \times [1 - 2 \times 0.05 + 2 \times 0.05^2] \times 1.96^2}{0.1^2[1 - 2 \times 0.05]^2} = 40.78.$$

This implies that the observer should repeat his assessments on approximately 40 specimens. Alternatively direct entry into **Table 14.2** gives $m_{Repeat} = 41$ as does SS_S.

Tables 14.2, 14.3 and Equations 14.5, 14.9 and 14.11

Example 14.3—observer error and disagreement—urothelial dysplasia

In a study to determine agreement with respect to the presence of urothelial dysplasia, as determined from of biopsies, Richards, Parmar, Anderson *et al.* (1991) suggest design values of individual observer error as 0.15 and of true disagreement as 0.2. Suppose they require the width of the 95% *CI* for the observer error to be 0.15 and that for the true disagreement 0.2. How many specimens should they assess?

For a 95% two-sided confidence interval, $\alpha = 0.05$ and from **Table 2.2** $z_{0.975} = 1.96$.

Here, $\alpha = 0.05$ the observer error $\xi = 0.15$ and the set width for the confidence interval, $w_\xi = 0.15$. The planning value for disagreement between observers is $\Theta_{Dis} = 0.2$ and the width of the confidence interval, $w_\Theta = 0.2$.

From Equation 14.5, the appropriate number of specimens required with replicate assessments is $m_{Repeat} = \dfrac{2 \times 0.15 \times (1 - 0.15) \times (1 - 2 \times 0.15 + 2 \times 0.15^2) \times 1.96^2}{0.15^2 \times (1 - 2 \times 0.15)^2} = 66.20$ or 67 which can be obtained directly from SS_S or from **Table 14.2**.

Use of Equation 14.9 with $m_{Repeat} = 67$, leads to a total number of patients $N = 1163.9$ or approximately 1170.

Alternatively, from **Table 14.3** or SS_S, with $\xi = 0.15$, $\Theta_{Dis} = 0.2$, $w_\Theta = 0.2$ and $\alpha = 0.05$, the desired precision for Θ_{Dis} can be obtained from $N_{Equal} = 171$ patients each assessed twice. Using Equation 14.11 gives a value of $m_{Optimal} > 172$. This implies that assessing each patient twice minimises the total number of assessments.

Table 14.4 and Equation 14.14

Example 14.4—Cohen's kappa

Suppose we believe that $\pi_{Dis} = 0.3$, we anticipate $\kappa_{Plan} = 0.4$ and we wish to determine this with $W_\kappa = 0.1$ for a two-sided 95% *CI*.

For a 95% two-sided confidence interval, $\alpha = 0.05$ and from **Table 2.2** $z_{0.975} = 1.96$.

Then from Equation 14.14 $m_\kappa = 4 \times \dfrac{(1 - 0.4)}{0.1^2}\left((1 - 0.4)[1 - (2 \times 0.4)] + \dfrac{0.4(2 - 0.4)}{2 \times 0.3 \times 0.7} \right) \times 1.96^2$

$= 1515.6$. This suggests that about 1600 specimens are needed. Using **Table 14.4** or SS_S gives 1516.

Table 14.5 and Equation 14.16

Example 14.5—intra-class correlation—confidence interval approach

Walter, Eliasziw and Donner (1998) describe a study in which therapists are assessing children with Down's syndrome using the gross motor functional measure (GMFM). This has been validated for use in children with cerebral palsy and it was felt necessary to check its validity in children with a different disease. Suppose we wished to estimate the intra-class correlation coefficient, ρ, to within ± 0.1, or a 95% CI width of $W_\rho = 0.2$. If we assume that $\rho_{Plan} = 0.85$ and that we had $k = 4$ raters.

$$\text{Equation 14.16 suggests } m_{Children} = 1 + \frac{8 \times 1.96^2(1 - 0.85)^2[(1 + (4 - 1) \times 0.85]^2}{4 \times (4 - 1) \times 0.2^2} = 19.2 \text{ or}$$

20 children are required. This is confirmed by the use of **Table 14.5** or $\boxed{^S\!S_S}$. Thus if the same four therapists rate a sample of 20 children, and if r, the estimate of ρ, is close to 0.85, then we would expect the 95% CI to range from 0.75 to 0.95.

Table 14.6, Equations 14.17 and 14.18

Example 14.6—intra-class correlation—hypothesis testing approach

Suppose the investigators were hoping for an inter-rater reliability of at least 0.85 in the above study of GMFM, and had determined that a reliability of 0.7 or higher would be acceptable. Hence, the null hypothesis $H_0 : \rho_0 = 0.7$ and the alternative $H_1 : \rho_1 = 0.85$. For practical reasons no child could be seen more than $k = 4$ times and approximately 30 children were available. Thus the design options were restricted to a choice of $k = 2, 3$ or 4.

> For a 5% two-sided test size, $\alpha = 0.05$, **Table 2.2** gives $z_{0.975} = 1.96$ while for a power of 80% a one-sided $1 - \beta = 0.80$, $z_{0.80} = 0.8416$ or direct use of **Table 2.3** to give $\theta = 7.849$.

For $\rho_0 = 0.7$, $\rho_{Plan} = 0.85$ and $k = 2, 3$ and 4, Equation 14.17 gives the respective effect sizes $C_0 = \dfrac{1 + 2 \times [0.7/0.3]}{1 + 2 \times [0.85/0.15]} = 0.4594, 0.4444$ and 0.4366. For two-sided significance of 5% and 80% power we find from Equation 14.18 when $k = 2$, $m_{Children} = 1 + \dfrac{2 \times 7.849 \times 2}{(\log 0.4594)^2(2 - 1)} = 52.9$ and so $N_{Observations} = km_{Children} \approx 106$, while for $k = 3$, $m_{Children} = 36.8$ and $N_{Observations} \approx 110$ and when $k = 4$, $m_{Children} = 31.5$ and $N_{Observations} = km_{Specimens} \approx 120$. The values for $m_{Children}$ can also be obtained directly from $\boxed{^S\!S_S}$.

In the design with the minimum number of observations, $N_{Observations} = 106$, and so 53 children would each be seen twice. However, the restriction in numbers of children possible to 30 eliminates the possibility of this design. In which case, the investigators would opt for $k = 4$ observations per child in all 30 children.

Note that **Table 14.6** does not tabulate values for $\rho_1 = 0.85$. But supposing $\rho_1 = 0.9$ had been used instead, then from Table 14.6, we would get $m_{Children} = 23, 17$ and 14 for $k = 2, 3$ and 4 respectively.

14.5 References

Baker SG, Freedman LS and Parmar MKB (1991). Using replicate observations in observer agreement studies with binary assessments. *Biometrics*, **47**, 1327–1338. Erratum (1996). *Biometrics*, **52**, 1530.

Bonett DG (2002). Sample size requirements for estimating intraclass correlations with desired precision. *Statistics in Medicine*, **21**, 1331–1335.

Cantor AB (1996). Sample size calculations for Cohen's kappa. *Psychological Methods*, **2**, 150–153.

Cicchetti DV (2001). The precision of reliability and validity estimates re-visited: distinguishing between clinical and statistical significance of sample size requirements. *Journal of Clinical and Experimental Neuropsychology*, **23**, 695–700.

Donner A and Eliasziw M (1992). A goodness-of-fit approach to inference procedures for the kappa statistic: confidence interval construction, significance-testing and sample size estimation. *Statistics in Medicine*, **11**, 1511–1519.

Freedman LS, Parmar MKB and Baker SG (1993). The design of observer agreement studies with binary assessments. *Statistics in Medicine*, **12**, 165–179.

Richards B, Parmar MK, Anderson, CK, Ansell ID, Grigor K, Hall RR, Morley AR, Mostofi FK, Risdon RA and Uscinska BM (1991). The interpretation of biopsies of 'normal' urothelium in patients with superficial bladder cancer. *British Journal of Urology*, **67**, 369–375.

Walter SD, Eliasziw M and Donner A (1998) Sample size and optimal designs for reliability studies. *Statistics in Medicine*, **17**, 101–110.

Table 14.1 Sample sizes required to observe a given confidence interval to estimate the proportion of disagreements between two observers. Each cell gives the number of specimens, m_{Two}.

π_{Dis}	Confidence intervals (CI)							
	90%				95%			
	Width of CI, W_{Dis}				Width of CI, W_{Dis}			
	0.05	0.1	0.15	0.2	0.05	0.1	0.15	0.2
0.01	43	11	5	3	61	16	7	4
0.02	85	22	10	6	121	31	14	8
0.03	126	32	14	8	179	45	20	12
0.04	167	42	19	11	237	60	27	15
0.05	206	52	23	13	292	73	33	19
0.06	245	62	28	16	347	87	39	22
0.07	282	71	32	18	401	101	45	26
0.08	319	80	36	20	453	114	51	29
0.09	355	89	40	23	504	126	56	32
0.1	390	98	44	25	554	139	62	35
0.11	424	106	48	27	602	151	67	38
0.12	458	115	51	29	650	163	73	41
0.13	490	123	55	31	696	174	78	44
0.14	522	131	58	33	741	186	83	47
0.15	552	138	62	35	784	196	88	49
0.16	582	146	65	37	827	207	92	52
0.17	611	153	68	39	868	217	97	55
0.18	639	160	71	40	908	227	101	57
0.19	667	167	75	42	946	237	106	60
0.2	693	174	77	44	984	246	110	62
0.25	812	203	91	51	1153	289	129	73
0.3	910	228	102	57	1291	323	144	81
0.35	985	247	110	62	1399	350	156	88
0.4	1039	260	116	65	1476	369	164	93
0.45	1072	268	120	67	1522	381	170	96
0.5	1083	271	121	68	1537	385	171	97

Table 14.2 Sample sizes required to observe a given confidence interval to estimate the within observer variation. Each cell gives the number of specimens, m_{repeat}.

	Confidence intervals (CI)							
	90%				95%			
	Width of CI, w_ξ				Width of CI, w_ξ			
ξ	0.05	0.1	0.15	0.2	0.05	0.1	0.15	0.2
0.01	22	6	3	2	32	8	4	2
0.02	45	12	5	3	63	16	7	4
0.03	68	17	8	5	96	24	11	6
0.04	91	23	11	6	129	33	15	9
0.05	115	29	13	8	164	41	19	11
0.06	140	35	16	9	199	50	23	13
0.07	166	42	19	11	236	59	27	15
0.08	193	49	22	13	274	69	31	18
0.09	221	56	25	14	314	79	35	20
0.1	250	63	28	16	355	89	40	23
0.11	281	71	32	18	398	100	45	25
0.12	313	79	35	20	444	111	50	28
0.13	346	87	39	22	492	123	55	31
0.14	382	96	43	24	542	136	61	34
0.15	420	105	47	27	596	149	67	38
0.16	461	116	52	29	654	164	73	41
0.17	504	126	56	32	715	179	80	45
0.18	550	138	62	35	781	196	87	49
0.19	600	150	67	38	852	213	95	54
0.2	655	164	73	41	929	233	104	59
0.25	1015	254	113	64	1441	361	161	91
0.3	1648	412	184	103	2340	585	260	147
0.35	2982	746	332	187	4234	1059	471	265
0.4	6754	1689	751	423	9589	2398	1066	600
0.45	27 053	6764	3006	1691	38 411	9603	4268	2401

Table 14.3 Sample sizes required to observe a given confidence interval to minimise the number of subjects required to achieve the desired precision in the probability of their disagreement, Θ_{Dis}. Each cell gives the number of specimens, $m_{Specimens}$.

		Confidence intervals (CI)							
		90%				95%			
		Width of CI, W_Θ				Width of CI, W_Θ			
Θ_{Dis}	ξ	0.05	0.1	0.15	0.2	0.05	0.1	0.15	0.2
0.1	0.05	515	129	58	33	732	183	82	46
	0.1	804	201	90	51	1142	286	127	72
	0.15	1464	366	163	92	2078	520	231	130
	0.2	3032	758	337	190	4305	1077	479	270
	0.25	7111	1778	791	445	10 096	2524	1122	631
	0.3	19 438	4860	2160	1215	27 599	6900	3067	1725
0.2	0.05	881	221	98	56	1251	313	139	79
	0.1	1230	308	137	77	1746	437	194	110
	0.15	1918	480	214	120	2723	681	303	171
	0.2	3395	849	378	213	4820	1205	536	302
	0.25	6959	1740	774	435	9881	2471	1098	618
	0.3	17 156	4289	1907	1073	24 358	6090	2707	1523
0.3	0.05	1142	286	127	72	1622	406	181	102
	0.1	1534	384	171	96	2178	545	242	137
	0.15	2243	561	250	141	3184	796	354	199
	0.2	3654	914	406	229	5188	1297	577	325
	0.25	6851	1713	762	429	9727	2432	1081	608
	0.3	15 526	3882	1726	971	22 044	5511	2450	1378
0.4	0.05	1299	325	145	82	1844	461	205	116
	0.1	1716	429	191	108	2437	610	271	153
	0.15	2437	610	271	153	3460	865	385	217
	0.2	3810	953	424	239	5409	1353	601	339
	0.25	6786	1697	754	425	9635	2409	1071	603
	0.3	14 548	3637	1617	910	20 655	5164	2295	1291
0.5	0.05	1351	338	151	85	1919	480	214	120
	0.1	1777	445	198	112	2523	631	281	158
	0.15	2502	626	278	157	3553	889	395	223
	0.2	3862	966	430	242	5483	1371	610	343
	0.25	6764	1691	752	423	9604	2401	1068	601
	0.3	14 222	3556	1581	889	20 192	5048	2244	1262

Table 14.4 Sample sizes required to observe a given confidence interval width for inter-observer agreement using Cohen's Kappa, κ. Each cell gives the number of specimens, m_κ.

		Confidence intervals (CI)							
		90%				95%			
		Width of CI, W_κ				Width of CI, W_κ			
π_{Dis}	κ	0.05	0.1	0.15	0.2	0.05	0.1	0.15	0.2
0.05	0.4	17 810	4453	1979	1114	25 287	6322	2810	1581
	0.6	15 173	3794	1686	949	21 542	5386	2394	1347
	0.8	8645	2162	961	541	12 275	3069	1364	768
0.1	0.4	9547	2387	1061	597	13 555	3389	1507	848
	0.6	7943	1986	883	497	11 277	2820	1253	705
	0.8	4514	1129	502	283	6409	1603	713	401
0.15	0.4	6831	1708	759	427	9699	2425	1078	607
	0.6	5566	1392	619	348	7903	1976	879	494
	0.8	3156	789	351	198	4481	1121	498	281
0.2	0.4	5507	1377	612	345	7819	1955	869	489
	0.6	4407	1102	490	276	6257	1565	696	392
	0.8	2494	624	278	156	3541	886	394	222
0.25	0.4	4745	1187	528	297	6737	1685	749	422
	0.6	3741	936	416	234	5311	1328	591	332
	0.8	2113	529	235	133	3000	750	334	188
0.3	0.4	4270	1068	475	267	6063	1516	674	379
	0.6	3325	832	370	208	4721	1181	525	296
	0.8	1876	469	209	118	2663	666	296	167
0.4	0.4	3775	944	420	236	5360	1340	596	335
	0.6	2892	723	322	181	4106	1027	457	257
	0.8	1628	407	181	102	2312	578	257	145
0.5	0.4	3637	910	405	228	5163	1291	574	323
	0.6	2771	693	308	174	3934	984	438	246
	0.8	1559	390	174	98	2213	554	246	139
0.6	0.4	3775	944	420	236	5360	1340	596	335
	0.6	2892	723	322	181	4106	1027	457	257
	0.8	1628	407	181	102	2312	578	257	145
0.7	0.4	4270	1068	475	267	6063	1516	674	379
	0.6	3325	832	370	208	4721	1181	525	296
	0.8	1876	469	209	118	2663	666	296	167
0.8	0.4	5507	1377	612	345	7819	1955	869	489
	0.6	4407	1102	490	276	6257	1565	696	392
	0.8	2494	624	278	156	3541	886	394	222
0.9	0.4	9547	2387	1061	597	13 555	3389	1507	848
	0.6	7943	1986	883	497	11277	2820	1253	705
	0.8	4514	1129	502	283	6409	1603	713	401

Table 14.5 Sample sizes required to observe a given intra-class correlation, ρ, using the confidence interval approach. Each cell gives the number of specimens, $m_{Specimens}$. Hence, the total number of observations for the study is $N_{observations} = km_{Specimens}$, where k is the number of observers.

Confidence interval (%)	k	ρ	Width of confidence interval, W_ρ			
			0.05	0.1	0.15	0.2
90	2	0.6	1775	445	199	112
		0.65	1445	362	162	92
		0.7	1127	283	127	72
		0.75	830	209	94	53
		0.8	563	142	64	37
		0.85	335	85	39	22
	3	0.6	1119	281	126	71
		0.65	937	235	105	60
		0.7	750	189	85	48
		0.75	565	142	64	37
		0.8	392	99	45	26
		0.85	238	61	28	16
	4	0.6	907	228	102	58
		0.65	771	194	87	50
		0.7	626	158	71	41
		0.75	478	121	54	31
		0.8	335	85	39	22
		0.85	206	53	24	14
95	2	0.6	2519	631	281	159
		0.65	2051	514	229	130
		0.7	1600	401	179	101
		0.75	1178	296	132	75
		0.8	798	201	90	51
		0.85	475	120	54	31
	3	0.6	1588	398	178	101
		0.65	1329	333	149	84
		0.7	1064	267	120	68
		0.75	802	202	90	52
		0.8	555	140	63	36
		0.85	338	86	39	23
	4	0.6	1286	323	144	82
		0.65	1094	275	123	70
		0.7	887	223	100	57
		0.75	678	171	77	44
		0.8	475	120	54	31
		0.85	292	74	34	20

Table 14.6 Sample sizes required to observe a given intra-class correlation using the hypothesis testing approach with two-sided $\alpha = 0.05$. Each cell gives the number of specimens, $m_{Specimens}$. Hence, the total number of observations for the study is $N_{observations} = km_{Specimens}$.

		Power $1 - \beta = 0.8$			Power $1 - \beta = 0.9$		
		Number of observers, k			Number of observers, k		
ρ_0	ρ_1	2	3	4	2	3	4
0.1	0.2	750	320	199	1004	428	266
	0.3	181	83	54	242	110	72
	0.4	77	37	26	102	49	34
	0.5	40	21	15	54	28	20
	0.6	24	13	10	31	17	13
	0.7	15	9	7	19	11	9
	0.8	9	6	5	12	8	6
	0.9	6	4	3	7	5	4
0.2	0.3	690	332	226	923	443	302
	0.4	162	83	58	217	110	78
	0.5	67	36	26	89	48	35
	0.6	34	19	15	45	26	19
	0.7	19	12	9	25	15	12
	0.8	11	7	6	15	9	8
	0.9	6	5	4	8	6	5
0.3	0.4	604	320	233	808	428	311
	0.5	138	77	58	184	102	77
	0.6	55	32	25	73	42	33
	0.7	27	17	13	35	22	17
	0.8	14	9	8	18	12	10
	0.9	7	5	5	9	7	6
0.4	0.5	499	286	219	667	382	293
	0.6	110	66	52	146	87	69
	0.7	41	26	21	55	34	28
	0.8	19	12	10	25	16	13
	0.9	9	6	5	11	8	7
0.5	0.6	381	234	186	509	312	249
	0.7	79	51	41	105	67	55
	0.8	28	18	15	36	24	20
	0.9	11	8	7	14	10	8
0.6	0.7	260	169	139	348	226	186
	0.8	49	33	28	65	44	37
	0.9	14	10	9	19	13	12
0.7	0.8	148	101	86	198	135	115
	0.9	23	17	14	30	22	19
0.8	0.9	58	41	36	77	55	48

15 Dose finding studies

SUMMARY

The object of this chapter is to describe clinical trial designs for determining, from a pre-selected range of doses of a drug, that which will be used for further testing in studies to determine activity. The dose finding trials determine, in each subject given the compound, the presence or absence of the dose limiting toxicity (DLT). On the basis of the DLT observed, the acceptable dose, the maximum tolerated dose (MTD), is determined. One approach to designing dose finding studies, which includes the 'Cumulative 3 + 3 (C33D)' and the 'Best-of–5' designs, involves no detailed computational methods, whereas, the 'Continual reassessment method (CRM)', entails quite complex assumptions and specialist computer software for implementation and this is provided within the $^S\!S_S$ software. In contrast to other chapters, no sample-size calculations are provided as the number of patients to be recruited is often dependent on the accumulating results from the study, up to a maximum number of patients which is specified in advance.

15.1 Introduction

For patients with a specific disease, one objective of treatment may be to reduce (ideally eradicate) the disease burden. However, it is recognised that any attack on the disease itself for example by a chemotherapeutic or other agent may bring collateral damage to normal tissue and vital organs. The usual strategy is to attempt to balance the two by first establishing the concept of dose limiting toxicity (DLT) which then helps identify the maximum tolerated dose (MTD) of the drug concerned.

Thus the aim of a dose finding study is to establish the MTD of a particular compound or treatment modality so that it can then be tested at that dose in a subsequent (Phase II) trial to assess activity.

In contrast to other situations, for dose finding designs, the number of patients to be recruited is dependent of the accumulating results from the study, with a maximum number of patients often stated in advance. In many cases, there is often very little knowledge about the MTD, and one could only suggest a starting dose based on animal studies. The early doses are usually chosen to be conservative.

In using $^S\!S_S$, should the investigator depart from the original design specification of the design, a warning will be given and the design implementation algorithm will cease. However, the database will remain operational.

Sample Size Tables for Clinical Studies, 3rd edition. By David Machin, Michael J. Campbell, Say Beng Tan, and Sze Huey Tan. Published 2009 by Blackwell Publishing, ISBN: 978-1-4051-4650-0

15.2 Choosing which doses to test

In advance of the patients being recruited in a dose finding study, the investigators first identify the range of the doses to consider and all the specific-dose levels, within this range, to test. Thus the first dose given to any patient, d_{START}, will be one of these options as will be the ultimately identified MTD.

Once the minimum dose to investigate, $d_{MINIMUM}$, is determined, the therapeutic range identified and the maximum dose, $d_{MAXIMUM}$, for the study fixed, we label the k doses finally chosen as $d_1 = d_{MINIMUM}$, d_2, d_3, ..., $d_k = d_{MAXIMUM}$. However, we still need to choose k and the specific values for each of the intermediate doses. Statistical design considerations may suggest that these should be chosen equally spaced between $d_{MINIMUM}$ and $d_{MAXIMUM}$ on either a linear or a logarithmic scale.

However, practice has often recognised that as the dose increases in equal steps it may become sequentially more-and-more toxic and hence possibly dangerous for the well-being of the patient. This caution has then led many investigators to decrease the step sizes as the dose increases. One method uses the Fibonacci (c. 1180–1250) series named after the Italian mathematician who first studied the following mathematical series: $a_0 = a_1 = 1$, then from a_2 onwards $a_{n+1} = a_n + a_{n-1}$. This gives the series: 1, 1, 2, 3, 5, 8, 13, 21, 34, etc. There is no theoretical reason why this or any other mathematical series should be chosen for this purpose—they are merely empirical devices. The corresponding Fibonacci ratios of successive terms are: $1/1 = 1$, $2/1 = 2$, $3/2 = 1.5$, $5/3 = 1.667$, $8/5 = 1.600$, $13/8 = 1.625$, $21/13 = 1.615$, $34/21 = 1.619$, ..., and eventually as n gets larger and larger this approaches $1.618 = (1 + \sqrt{5})/2$. These ratios are shown in **Figure 15.1** and, for relatively small n appropriate to the number of dose levels in a Phase I study, the ratio oscillates up and down. In mathematical terminology the series of ratios is not monotonically decreasing and so in fact do not provide successively decreasing step sizes.

Nevertheless, it is usually regarded as desirable that successive doses are a decreasing multiplier of the preceding dose and thus (often without a clear explanation provided) 'modified'

| Dose | Fibonacci multiplier | | Nolatrexed dihydrochloride | |
	Full	'Modified'	Escalation	Dose (mg/m²/day)
d_1	1.0	1.0	1.0	600
d_2	2.0	2.0	**1.33**	800
d_3	1.50	1.67	1.20	960
d_4	1.67	1.50	1.17	1120
d_5	1.60	1.40	1.07	1200
d_6	1.63	1.33	1.20	1440
d_7	1.62	1.33	1.11	1600
...	...	...		
d_∞	**1.62**	**1.33**		

Figure 15.1 Dose-escalation methods based on the Fibonacci series and that used for a dose finding study of nolatrexed dihydrochloride conducted by Estlin, Pinkerton, Lewis *et al.* (2001).

Fibonacci multipliers like those of **Figure 15.1** are substituted in practice. However, it is usually pragmatic considerations that determine the modifications and no consistent rationale across studies underlies the changes.

15.3 Step-by-step designs

The basic design consists of giving one or more subjects a specific starting dose then, depending on the number of DLTs observed amongst them, stepping up to the next higher preset dose level, or stepping down to the nearest lower level. At this new dose level the process is then repeated. Standard design options are 1, 3 and 5 patients at each dose.

Storer (precursor design)

This design usually starts at $d_{MINIMUM}$, and gives successive (single) patients increasing doses of the compound under investigation, and monitors whether or not they experience DLT with each dose. The dose given depends on the experience of the immediately preceding patient; an absence of DLT will increase the dose for the next patient, while the presence of a DLT will suggest that the immediate prior (and lower) dose will be the MTD. In fact, this is not usually regarded as establishing the MTD but rather to determine the suggested d_{START} for a second stage comprising one of the full C33D, Best-of-5 or CRM designs described below. The strategy is essentially to enable the start of the alternative designs to begin at a more informative dose than $d_{MINIMUM}$. Clearly if a DLT occurs at $d_{MINIMUM}$, the investigators would have to reconsider their whole dose level choice strategy as they would in the absence of a DLT at all doses up to and including $d_{MAXIMUM}$.

Although we have termed Storer as a 'precursor' design, as its objective is to determine a starting dose for other designs, it may be used as a 'stand-alone' examining a different dose range (perhaps wider or with intermediate steps) than might have been considered if one of the 'full' designs had been initiated. Conducted in this way, it may be used to guide the ultimate choice of the doses to be investigated in the more detailed study planned for the next stage of the investigation.

C33D

A common dose finding study design is termed the 'three-subjects-per-cohort design', or 'Cumulative 3 + 3 Design' (C33D). This design chooses a 'low' starting dose perhaps with $d_{START} = d_{MINIMUM}$ (or one suggested by the Storer precursor) and has 3 replicates at each dose. The choice of the next dose, d_{NEXT}, then depends on the number of patients (0, 1, 2 or 3) experiencing DLT. Clearly if no patients experience DLT then the subsequent dose to investigate will be higher than the one just tested. This process continues until either the stopping level of DLT is attained in the successive groups of 3 patients or $d_{MAXIMUM}$ has been tested. In circumstances where the first 2 patients both experience DLT at a particular dose, it is not usual to give the third patient this same dose but to change the dose chosen to a lower one from the pre-specified dose range.

Although this process will (in general) establish the MTD it is only a pragmatic consideration that dictates that a dose finding study should have tested at least 6 patients at d_{MTD}.

Commencing with dose h:

(**A**) Evaluate 3 patients at d_h:

  (**A1**) If 0 of 3 experience DLT, then escalate to d_{h+1}, and go to (**A**).

  (**A2**) If 1 of 3 experience DLT, then go to (**B**).

  (**A3**) If at least 2 of 3 experience DLT, then go to (**C**).

(**B**) Evaluate an additional 3 patients at d_h:

  (**B1**) If 1 of 6 experience DLT, then escalate to d_{h+1}, and go to (**A**).

  (**B2**) If at least 2 of 6 experience DLT, then go to (**C**).

(**C**) Discontinue dose escalation.

Figure 15.2 Establishing the maximum tolerated dose (MTD) in a C33D for a Phase I trial (after Storer 2001).

This usually implies that, once the MTD is first identified, extra patients are then recruited and tested at this provisional d_{MTD} until 6 patients in total have experienced this dose. It is also based on the premise that an acceptable probability of DLT will be somewhere between 1 in 6 (17%) and 1 in 3 (33%) of patients.

However, practical issues often constrain the size of dose finding studies and a maximum size in the region of 24 (8×3) is often chosen. This implies that if pre-determined doses are to be used, and the final dose chosen will have 3 extra patients tested, then $k = 7$ dose options are the maximum that can be chosen for the design as $(k \times 3) + 3 = 24$ patients although the precise numbers included will be dependent on the DLT experience observed.

The C33D design, with or without the Storer (2001) modification, has no real statistical basis, and more efficient alternatives have been sought. Efficiency here can be thought of as achieving the right MTD and with as few patients as possible. However, the design is easy to implement and requires little (statistical) manipulation—only keeping a count of the number of patients experiencing DLT at each dose tested.

The full strategy is described by Storer (2001) and is implemented by following the rules of **Figure 15.2** to determine whether dose-escalation should, or should not, occur.

'Best-of-5'

This follows the same format as C33D except that 5 replicates is used rather than 3. The process is summarised in **Figure 15.3**.

15.4 Continual reassessment method

This design gives successive groups of patients differing doses of the compound under investigation, and monitors the number who experience DLT with each dose. The dose given to the next patient at any one time depends on the experience of *all* the preceding patients. In general an unacceptable level of DLT in the preceding group will lower the dose, while an acceptable level will increase the dose.

There are several variants of the continual reassessment method (CRM). We discuss two of these: the first involves a Bayesian approach and the second a combined Bayesian/Maximum Likelihood approach.

Commencing with dose, h:

(**A**) Evaluate 3 patients at d_h:

   (**A1**) If 0 of 3 experience DLT, then escalate to d_{h+1}, and go to (**A**).

   (**A2**) If 1 or 2 of 3 experience DLT, then go to (**B**).

   (**A3**) If 3 of 3 experience DLT, then go to (**D**).

(**B**) Evaluate an additional 1 patient at d_h:

   (**B1**) If 1 of 4 experience DLT, then escalate to d_{h+1}, and go to (**A**).

   (**B2**) If 2 of 4 experience DLT, then go to (**C**).

   (**B3**) If 3 of 4 experience DLT, then go to (**D**).

(**C**) Evaluate an additional 1 patient at d_h:

   (**C1**) If 2 of 5 experience DLT, then escalate to d_{k+1}, and go to (**A**).

   (**C2**) If 3 of 5 experience DLT, then go to (**D**).

(**D**) Discontinue dose escalation.

Figure 15.3 Establishing the maximum tolerated dose (MTD) in a 'Best-of-5' design for a Phase I trial (after Storer 2001).

Dose level, i	1	2	. . .	k
Actual dose, d_i	d_1	d_2	. . .	d_k
Working dose, z_i	z_1	z_2	. . .	z_k
Probability of DLT, θ_i	θ_1	θ_2	. . .	θ_k

Figure 15.4 Tabulation of the actual dose, corresponding working dose and probability of dose limiting toxicity (DLT).

The same process of selecting the range and actual doses for the step-by-step designs is necessary for the CRM design. In addition, however, it is also necessary to attach to each of these doses (based on investigator opinion and/or on more objective information if available) the anticipated probability of patients experiencing DLT at that dose. We label these *prior* probabilities θ_1, θ_2, θ_3, . . . , θ_k. as in **Figure 15.4**. Once the investigator prior probabilities are attached to each dose that has been selected for investigation, they provide an initial dose-response plot such as that of **Figure 15.5**.

It is implicit in the method of selecting these probabilities that, once they are assigned, then a 'reasonable' starting dose, d_{START}, would correspond to the dose that gives a value of θ_{START} close to some predefined 'acceptable' value, termed the target value and denoted, θ_0. This probability is often chosen to be less than 0.3. The chosen d_{START} would not usually correspond to the extremes $d_{MINIMUM}$ or $d_{MAXIMUM}$ of the dose range cited.

CRM assumes a continuous dose-toxicity model like **Figure 15.6** such that as the dose increases the probability of DLT also increases.

CRM uses a mathematical model for the idealised dose-response curve of the type of **Figure 15.6** that is increasing with increasing dose. One model for this defines the probability of DLT, at working dose z, as

$$\theta(z, q) = \left(\frac{\tanh z + 1}{2} \right)^q = \left(\frac{1}{1 + \exp(-2z)} \right)^q, q > 0. \tag{15.1}$$

where $\tanh z = \dfrac{e^z - e^{-z}}{e^z + e^{-z}}$. Thus $\theta(z, q)$ is the probability of DLT at 'working' dose z and q is a parameter to be estimated.

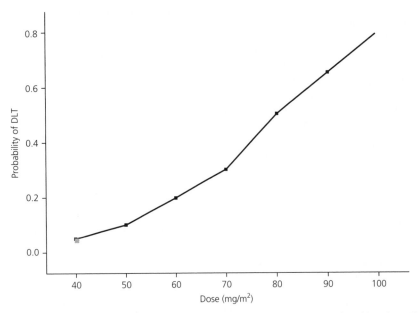

Figure 15.5 Empirical dose-response curve of dose limiting toxicity (DLT) against dose (data from Flinn, Goodman, Post *et al*. 2000).

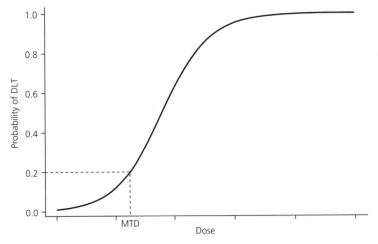

Figure 15.6 Hypothetical dose-response curve of the probability of dose limiting toxicity (DLT) against received dose. MTD, maximum tolerated dose.

It is important to note that z does not correspond to the actual dose of the drug (chosen at the design stage), d, but the so-called working dose level (as patient information accumulates) and, if Equation 15.1 is chosen, the working doses z are determined by

$$z = \frac{1}{2}\log\left(\frac{\theta^{1/q}}{1 - \theta^{1/q}}\right). \tag{15.2}$$

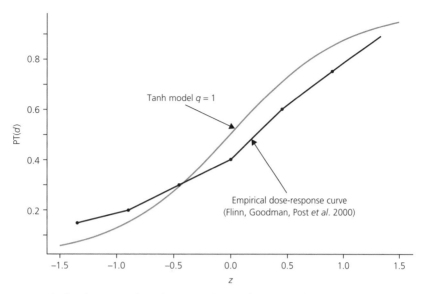

Figure 15.7 The first (no patient data—hence $q = 1$) model for the dose finding trial design of Flinn, Goodman, Post, *et al.* (2000).

Thus from Equation 15.2, for example, with $q = 1$, if $\theta = 0.5$, $z = 0$, $\theta = 0.025$, $z = -1.83$, whereas if $\theta = 0.975$, $z = 1.83$.

An alternative to Equation 15.1 is the logistic function

$$\theta(z, q) = \frac{\exp(qz + 3)}{1 + \exp(qz + 3)}.$$ (15.3)

If Equation 15.3 is chosen, the working doses z are determined by

$$z = \frac{1}{q}\left[\log\left(\frac{\theta}{1 - \theta}\right) - 3\right].$$ (15.4)

Thus from, Equation 15.4, for example, again with $q = 1$, if $\theta = 0.5$, $z = -3$, $\theta = 0.025$, $z = -6.664$, whereas if $\theta = 0.975$, $z = 0.664$.

To begin the implementation of the CRM design, the parameter q is set to 1 in the (investigator) chosen model of either Equations 15.1 or 15.3. A tanh model 'fitted' to the 'subjective probability' data that were illustrated in **Figure 15.5** is shown in **Figure 15.7**.

The uncertainty with respect to the value of q is expressed via a *prior* distribution, $g(q)$. There are several options for this but all can be chosen to have the same mean for q but with increasing variance reflecting the uncertainty about q. These prior distributions are summarised in **Figure 15.8**. Thus if the investigators had a lot of 'experience' of similar drugs in similar patients to that under study then the Exponential distribution might be chosen. In the opposite extreme, Gamma 2 might be chosen. In broad terms this would imply more patients would be needed to determine a suitable value for q.

Once this distribution has been selected, patients have entered the trial and have provided toxicity data, then the value for q can be updated following each successive patient outcome.

Type of prior distribution	$g(q)$	Mean	Variance	Prior
Exponential*	$\lambda \exp(-\lambda q)$	$1/\lambda = 1$	$1/\lambda^2 = 1$	$\exp(-q)$
Gamma 1	$\dfrac{\lambda^r}{\Gamma(r)} q^{r-1} \exp(-\lambda q)$	$r/\lambda = 1$	$r/\lambda^2 = 5$	$\dfrac{0.2^{0.2}}{\Gamma(0.2)} q^{0.2-1} \exp(-0.2q)$
Gamma 2	$\dfrac{\lambda^r}{\Gamma(r)} q^{r-1} \exp(-\lambda q)$	$r/\lambda = 1$	$r/\lambda^2 = 10$	$\dfrac{0.1^{0.1}}{\Gamma(0.1)} q^{0.1-1} \exp(-0.1q)$

*The Gamma distribution with $r = 1$ is the Exponential distribution.

Figure 15.8 Prior distributions for q.

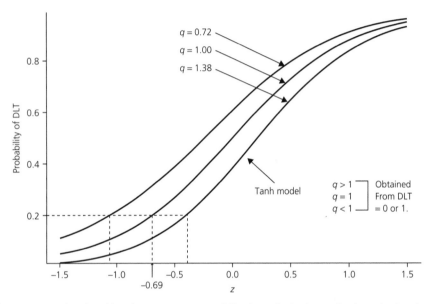

Figure 15.9 Updated working dose response curves following a single observation investigating dose limiting toxicity (DLT) ($y_1 = 0$ or 1) at first working dose $z = -0.69$.

This then allows $\theta(z, q)$ to be calculated and this can be 'fitted' onto the subjective probability data. **Figure 15.9** shows one such example (compare with **Figure 15.7**) in which if the latest patient experiences toxicity the 'curve' moves 'Up' otherwise 'Down'. A move 'Up' implies a *more* 'toxic' dose and hence we would move down the dose options for the next patient.

Bayes and Maximum Likelihood

The object of CRM is to estimate q and find the value of z, hence of d, which corresponds to $\theta(z_{\mathrm{MTD}}, q) = \theta_0$.

At the start of the trial, the first entered patient would be treated at a level chosen by the investigator, d_{START}, believed in the light of all current available knowledge to be the dose closest to the target probability of DLT level, θ_0. As indicated above, once given that dose, whether or not a DLT occurs is noted (we denote this as $y_1 = 0$ or 1). On the basis of this (single) observation q (originally set equal to 1) is then estimated.

There are two methods by which this updating is carried out. One involves a maximum likelihood and the other uses a Bayesian approach. To implement the likelihood method, a number of patients (at least 2) have to be recruited as the method intrinsically needs at least 1 patient to give $y = 0$ and one $y = 1$. The Bayesian approach does not rely on this (early) heterogeneity of responses and so will 'work' even for the first patient. In ^SS_S, users may choose either the Bayesian or Likelihood approach. However both approaches start by implementing the Bayesian approach until heterogeneity of responses is achieved. From there the approaches differ.

Whichever method chosen, after each patient is treated and the presence or absence of DLT observed, the current (prior) distribution $g(q)$ is updated along with the estimated probabilities of toxicity at each dose level. The next patient is then treated at the dose level minimising a measure of the distance between the current estimate of the probability of toxicity and θ_0. After a fixed number, n, of patients have been entered sequentially in this fashion, the dose level selected as the MTD is the one that would be chosen for a hypothetical patient number $(n + 1)$. Alternatively a stopping rule could be set-up whereby the trial would terminate after a minimum number of patients have been recruited at the MTD or when the pre-specified maximum number of patients have been recruited, whichever comes first.

In order to save time during the course of a study, at the time the current patient is being recruited, ^SS_S calculates the recommended dose for the next cohort. If whatever the outcome for the current patient (DLT or no DLT), although not yet observed, would still recommend the same dose then the ^SS_S indicates that fact. This would enable the next cohort of patients to be recruited immediately without waiting for the current patient outcome. This is termed the 'Look-Ahead' option.

The CRM starts with a dose close to that which is expected to give the target probability of DLT, although this is not essential, and then escalates or de-escalates following the result observed at that dose in a single patient (or more generally, in a pre-specified cohort of patients). Once the results from a second patient (or cohort) is obtained then the recommendation for the third patient is based on the results of all two to date and so on. This process can result in jumping over intermediate doses and hence runs the risk of challenging a patient with a (high) dose with no information available on the immediate preceding (lower) dose. Further, if Patient 1 does not experience a DLT then automatically the next higher dose will be recommended. These difficulties can be overcome, by using ^SS_S with the option 'Start at lowest dose' and 'Always escalate by one'.

15.5 Which design?

Although the CRM method is more efficient than the C33D and Best-of-5 designs it is considerably more difficult to implement, as the (statistical) manipulation required to determine the next dose to use is technically complex and requires specialist computer statistical software.

The CRM design reduces the number of patients receiving the (very) low dose options. O'Quigley, Pepe and Fisher (1990) argue this avoids patients receiving doses at which there is little prospect of them deriving benefit but the design has been criticised by Korn, Midthune, Chen et al. (1994) for exposing patients to the risk of receiving potentially very toxic doses.

However, the use of the Storer (2001) precursor prior to the original design allows both these difficulties (too low or too high) to be overcome. Other modifications proposed by Goodman, Zahurak and Piantadosi (1995), and which can be implemented in ^SS_S, also help deal with these.

15.6 Bibliography

Despite the fact that the traditional C33D (and implicitly the Best-of-5) method for dose escalation has been criticised by Heyd and Carlin (1999) and others for the tendency to include too many patients at suboptimal dose levels and give a poor estimate of the MTD, it is still widely used in practice because of its algorithm-based simplicity.

O'Quigley, Pepe and Fisher (1990) and O'Quigley (2001) proposed the CRM with the goal to improve the (statistical) performance of dose escalation designs in determining the MTD. The choice, of the '3' in Equation 15.3, follows from the empirical study conducted by Chevret (1993) who 'fine-tuned' the CRM model by examining a range of possible values that might be placed in the equation. A modification, to the CRM design itself by Goodman, Zahurak and Piantadosi (1995) suggests assigning more than 1 patient to each dose level chosen, and only allowing escalation by one dose level at a time. For de-escalation, the dose recommended by CRM is chosen.

A number of dose finding designs involving the use of Bayesian decision theoretic procedures have been proposed by Whitehead and Williamson (1998); Loke, Tan, Cai and Machin (2006); and Zhou, Whitehead, Bonvini and Stevens (2006). Various other designs have also been suggested, including those by Piantadosi and Liu (1996) which incorporate pharmacokinetic measurements, and by Thall and Russell (1998), O'Quigley, Hughes and Fenton (2001) as well as others who look at designs with bivariate outcomes. However none of these designs appear to have been commonly used to the same extent as the C33D and even the CRM options.

15.7 Examples

Example 15.1—design—nolatrexed dihydrochloride in advanced paediatric cancer
Estlin, Pinkerton, Lewis *et al.* (2001) report on the dose finding study conducted in children with advanced cancer the design of which was described earlier in **Figure 15.1**. The three doses actually tested are given in **Figure 15.10** and were not those specified in the design. At the conclusion of this study, a MTD of 640 mg/m^2/day of nolatrexed dihydrochloride was recommended. However, it is clear from their report that DLT was observed with a dose of 768 mg/m^2/day although only 4 rather than 6 patients required of the C33D design were accumulated at the MTD of 640 mg/m^2/day.

Example 15.2—non-Hodgkins' lymphoma
In the study of Flinn, Goodman, Post *et al.* (2000) a dose escalation strategy was utilised with decreasing multiples of the previous dose used. Their design was the CRM of O'Quigley, Pepe and Fisher (1990) as modified by Goodman, Zahurak and Piantadosi (1995). They defined minimum, $d_{\text{MINIMUM}} = 40$, and maximum, $d_{\text{MAXIMUM}} = 100$, doses with six 10 mg/m^2 steps and

Patient	Dose (mg/m²/day)	Dose escalation	DLT (0 = No, 1 = Yes)
1, 2, 3	480	–	0/3
4, 5, 6, 7	640	1.33	0/4
8, 9, 10, 11	768	1.20	3/4

DLT, dose limiting toxicity.

Figure 15.10 Results of Phase I study of nolatrexed dihydrochloride in childhood cancer (adapted from Estlin, Pinkerton, Lewis *et al.*, 2001, Table 2).

Liposomal daunorubicin (mg/m²)	Dose escalation multiplier	Prior probability of DLT, θ	Number of patients recruited	Number of patients with DLT
40	–	0.05	–	–
50 (start)	1.25	0.10	4	0
60	1.20	0.20	4	1
70	1.17	0.30	3	0
80	1.14	0.50	7	2
90	1.13	0.65	2	2
100	1.11	0.80	–	–

DLT, dose limiting toxicity.

Figure 15.11 DLT observed in patients with advanced non-Hodgkins' lymphoma treated with liposomal daunorubicin with constant doses of the combination cyclophosphamide, vincristine and prednisone (after Flinn, Goodman, Post *et al.*, 2000).

investigator prior probabilities, θ, attached to each dose as given in **Figure 15.11**. As would be expected, as the dose is increased the anticipated (subjective) probability of DLT increases, so that with dose 40 mg/m², θ is only 0.05 (or anticipated to be seen in 1 in every 20 patients with this dose) whereas at dose 100 mg/m² θ is 0.8 (4 in every 5 patients).

The $d_{START} = 50$ mg/m² chosen corresponds to a prior probability of toxicity θ close to 0.1 and not the 0.3 we indicated as a common value to be used. A total of 20 patients were eventually included in total. Their final conclusion was that in patients with advanced non-Hodgkins' lymphoma (NHL) the MTD for liposomal daunorubicin was 70–80 mg/m².

15.8 References

Chevret S (1993). The continual reassessment method for phase I clinical trials: A simulation study. *Statistics in Medicine*, **12**, 1093–1108.

Estlin EJ, Pinkerton CR, Lewis IJ, Lashford L, McDowell H, Morland B, Kohler J, Newell DR, Boddy AV, Taylor GA, Price L, Ablett S, Hobson R, Pitsiladis M, Brampton M, Cledeninn N, Johnston A and Pearson AD (2001). A Phase I study of nolatrexed dihydrochloride in children with advanced cancer. A United Kingdom Children's Cancer Study Group Investigation. *British Journal of Cancer*, **84**, 11–18.

Flinn IW, Goodman SN, Post L, Jamison J, Miller CB, Gore S, Diehl L, Willis C, Ambinder RF and Byrd JC (2000). A dose-finding study of liposomal daunorubicin with CVP (COP-X) in advanced NHL. *Annals of Oncology*, 11, 691–695.

Goodman SN, Zahurak ML and Piantadosi S (1995). Some practical improvements in the continual reassessment method for Phase I studies. *Statistics in Medicine*, 14, 1149–1161.

Heyd JM and Carlin BP (1999). Adaptive design improvements in the continual reassessment method for Phase I studies. *Statistics in Medicine*, 18, 1307–1321.

Korn EL, Midthune D, Chen TT, Rubinstein LV, Christian MC and Simon RM (1994). A comparison of two Phase I trial designs. *Statistics in Medicine*, 13, 1799–1806.

Loke YC, Tan SB, Cai Y and Machin D (2006). A Bayesian dose finding design for dual endpoint Phase I trials. *Statistics in Medicine*, 25, 3–22.

O'Quigley J (2001). Dose-finding designs using continual reassessment method. In Crowley J (ed) *Handbook of Statistics in Clinical Oncology*, Marcel Dekker Inc, New York, pp. 35–72.

O'Quigley J, Hughes MD and Fenton T (2001). Dose finding designs for HIV studies. *Biometrics*, 57, 1018–1029.

O'Quigley J, Pepe M and Fisher L (1990). Continual reassessment method: a practical design for Phase I clinical trials in cancer. *Biometrics*, 46, 33–48.

Piantadosi S and Liu G (1996). Improved designs for dose escalation studies using pharmacokinetic measurements. *Statistics in Medicine*, 15, 1605–1618.

Storer BE (2001). Choosing a Phase I design. In Crowley J (ed) *Handbook of Statistics in Clinical Oncology*, Marcel Dekker Inc, New York, pp. 73–91.

Thall PF and Russel KE (1998). A strategy for dose-finding and safety monitoring based on efficacy and adverse outcomes in Phase I/II clinical trials. *Biometrics*, 54, 251–264.

Whitehead J and Williamson D (1998). An evaluation of Bayesian decision procedures for dose-finding studies. *Journal of Biopharmaceutical Medicine*, 8, 445–467.

Zhou Y, Whitehead J, Bonvini E and Stevens JW (2006). Bayesian decision procedures for binary and continuous bivariate dose-escalation studies. *Pharmaceutical Statistics*, 5, 125–133.

16 Phase II trials

SUMMARY

In this chapter we describe single and two-stage designs for Phase II trials. The single-stage designs include that of Fleming–A'Hern, which considers a single compound for test, and the randomised design of Simon–Wittes–Ellenberg when two or more compounds are under consideration. The two-stage designs described are those of Gehan, the Simon–optimal and the Simon–Minimax. The designs by Tan–Machin and Mayo–Gajewski are based on Bayesian methods and have two options: single and dual threshold. These designs use response criteria as the endpoint of concern, while the Case–Morgan design considers survival time endpoints, and Bryant–Day the dual endpoints of response and toxicity.

16.1 Introduction

Before embarking on large-scale randomised Phase III clinical trials, investigators will often first conduct conduct a Phase II trial to investigate the activity of the compound under consideration. The primary goal is to decide if it warrants further investigation.

There are a relatively large number of alternative designs for Phase II trials. These include single-stage designs, in which a pre-determined number of patients are recruited and two-stage designs, in which patients are recruited in two stages with the move to Stage 2 being conditional on the results observed in Stage 1. A key advantage of a two-stage design is that the trial may stop, after relatively few patients have been recruited, should the response rate appear to be (unacceptably) low. Multi-stage designs have been proposed but the practicalities of having several decision points have limited their use.

16.2 Theory and formulae

A common feature of many of the designs are the requirements that the investigators set the largest response proportion as π_0, which, if true, would clearly imply that the treatment does not warrant further investigation. The investigators then judge what is the smallest response proportion, π_{New}, that would imply the treatment clearly warrants further investigation. This implies that the one-sided hypotheses to be tested are: $H_0 : \pi \leq \pi_0$ versus $H_A : \pi \geq \pi_{New}$, where π is the actual probability of response which is to be estimated.

Sample Size Tables for Clinical Studies, 3rd edition. By David Machin, Michael J. Campbell, Say Beng Tan, and Sze Huey Tan. Published 2009 by Blackwell Publishing, ISBN: 978-1-4051-4650-0

It is typically also necessary to specify α, the probability of rejecting H_0 when it is true, together with β, the probability of rejecting H_A when that is true.

In practice, for a two-stage design, the appropriate number of patients is recruited to Stage 1 and once all their responses are observed, a decision whether or not to proceed to Stage 2 is taken. If Stage 2 is implemented then once recruitment is complete and all assessments made the response rate (and corresponding confidence interval, CI) is calculated. A decision with respect to efficacy is then made. If Stage 2 is not activated, the response rate (and CI) can still be calculated for the Stage 1 patients despite failure to demonstrate sufficient activity.

Single-stage procedure
Fleming–A'Hern
The Fleming (1982) single-stage design for Phase II trials recruits a pre-determined number of patients and a decision about activity is obtained from their responses.

If N_{Fleming} patients are recruited then the observed number of patient responses r will have a Binomial distribution with parameter π. For N_{Fleming} reasonably large and π not too small, the sample size required for the single-stage procedure is approximately

$$N_{\text{Fleming}} = \frac{\left\{ z_{1-\alpha}\sqrt{[\pi_0(1-\pi_0)]} + z_{1-\beta}\sqrt{[\pi_{\text{New}}(1-\pi_{\text{New}})]} \right\}^2}{(\pi_{\text{New}} - \pi_0)^2}. \tag{16.1}$$

where $z_{1-\alpha}$ and $z_{1-\beta}$ are the standardised Normal deviates of **Table 2.1**. However, A'Hern (2001) has used the exact Binomial probabilities to calculate the sample size and, in general, these are marginally greater than those given by Equation 16.1.

The design would reject the null hypothesis $\pi \le \pi_0$ if the observed number of responses R is $\ge C$ and would then conclude $\pi \ge \pi_{\text{New}}$. Fleming determined the critical number of responses as

$$C_{\text{Fleming}} = 1 + N_{\text{Fleming}}\pi_0 + z_{1-\alpha}\sqrt{N_{\text{Fleming}}\pi_0(1-\pi_0)} \tag{16.2}$$

but this was modified by A'Hern to

$$C_{\text{A,Hern}} = N_{\text{A,Hern}} \times \left(\pi_0 + \left(\frac{z_{1-\alpha}}{z_{1-\alpha} + z_{1-\beta}} \right)(\pi_{\text{New}} - \pi_0) \right). \tag{16.3}$$

Note
Although the A'Hern calculations should supersede Fleming's, $^S\!S_S$ also provides sample sizes according to the Fleming approximation. This is because the design has been very widely used and so this option is intended to facilitate comparisons with these earlier studies.

Two-stage designs
Gehan
In this design only a minimum requirement of efficacy, π_{New}, is set and patients are recruited in two stages. If no responses are observed in the Stage 1, then the trial terminates. On the other hand, if one or more responses are observed then the size of Stage 2 depends on their actual number.

If the probability of response to a particular treatment is π_{New}, then the probability of n_{G1} successive patients *failing* to respond is

$$\eta = (1 - \pi_{\text{New}})^{n_{\text{G1}}}. \tag{16.4}$$

For a specified η, the Stage 1 rejection error, this can be solved to give the number of patients for this stage as

$$n_{\text{G1}} = \frac{\log \eta}{\log(1 - \pi_{\text{New}})}. \tag{16.5}$$

Assuming r_{G1} (> 0) responses are observed in these n_{G1} patients, then n_{G2} patients are recruited to the Stage 2 to give a total of $N_{\text{Gehan}} = n_{\text{G1}} + n_{\text{G2}}$ in all. The value of n_{G2} is chosen to give a specified standard error, $SE(p) = \gamma$, for the final estimate of the activity obtained. This implies that

$$SE(p) = \sqrt{\frac{p(1 - p)}{n_{\text{G1}} + n_{\text{G2}}}} = \gamma. \tag{16.6}$$

If r_{G2} is the number of responses in Stage 2 then $p = (r_{\text{G1}} + r_{\text{G2}})/(n_{\text{G1}} + n_{\text{G2}})$ is the estimate of the efficacy of the drug. Rearranging Equation 16.6 we obtain the required number of patients for Stage 2 as

$$n_{\text{G2}} = \frac{p(1 - p)}{\gamma^2} - n_{\text{G1}}. \tag{16.7}$$

However, at the end of Stage 1 we only know $p_{\text{G1}} = r_{\text{G1}}/n_{\text{G1}}$, the proportion of successes in Stage 1. Thus, to estimate n_{G2} from Equation 16.7, we must use p_{G1} rather than p since the latter is not available to us. However, n_{G1} is usually so small that the resulting p_{G1} will be rather imprecise. As a consequence, rather than using p_{G1} to estimate p in Equation 16.7, Gehan (1961) estimated this by π_{U}, the one-sided upper 75% confidence limit for π, which is the solution of

$$B(r_{\text{G1}}; \pi_{\text{U}}, n_{\text{G1}}) = 0.25. \tag{16.8}$$

Here $B(.)$ is the cumulative Binomial distribution of Equation 2.9 with $R = r_{\text{G1}}$, $\pi = \pi_{\text{U}}$ and $m = n_{\text{G1}}$.

The final estimate for the sample size of Stage 2 is therefore

$$n_{\text{G2}} = \frac{\pi_{\text{U}}(1 - \pi_{\text{U}})}{\gamma^2} - n_{\text{G1}}. \tag{16.9}$$

This number depends rather critically on the number of successes r_{G1} observed in Stage 1.

Simon–Optimal and Simon–Minimax

As with Fleming–A'Hern, for the Simon (1989) design the investigators set π_0 and π_{New} as we have described previously. The trial proceeds by recruiting n_{S1} patients in Stage 1 from which r_{S1} responses are observed. A decision is then made to recruit n_{S2} patients to Stage 2 if $r_{\text{S1}} \geq R_{\text{S1}}$ otherwise the trial is closed at the end of Stage 1. At the end of the second stage, the drug is recommended for further use if a predetermined $R_{\text{Simon}} = (R_{\text{S1}} + R_{\text{S2}})$ or more responses are observed.

In such a design, even if $\pi > \pi_0$ there is a possibility that the trial once conducted will *not* go into the Stage 2. The probability that the trial is terminated after Stage 1, that is there are fewer than R_{S1} responses observed, is

$$P_{\text{Early}} = B(R_{S1} - 1; \pi, n_{S1}), \tag{16.10}$$

where $B(.)$ is the cumulative Binomial distribution of Equation 2.9 with $R = R_{S1} - 1$, $\pi = \pi$ and $m = n_{S1}$. The expected sample size is

$$N_{\text{Expected}} = n_{S1} + (1 - P_{\text{Early}})n_{S2}. \tag{16.11}$$

In this context, *expected* means the average sample size that would turn out to have been used had a whole series of studies been conducted with the same design parameters in situations where the true activity is the same.

Optimal design

By not continuing to Stage 2, the Simon–Optimal design attempts to ensure that as few patients as possible receive what appears to be an ineffective drug at the end of Stage 1.

A computer search is necessary to determine sample size. Essentially for each potential (Stage 1 plus Stage 2) sample size N_{Simon} and each value of n_{S1} in the range $(1, N_{\text{Simon}} - 1)$, values of R_{S1} and R_{S2} are found corresponding to the specified values of π_0, π_{New}, α and β, and which minimise the expected sample size of Equation 16.11 when $\pi = \pi_0$.

Minimax design

In the Simon–Minimax design, the total size of the trial, that is the sum of patients required for Stage 1 and Stage 2 together, is chosen to minimise the maximum trial size.

Again a computer search is necessary to determine sample size. The search strategy is the same as for the optimal design, except that the values of n_{S1}, n_{S2}, R_{S1} and R_{S2} that result in the smallest total sample size are determined.

Bayesian two-stage designs

In the Phase II designs discussed so far, the final response rate is estimated by R/N, where R is the total number of responses observed from the total number of patients recruited N (whether obtained from a single-stage design or one or both stages of a two-stage design). This response rate, together with the corresponding 95% *CI*, provide the basic information for the investigators to decide if a subsequent Phase III trial is warranted. However, as Phase II trials are usually of modest size, the resulting *CI*s will usually be rather wide—encompassing a wide range of options for π. This inevitable uncertainty arising from small sample sizes led Tan and Machin (2002) and others to propose Bayesian designs. In their approach, the focus of the design is to estimate the (so-called) posterior probability that $\pi > \pi_{\text{New}}$, denoted Prob$(\pi > \pi_{\text{New}})$. If this probability is high (a threshold level is set by the design) at the end of the trial, the investigators can be reasonably confident in recommending the compound for Phase III trial.

Single threshold design

In the two-stage single threshold design (STD) the investigator first sets the minimum interest response rate π_{New} as for other designs but now specifies π_{Prior} (not π_0) the *anticipated* response rate of the drug under test. Further, in place of α and β, λ_1 the required threshold probability following Stage 1 that $\pi > \pi_{\text{New}}$, denoted $\text{Prob}_{\text{Stage-1}}(\pi > \pi_{\text{New}})$, and λ_2 the required threshold $\text{Prob}_{\text{End}}(\pi > \pi_{\text{New}})$ after completion of Stage 2 are specified. Here λ_2 is set to be greater than λ_1. Once Stage 1 of the trial is completed, the estimated value of λ_1, that is u_1, is computed and a decision is made to proceed to Stage 2 if $u_1 \geq \lambda_1$. Should the trial continue to Stage 2 then, on trial completion, u_2 is computed and a recommendation to proceed to Phase III if $u_2 \geq \lambda_2$.

The design determines the sample sizes for the trial based on the following principle. Suppose also that the (hypothetical) response proportion is just larger than the pre-specified π_{New}, say $\pi_{\text{New}} + \varepsilon$, with $\varepsilon > 0$ being small. We then want the smallest overall sample size, $N_{\text{T-M}}$, that will enable $\text{Prob}_{\text{End}}(\pi > \pi_{\text{New}})$ to be at least λ_2. At the same time, we also want the smallest possible Stage 1 sample size $n_{\text{T-M1}}$ which is just large enough so that $\text{Prob}_{\text{Stage-1}}(\pi > \pi_{\text{New}})$ is at least λ_1.

Dual threshold design

The dual threshold design (DTD) is identical to the STD except that the Stage 1 sample size is determined, not on the basis of the probability of exceeding π_{New}, but on the probability that π will be less than the 'no further interest' proportion, π_0. Thus π_0 functions as a lower threshold on the response rate. The rationale behind this aspect of the DTD is that we want our Stage 1 sample size to be large enough so that, if the trial data really does suggest a response rate that is below π_0, we want the posterior probability of π being below π_0, to be at least λ_1. The design determines the smallest Stage 1 sample size that satisfies this criterion.

The DTD requires the investigators to set π_{Prior} as the anticipated value of π for the drug being tested. A convenient choice may be $(\pi_0 + \pi_{\text{New}})/2$ but this is not a requirement. Further λ_1 is set as the required threshold probability following Stage 1, that $\pi < \pi_0$, while λ_2 is the required threshold probability that, after completion of Stage 2, $\pi > \pi_{\text{New}}$. [Note that unlike the STD, it is no longer a requirement that $\lambda_1 < \lambda_2$.] Once Stage 1 of the trial is completed, the estimated value of λ_1, that is l_1, is computed and should the trial continue to Stage 2 then on its completion, u_2 is computed. The latter is then used to help make the decision whether or not a Phase III trial is suggested.

Prior distributions

In the original version of the designs proposed by Tan and Machin (2002), the designs work on the basis of having a 'vague' prior distribution. Mayo and Gajewski (2004) extended the designs to allow for the inclusion of informative prior distributions. In $^{S}S_{S}$ users have the option of using such informative prior distributions (which could also be set to be equivalent to the vague priors used by Tan and Machin). Moreover Tan and Machin imposed some practical constraints on their designs, so as to encourage the adoption of the designs into practice. In particular, they constrained the total study size, $N_{\text{T-M}}$, to be a minimum of 10 and a maximum of 90, with Stage 1 size, $n_{\text{T-M1}}$, having a minimum size of 5 and a maximum of $N_{\text{T-M}} - 5$. These constraints are not applied in $^{S}S_{S}$.

Survival time and survival proportion endpoints

Although many Phase II trials have disease response as a (binary) outcome, survival times or at least survival proportions at a fixed time are sometimes more relevant.

Case–Morgan

In the Case and Morgan (2003) two-stage Phase II trial designs, 'survival' times are utilised in place of binary response variables. The 'survival' times usually correspond to the interval between commencement of the Phase II treatment and when the 'event' of primary concern occurs.

In these designs, patients are observed from a fixed point in time to, for example, recurrence of the disease, death or either of these. However, to implement these designs, it is important to distinguish between *chronological* time, that is the date (day, month, year) in which the trial recruits its first patient, the date of the planned interim analysis (end of Stage 1), the date the trial closes recruitment (end of Stage 2), and the date all patient follow-up ends from the time *interval* between start of therapy and the occurrence of the event for the individual patients. Trial conduct is concerned with *chronological* time while trial analysis is concerned with *interval* time. We denote the former by D and the latter by t.

Survival data are typically summarised by the Kaplan–Meier (*K-M*) survival curve, which takes into account censored observations. Censored survival time observations arise when a patient, although entered on the study and followed for a period of time, has not as yet experienced the 'event' defined as the outcome for the trial. For survival itself 'death' will be the 'event' of concern whereas if event-free survival was of concern the 'event' may be recurrence of the disease.

Technical details

(*Note* The description that follows is not a precise summary of the technical details as set out by Case and Morgan (2003) but attempts to summarise the rationale behind the designs. For example, Case and Morgan do not use the *K-M* estimate of survival in their description, and their estimate of the standard error differs from that indicated here.)

The *K-M* estimate of the proportion alive at any follow-up time t, is denoted $S(t)$. Thus, for example, when $t = 1$ year, the *K-M* estimate at that time-point is denoted $S(1)$. In general, a convenient time-point, which we denote by $T_{Summary}$, is chosen by the investigators and the corresponding $S(T_{Summary})$ estimates the proportion of patients experiencing the event by that time-point.

To implement the design, the investigators set for interval time, $T_{Summary}$, the largest survival proportion as $S_0(T_{Summary})$ which, if true, would clearly imply that the treatment does not warrant further investigation. The investigators then judge what is the smallest survival proportion, $S_{New}(T_{Summary})$, that would imply the treatment warrants further investigation. This implies that the one-sided hypotheses to be tested are: $H_0 : S(T_{Summary}) \leq S_0(T_{Summary})$ versus $H_{New} : S(T_{Summary}) \geq S_{New}(T_{Summary})$, where $S(T_{Summary})$ is the actual probability of survival which is to be estimated at the close of the trial. In addition, it is necessary to specify α, and β.

The Case–Morgan design assumes that the survival times follow an exponential distribution and this implies that

$$S(t) = \exp(-\lambda t). \tag{16.12}$$

Here λ is termed the instantaneous event rate and is assumed to have the same constant value for all those entering the trial.

It then follows from Equation 16.12 that

$$CL(t) = \log[-\log S(t)] = \log \lambda + \log t. \tag{16.13}$$

This transformation results in $CL(t)$ having an approximately Normal distribution with standard error,

$$SE[CL(t)] = SE[\log \lambda] = 1/\sqrt{E}, \tag{16.14}$$

where E is the corresponding number of events observed by time t.

The assumption of Exponential survival times implies $S_0(T_{Summary}) = \exp(-\lambda_0 T_{Summary})$ and $S_{New}(T_{Summary}) = \exp(-\lambda_{New} T_{Summary})$ where λ_0 and λ_{New} are essentially the 'event' rates under the two hypotheses (the event rate will be less under H_{New}). This implies that the two one-sided hypotheses discussed above can be alternatively expressed as: $H_0 : \lambda \geq \lambda_0$ and $H_{New} : \lambda \leq \lambda_{New}$.

Stage 1 and interim analysis

To implement a two-stage design, n_{C-M1} patients are recruited in Stage 1 whose duration $D_{Stage1} (= D_{Interim})$ is set to coincide with the interim analysis which implies a recruitment rate of $R = n_{C-M1}/D_{Stage1}$ for this period. The duration of Stage 1 and hence the date of the interim analysis, can potentially be at any time after a period equal to $T_{Summary}$ has elapsed from the date the first patient is treated. At this analysis, $E_{C-M1} (\leq n_{C-M1})$ events will have been observed while other patients will have been on the trial for a time-period less than $T_{Summary}$ without experiencing the event. These patients will be censored, as will those who have a 'survival' time greater than $T_{Summary}$ but have not yet experienced the event. Thus at chronological time $D_{Interim}$ for interval time $T_{Summary}$ the one-sided hypothesis, H_0 can be tested by

$$z_{Interim} = \frac{CL_{Interim}(T_{Summary}) - CL_0(T_{Summary})}{SE[CL_{Interim}(T_{Summary})]}. \tag{16.15}$$

The components of this equation are obtained by use of Equations 16.13 and 16.14. This $z_{Interim}$ test has a standard Normal distribution with mean 0 and standard deviation 1 if H_0 is true. If $z_{Interim} < C_1$ (see below) then recruitment to the trial is stopped, that is, the hypothesis $H_0 : S(T_{Summary}) \leq S_0(T_{Summary})$ is *accepted*.

Otherwise, if the decision is to recruit a further n_{C-M2} patients over a period D_{Stage2}, then the last of these patients so recruited will be followed for the minimum period of $T_{Summary}$. With the same recruitment rate R as for Stage 1, $D_{Stage2} = n_{C-M2}/R$. The final analysis will then be conducted at $D_{Final} = D_{Interim} + D_{Stage2} + T_{Summary} = D_{Accrual} + T_{Summary}$. By that time, and in addition to the events of some of the Stage 2 patients, there may be more events from the Stage 1 patients than were observed at $D_{Interim}$.

At chronological time D_{Final}, Equation 16.15 is adapted to that involving the alternative hypothesis H_{New}. Thus

$$z_{Final} = \frac{CL_{Final}(T_{Summary}) - CL_{New}(T_{Summary})}{SE[CL_{Final}(T_{Summary})]}. \tag{16.16}$$

This z_{Final} has a standard Normal distribution with mean 0 and standard deviation, 1 if H_{New} is true. If $z_{Interim} > C_2$ (see below) then the alternative hypothesis $H_{New} : S(T_{Summary}) \geq S_{New}(T_{Summary})$ is *accepted* and activity is claimed.

Determining C_1 and C_2

At the design stage of the trial, the values of the survival rates λ_0 and λ_{New} under each hypothesis are specified by the investigators, as are the corresponding error rates α and β. The values of C_1 and C_2 are determined as the solutions to the following equations

$$1 - \Phi_2(C_1, C_2) = \alpha \tag{16.17}$$

and

$$1 - \Phi_2(C_1 - \rho u, C_2 - u) = 1 - \beta, \tag{16.18}$$

which can only be found by computer search methods.

In these equations, $\Phi_2(.,.)$ is the cumulative form of the bivariate Normal distribution while

$$u = \frac{CL_{New}(T_{Summary}) - CL_0(T_{Summary})}{\sigma_{C-M}/\sqrt{N_{C-M}}} = \frac{\log \lambda_{New} - \log \lambda_0}{\sigma_{C-M}/\sqrt{N_{C-M}}}. \tag{16.19}$$

When planning a two-stage trial, one cannot be certain that Stage 2 will be activated as this will depend on the patient outcomes from Stage 1, and so Case and Morgan (2003) take the probability of stopping at the end of Stage 1 (P_{Early}) into their design considerations. This then leads to the expected duration of accrual

$$EDA = D_{Stage1} + (1 - P_{Early})\,D_{Stage2}, \tag{16.20}$$

where $D_{Accrual} = D_{Stage1} + D_{Stage2}$. In this context, *expected* means the average duration of accrual that would have occurred had a whole series of studies been conducted with the same design parameters.

Using the notation of Equation 2.2

$P_{Early} = \Phi_1(C_1)$, where $\Phi_1(.)$ is the cumulative form of the univariate standardised Normal distribution. $\tag{16.21}$

In a similar way, the expected total study length (duration) is

$$ETSL = D_{Stage1} + (1 - P_{Early})(D_{Stage2} + T_{Summary}). \tag{16.22}$$

Assuming there is a constant accrual rate, R, over the recruitment stages of the trial, then there are four unknowns, n_{C-M1} (or D_{Stage1}), n_{C-M2} (or D_{Stage2}), C_1 and C_2, but only two constraints, α and β. As a consequence there are more unknowns than constraints, hence, those design options that minimise either the *EDA* of Equation 16.20 or *ETSL* of Equation 16.22 are chosen.

Case–Morgan–EDA

To determine the expected duration of accrual (EDA) design, the search process assumes that the Fleming–A'Hern single-stage design is to be implemented with response rates of $S_0(T_{Summary})$ and $S_{New}(T_{Summary})$. This gives a sample size, $N_{F-A'H}$, for which the investigator then specifies how long these would take to recruit, $D_{F-A'H}$; once specified this is related to $T_{Summary}$. The final (two-stage) solutions from the computer search depend on the ratio $D_{F-A'H}/T_{Summary}$ (> 1). A search is then made for each total potential sample size N_{C-M}, to find the Stage 1/Stage 2 split amongst these with the specific design parameters for survival rates of $S_0(T_{Summary})$, $S_{New}(T_{Summary})$, and error constraints α and β, that minimises the *EDA*.

Case–Morgan–ETSL

To determine the *ETSL* design, the same procedures are followed as for *EDA* above, except that the final stage searches for designs that minimise *ETSL* rather than *EDA*.

For either design, patients are recruited until chronological time D_{Stage1} to a total of $n_{\text{C-M1}}$. At this time the Kaplan–Meier estimate of $S(T_{\text{Summary}})$ and its *SE* are estimated using a standard statistical package or by CIA (confidence interval analysis) provided by Altman, Machin, Bryant and Gardner (2000). From these z_{Interim} is calculated. If the decision is made to continue, repeat the process after a further $n_{\text{C-M2}}$ patients have been recruited and a further additional T_{Summary} of time has elapsed since the last patient.

Randomised design

Simon–Wittes–Ellenberg

When there are several compounds available for potential Phase III testing in the same type of patients but practicalities imply that only one of these can go forward for this subsequent assessment, then the randomised (single-stage) Simon, Wittes and Ellenberg (1985) design selects the candidate drug with the highest level of activity. Although details of the random allocation process are not outlined below this is a vital part of the design implementation. Details are provided by, for example, Machin and Campbell (2005).

The approach chooses the observed best treatment for the Phase III trial, however small the advantage over the others. The trial size is determined in such a way that if a treatment exists for which the underlying efficacy is superior to the others by a specified amount, then it will be selected with a high probability.

When the difference in true response rates of the best and next best treatment is δ, then the probability of correct selection, P_{cs}, is smallest when there is a single best treatment and the other $g - 1$ treatments are of equal but lower efficacy. The response rate of the worst treatment is denoted π_{Worst}.

For a specified response π, the probability that the best treatment produces the highest observed response rate is

$$\text{Prob(Highest)} = \sum_{i=0}^{m} f(i)[1 - B(i; \pi_{\text{Worst}} + \delta, m)], \tag{16.23}$$

where $R = i$, $\pi = \pi_{\text{Worst}} + \delta$ in Equation 2.9 and

$$f(i) = [B(i; \pi_{\text{Worst}}, m)]^{g-1} - [B(i - 1; \pi_{\text{Worst}}, m)]^{g-1}, \tag{16.24}$$

where $R = i - 1$ and $\pi = \pi_{\text{Worst}}$ in Equation 2.9.

If there is a tie among the treatments for the largest observed response rate, then one of the tied treatments is randomly selected. Hence, in calculating the probability of correct selection, it is necessary to add to Expression 16.23 the probability that the best treatment was selected after being tied with one or more of the other treatments for the greatest observed response rate. This is

$$\text{Prob(Tie)} = \sum_{i=0}^{m} \left[b(i; \pi_{\text{Worst}} + \delta, m) \sum_{j=1}^{g-1} \left(\frac{1}{j+1} \right) k(i, j) \right], \tag{16.25}$$

where $k(i, j) = \dfrac{(g - 1)!}{j!(g - 1 - j)!} [b(i; \pi_{\text{Worst}}, m)]^j [B(i - 1; \pi_{\text{Worst}}, m)]^{g-1-j}$.

The quantity $k(i, j)$ represents the probability that exactly j of the inferior treatments are tied for the largest number of observed responses among the $g - 1$ inferior treatments, and this number of responses is i. The factor $\left(\dfrac{1}{j+1}\right)$ in Equation 16.25 is the probability that the tie between the best and the j inferior treatments, is randomly broken by selecting the best treatment.

The sum of Expressions 16.23 and 16.25 gives the probability of correct selection, that is

$$P_{CS} = \text{Prob(Highest)} + \text{Prob(Tie)}. \tag{16.26}$$

The corresponding tables for the number of patients per treatment group required, is determined by searching for specified values of π_{Worst}, δ, and g, the value of m which provides a probability of correct selection equal to a set value for P_{CS}.

Except in extreme cases, when π_{Worst} is small or large, the sample size is relatively insensitive to these baseline response rates. Since precise knowledge of these may not be available, Liu (2001) propose a conservative approach to trial design which involves using the largest sample size for each g and δ. Unfortunately, with $g \geq 4$ groups these designs lead to relatively large randomised trials and this may limit their usefulness.

Response and toxicity endpoints

Bryant–Day

Bryant and Day (1995) point out that a common situation when considering Phase I and Phase II trials is that although the former primarily focuses on toxicity and the later on efficacy, each in fact considers both. This provides the rationale for their Phase II design which incorporates toxicity and activity considerations. Essentially they combine a design for activity with a similar design for toxicity in which one is looking for both *acceptable* toxicity and *high* activity.

The Bryant and Day (1995) design implies that two, *one-sided* hypotheses, are to be tested. These are that the true response rates π_R is either $\leq \pi_{R0}$, the maximum response rate of no interest, or $\geq \pi_{RNew}$, the minimum response rate of interest. Further the probability of incorrectly rejecting the hypothesis $\pi_R \leq \pi_{R0}$ is set as α_R. Similarly α_T is set for the hypothesis $\pi_T \leq \pi_{T0}$ where π_T is the maximum non-toxicity rate of no interest. In addition, the hypothesis $\pi_T \geq \pi_{TNew}$ has to be set together with β, the probability of failing to recommend a treatment that is acceptable with respect to both activity and (non-) toxicity. [The terminology is a little clumsy here as it is more natural to talk in terms of 'acceptable toxicity' rates rather than 'acceptable non-toxicity' rates. Thus $1 - \pi_{T0}$ is the highest rate of toxicity above which the drug is unacceptable. In contrast, $1 - \pi_{TNew}$ is the lower toxicity level below which the drug would be regarded as acceptable on this basis.]

In the Bryant and Day design, toxicity monitoring is incorporated into the Simon (1989) design by requiring that the trial is terminated after Stage 1 if there is an inadequate number of observed responses or an excessive number of observed toxicities. The treatment under investigation is recommended at the end of Stage 2 only if there are both a sufficient number of responses and an acceptably small number of toxicities in total.

Since both toxicity and response are assessed in the same patient, the distributions of response and toxicity are not independent, and these two are linked by means of

$$\varphi = \frac{\eta_{00}\eta_{11}}{\eta_{01}\eta_{10}}. \tag{16.27}$$

Here η_{00} is the true proportion of patients who both fail to respond and also experience unacceptable toxicity, η_{01} is the proportion of patients who fail to respond but have acceptable toxicity, η_{10} is the proportion of patients who respond but who have unacceptable toxicity, and finally η_{11} is the proportion of patient who respond and also have acceptable toxicity.

The design parameters chosen will establish a particular design with Stage 1 and total sample sizes $(n_{\text{B-D1}}, n_{\text{B-D2}})$, cut-off values for response and toxicity (C_{R1} and C_{T1}) in order to move from Stage 1 to Stage 2, and finally cut-off values C_{R}, and C_{T} to declare sufficient activity with acceptable toxicity once the results from $N_{\text{B-D}} = n_{\text{B-D1}} + n_{\text{B-D2}}$ patients has been observed. We describe these collectively by $Q = \{n_{\text{B-D1}}, C_{\text{R1}}, C_{\text{T1}}, n_{\text{B-D2}}, C_{\text{R}}, C_{\text{T}}\}$ and this set of six quantities are then determined by minimising the *expected* patient accrual under hypotheses of unacceptable treatment characteristics (inadequate response, excessive toxicity, or both). In this context, *expected* refers to the average sample size that would turn out to have been used had a whole series of studies been conducted with the same design parameters in situations where the true activity, and true toxicity levels, remain constant.

In particular, suppose that the true response rate is indeed π_{R0} and the true non-toxicity rate is π_{T0}, then for the trial to proceed to Stage 2 both these response and toxicity criterion must be met.

In such a two-stage design, even if both $\pi_{\text{R}} \leq \pi_{\text{R0}}$ and $\pi_{\text{T}} \leq \pi_{\text{T0}}$ there is a possibility that the trial once conducted will go into the second stage if (by chance) many responses and few toxicities have been observed.

The probability of *not* moving to Stage 2 based on the response criterion is $B(C_{\text{R1}} - 1; \pi_{\text{R0}}, n_{\text{B-D1}})$, where $B(.)$ is the cumulative binomial distribution of Equation 2.9 with $R = C_{\text{R1}} - 1$, $\pi = \pi_{\text{R0}}$ and $m = n_{\text{B-D1}}$. Similarly, based on the toxicity criterion, the probability of *not* moving to Stage 2 is $B(C_{\text{T1}} - 1; \pi_{\text{T0}}, n_{\text{B-D1}})$. Thus if we assume response and toxicity are not associated within patients, that is they are statistically *independent*, then the overall probability that the trial does not proceed to Stage II is given by

$$P_{00} = P_{\text{Early}} = 1 - [1 - B(C_{\text{R1}} - 1; \pi_{\text{R0}}, n_{\text{B-D1}})] \times [1 - B(C_{\text{T1}} - 1; \pi_{\text{T0}}, n_{\text{B-D1}})]. \tag{16.28}$$

This independence is equivalent to assuming in Equation 16.27 that $\varphi = 1$.

The *expected* number of patients accrued given this situation is

$$N_{00} = N_{\text{Expected}} = n_{\text{B-D1}} + (1 - P_{00}) n_{\text{B-D2}}, \tag{16.29}$$

with similar expressions for N_{New0}, N_{0New} and $N_{\text{New,New}}$.

Now suppose that δ_{00} is the probability of recommending the treatment, then the probability of recommending the treatment based on the response criterion is:

$$\delta_{\text{R0}} = \sum_{y \geq C_{\text{R1}}} b(y; \pi_{\text{R0}}, n_{\text{B-D1}})[1 - B(C_{\text{R}} - 1 - y; \pi_{\text{RNew}}, N_{\text{B-D}} - n_{\text{B-D1}})], \tag{16.30}$$

where $b(y; \pi_{\text{R0}}, n_{\text{B-D1}})$ is Equation 2.8 with $r = y$, $\pi = \pi_{\text{R0}}$ and $m = n_{\text{B-D1}}$. Similarly for the toxicity criterion,

$$\delta_{\text{T0}} = \sum_{y \geq C_{\text{T1}}} b(y; \pi_{\text{T0}}, n_{\text{B-D1}})[1 - B(C_{\text{T}} - 1 - y; \pi_{\text{TNew}}, N_{\text{B-D}} - n_{\text{B-D1}})]. \tag{16.31}$$

Note that each of these expressions involve multiplying the probability that the trial proceeds to Stage II with the probability that the Stage II results eventually conclude 'success', that is a recommendation of the treatment. Thus the overall probability of recommending the treatment given that true response rate is π_{R0} and the true non-toxicity rate is π_{T0} is given by

$$\delta_{00} = \delta_{R0} \times \delta_{T0} \tag{16.32}$$

Similarly the corresponding values: $\delta_{New0} = \delta_{RNew} \times \delta_{T0}$, $\delta_{0New} = \delta_{R0} \times \delta_{TNew}$ and $\delta_{New,New} = \delta_{RNew} \times \delta_{TNew}$ are obtained.

The design then seeks the value of Q which minimises the maximum of $\{N_{0New}, N_{New0}\}$, subject to the conditions $\delta_{0New} \leq \alpha_R$, $\delta_{New0} \leq \alpha_T$ and $\delta_{New,New} \geq 1 - \beta$. This is done by a computer search of all the values of Q that satisfy the constraints and then choosing the appropriate one.

There is a corresponding set of (more complex) equations if the value of φ, of Equation 16.27, is not assumed equal to 1 and for which a similar such process can be conducted. However, assuming independence between response and toxicity, that is, $\varphi = 1$ gives designs which are close to optimal and so Bryant and Day (1995) recommend that this is adequate for general use and it is implemented in $^S\!S_S$.

16.3 Bibliography

Fleming (1982) and A'Hern (2001) provide further details of the single-stage design discussed. Gehan (1961) gives the theory and formulae for Equations 16.4 and 16.8 and corresponding tables. Simon (1989) describes two designs, one optimal for Stage I and the second to minimise the total recruitment from both stages. He provides tables for sample size and compares the two approaches. Tan, Machin, Tai *et al.* (2002) provide examples of two trials designed with the Simon–Minimax design, but reassessed using a Bayesian approach. Tan and Machin (2002) discuss the original versions of the Bayesian single and dual threshold designs and compare these with the Simon (1989) designs. Several other papers discuss the properties and expand on the ideas of Tan and Machin, including Mayo and Gajewski (2004), Tan, Wong and Machin (2004), Wang, Leung, Li *et al.* (2005) and Gajewski and Mayo (2006). Phase II designs with survival outcomes are discussed in detail by Case and Morgan (2003). Alternative designs for such endpoints have also been proposed by Mick, Crowley and Carroll (2000) as well as Cheung and Thall (2002), among others. As for the randomised designs as well as the designs looking at both response and toxicity, full details of these can be found in Simon, Wittes and Ellenberg (1985) and Bryant and Day (1995) respectively.

16.4 Examples and use of the tables

Table 16.1 Fleming–A'Hern
Example 16.1—sequential hormonal therapy in advanced and metastatic breast cancer
Iaffaioli, Formato, Tortoriello *et al.* (2005) used A'Hern's design for two Phase II studies of sequential hormonal therapy with first-line anastrozole (Study 1) and second-line exemestane (Study 2) in advanced and metastatic breast cancer.

For Study 1 they set $\alpha = 0.05$, $1 - \beta = 0.9$, $\pi_0 = 0.5$ and $\pi_{New} = 0.65$. With these inputs, $\boxed{SS}$ gives for the A'Hern design a sample size of 93, with 55 being the minimum number of responses required for a conclusion of 'efficacy'.

In the event 100 patients were recruited amongst whom eight complete responses and 19 partial responses were observed. These give an estimated response rate of 27% with 95% *CI* 19.3 to 36.4% calculated using Equation 2.14. This is much lower than the desired minimum of 65%.

For Study 2, the investigators set $\alpha = 0.05$, $1 - \beta = 0.9$, $\pi_0 = 0.2$ and $\pi_{New} = 0.4$, giving rise to a sample size of 47 with a minimum of 15 responses required.

In the event 50 patients were recruited amongst whom one complete response and three partial responses were observed. These give an estimated response rate of 8% (95% *CI* 3.2 to 18.8%). Again this is much lower than the desired minimum of 40%.

Tables 16.2 and 16.3 Gehan's design

Example 16.2—dexverapamil and epirubicin in non-responsive breast cancer
Lehnert, Mross, Schueller *et al.* (1998) used the Gehan design for a Phase II trial of the combination dexverapamil and epirubicin in patients with breast cancer. For Stage 1 they set $\pi_{New} = 0.2$ and $\beta = 0.05$, which corresponds to keeping the chance of rejecting a drug of efficacy at least 20% to below 0.05. This gives rise to a sample size of $n_{G1} = 14$. Using Equation 16.4 with $n_{G1} = 14$ and $\pi = 0.2$, gives the chance of rejecting the drug as 0.044. Of these 14 patients, $r_{G1} = 3$ responses were observed, then their requirement of $\gamma = 0.1$ implies a further $n_{G2} = 9$ patients were to be recruited.

Finally a total of four (17.4%) responses was observed from the $N_{Gehan} = n_{G1} + n_{G2} = 14 + 9 = 23$ patients. Using the 'recommended' method for calculating *CI*s of Equation 2.16 gives the corresponding 95% *CI* for π from 7 to 37%.

Table 16.4 Simon's Optimal and Minimax designs

Example 16.3—gemcitabine in metastatic nasopharyngeal carcinoma
In a trial of gemicitabine in previously untreated patients with metastatic nasopharyngeal carcinoma (NPC) Foo, Tan, Leong *et al.* (2002) utilised the Simon's Minimax design. The trial design assumed a desired overall response rate (complete and partial) of at least 30% and no further interest in gemicitabine if the response was as low as 10%.

Thus for $\alpha = 0.05$, $1 - \beta = 0.8$, $\pi_0 = 0.1$ and $\pi_{New} = 0.3$, $\boxed{SS}$ gives:
Stage 1 Sample size of 15 patients: if responses less than two, stop the trial and claim gemicitabine lacks efficacy.
Stage 2 Overall sample size of 25 patients for both stages, hence 10 more patients were to be recruited; if the total responses for the two stages combined is less than six, stop the trial as soon as this is evident and claim gemicitabine lacks efficacy.
Once the Phase II trial was conducted, the investigators observed $r_{S1} = 3$ and $r_{S2} = 4$ responses, giving $p = (3 + 4)/25$ or 28% (95% *CI* 14 to 48%).

Had the above trial been designed using the optimal design but with the same characteristics namely, $\alpha = 0.05$, $1 - \beta = 0.8$, $\pi_0 = 0.1$ and $\pi_{New} = 0.3$, then in $\boxed{SS}$ gives the following results:
Stage 1 Sample size of 10 patients: if responses less than two, stop the trial and claim gemicitabine lacks efficacy.

Stage 2 Overall sample size of 29 patients for both stages, hence 19 more patients to be recruited; if total responses for two stages combined is less than six, stop the trial as soon as this is evident and claim gemcitabine lacks efficacy.

In this case, for the same design parameters, the optimal design has 5 fewer patients in Stage 1 of the design, but 4 more patients if the trial goes on to complete Stage 2, than the corresponding minimax design. However, the number of responses to be observed are the same in each stage for both designs.

Example 16.4—paclitaxel for unresectable hepatocellular carcinoma

Chao, Chan, Birkhofer *et al.* (1998) state in their methods that a Simon (1989) design was used in which if the response rate was ≤ 3 of 19 in the first stage, then the trial would be terminated. The authors set $\alpha = 0.1$, $\beta = 0.1$ but did not specify π_0 or π_{New}. With a back calculation using $^S S_S$ it is possible to deduce that the minimax design was chosen with $\pi_0 = 0.2$, $\pi_{New} = 0.4$ and $n_{S1} = 19$.

In this trial zero responses were observed in Stage 1 and so Stage 2 was not implemented. This implies that the response rate π is estimated by $p = 0/17$ or 0% with 95% *CI* obtained from Equation 2.15 of 0 to $\dfrac{z^2_{1-\alpha/2}}{(n + z^2_{1-\alpha/2})} = \dfrac{1.96^2}{(19 + 1.96^2)} \approx \dfrac{4}{23}$ or approximately 0 to 17%. Thus even with an optimistic view of the true response rate as possibly close to 17% this is far below the expectations of the investigators who set $\pi_{New} = 0.4$ or 40%.

Tables 16.5 and 16.6 Bayesian STD and DTD

Example 16.5—combination therapy for nasopharyngeal cancer

A Phase II trial using a triplet combination of paclitaxel, carboplatin and gemcitabine in metastatic nasopharyngeal carcinoma was conducted by Leong, Tay, Toh *et al.* (2005).

The trial was expected to yield a minimum interest response rate of 80% and a no further interest response of 60%. The anticipated response rate was assumed to be equal to the minimum interest response rate and the overall threshold probability at the start and end of the trial was set to be 0.65 and 0.7 respectively. The sample size of the trial was calculated using the DTD.

Entering the no interest response rate $\pi_0 = 0.6$; minimum interest response rate $\pi_{New} = 0.8$; anticipated response rate $\pi_{Prior} = 0.8$; minimum desired threshold probability at the start of the trial $\lambda_1 = 0.65$; minimum desired threshold probability at the end of the trial $\lambda_2 = 0.7$, along with the default settings of $\varepsilon = 0.05$ and $n_{Prior} = 3$ (corresponding to a vague prior), $^S S_S$ gives the following design:

Stage 1 Sample size of 19 patients; if responses less than 15, stop the trial as soon as this becomes apparent and declare lack of efficacy. Otherwise complete Stage 1 and commence Stage 2.

Stage 2 Overall sample size of 32 patients for both stages, hence 13 Stage 2 patients to be recruited; if total responses for the two stages combined is less than 28, stop trial as soon as this becomes apparent and declare lack of efficacy. Otherwise complete the trial.

Had the investigators instead chosen the first STD design of **Table 16.5**, that is with $\pi_{Prior} = 0.1$ and $\pi_{New} = 0.3$; then the first row corresponding to, $\lambda_1 = 0.6$ and $\lambda_2 = 0.7$, suggests recruiting 5 patients to Stage 1 and if two or more responses are observed recruiting another

(24 − 5) = 19 patients. The corresponding DTD of **Table 16.6** for these same design specifications and $\pi_0 = 0.2$ suggests 15 patients for Stage 1 and 9 to Stage II to give the same total of 24. Only three responses would be sufficient to move into Stage II, but should such a low figure in practice occur, then all the 6 Stage II patients would have to respond to claim efficacy.

Tables 16.7 and 16.8 Case–Morgan EDA and ETSL designs

Example 16.6—gemcitabine and external beam radiotherapy for resectable pancreatic cancer
Case and Morgan (2003) consider the design of a Phase II trial of the effectiveness of adjuvant gemcitabine and external beam radiotherapy in the treatment of patients with resectable pancreatic cancer with null hypothesis that 1-year survival is 35% or less. They plan a 90% power at an alternative 1-year survival of 50%, for testing this hypothesis at 10% (one-sided) significance level.

In our notation, $T_{Summary} = 1, S_0(1) = 0.35, S_{New}(1) = 0.50$, from which $\lambda_0 = -\log 0.35 = 1.0498$ and if $S_{New}(1) = 0.5$ then $\lambda_{New} = -\log 0.5 = 0.6931$. Further $1 - \beta = 0.9$ and $\alpha = 0.1$. $\boxed{SS}$ begins by calculating the A'Hern single-stage sample size with design parameters set as $\pi_0 = S_0(1)$ and $\pi_{New} = S_{New}(1)$. This gives $N_{A'H} = 72$.

The investigators then decide on how long it would take to recruit this number of patients, and this is input into $\boxed{SS}$. We assume 3 years for this to be achieved, giving an accrual rate of 72/3 = 24 per year. Thus $D_{A'H} = 3$ and $T_{Summary} = 1$, so $R = D_{A'H}/T_{Summary} = 3$.

The *ETSL* design then suggests that Stage 1 recruits $n_{C-M1} = 54$, which will take 54/24 = 2.2 years. For Stage 2 $n_{C-M2} = 29$ patients, taking a further 29/24 = 1.2 years. Giving a total recruitment time of $D_{Accrual} = 2.2 + 1.2 = 3.4$ years. Thus the final analysis will occur 1 year later at 4.4 years.

With the *EDA* design the corresponding $n_{C-M1} = 46$, $n_{C-M2} = 79$, so $N_{C-M} = 79$ with a final analysis at (79/24) + 1 = 4.3 years post start of the trial.

Table 16.9 Simon–Wittes–Ellenberg design

Example 16.7—gemcitabine, vinorelbine or docetaxel for advanced non-small-cell lung cancer
Leong, Toh, Lim *et al.* (2007) conducted a randomised Phase II trial of single-agent gemcitabine, vinorelbine or docetaxel in the treatment of elderly and/or poor performance status patients with advanced non-small-cell lung cancer. The design was implemented with the probability of correctly selecting the best treatment assumed to be 90%. It was anticipated that the single-agent activity of each drug has a baseline response rate of approximately 20%. In order to detect a 15% superiority of the best treatment over the others, how many patients should be recruited per treatment for the trial?

For the difference in response rate $\delta = 0.15$, smallest response rate $\pi_{Worst} = 0.2$, probability of correct selection $P_{CS} = 0.90$ and treatment groups, $g = 3$, $\boxed{SS}$ gives a sample size of $m = 44$ per treatment group. Thus the total number of patients to be recruited is given as $N = 3 \times 44 = 132$. In the event, the trial proceeded to recruit 135 patients.

Example 16.8—non-Hodgkin's lymphoma
Itoh, Ohtsu, Fukuda *et al.* (2002) describe a randomised two-group Phase II trial comparing dose-escalated (DE) with biweekly (dose-intensified) CHOP (DI) in newly diagnosed patients with advanced-stage aggressive non-Hodgkin's lymphoma. Their design anticipated at least a

65% complete response rate (CR) in both groups. To achieve a 90% probability of selecting the better arm when the CR rate is 15% higher in one arm than the other, at least 30 patients would be required in each arm. [The more detailed tabulations of ^SS_S give 29 as opposed to 30.]

In the event, they recruited 35 patients to each arm and observed response rates with DE and DI of 51% and 60% respectively. Their follow on study, a randomised Phase III trial, compares DI CHOP with the Standard CHOP regimen.

Table 16.10 Bryant–Day design

Example 16.9—ifosfamide and vinorelbine in ovarian cancer

González-Martín, Crespo, García-López *et al.* (2002) used the Bryant and Day two-stage design with a cut-off point for the response rate of 10% and for severe toxicity, 25%. Severe toxicity was defined as grade 3–4 non-haematological toxicity, neutropenic fever or grade 4 thrombocytopenia. They do not provide full details of how the sample size was determined but their choice of design specified a Stage 1 of 14 patients and Stage 2 a further 20 patients. In the event, in these advanced platinum-resistant ovarian cancer patients, the combination of ifosfamide and vinorelbine was evidently very toxic. Hence the trial was closed after 12 patients with an observed toxicity level above the 25% contemplated.

In fact this corresponds to a design with $\alpha_R = \alpha_T = 0.1$, $\beta = 0.2$; $\pi_{R0} = 0.1$, $\pi_{RNew} = 0.3$; $\pi_{T0} = 0.25$ and $\pi_{TNew} = 0.45$. On this basis, the completed Stage 1 trial of 14 patients proceeds to Stage 2 if there are at least two responses *and* there are also 10 or fewer patients with high toxicity. The Stage 2 trial size is a further 20 patients, for a total of 34 for the whole trial, and sufficient efficacy with acceptable toxicity would be concluded if there were six or more responses observed *and* 22 or fewer with high toxicity.

Had they chosen instead the first design of **Table 16.10**, that is, $\alpha_R = \alpha_T = 0.1$, $\beta = 0.15$; $\pi_{R0} = 0.1$, $\pi_{RNew} = 0.3$; $\pi_{T0} = 0.6$ and $\pi_{TNew} = 0.8$, then Stage 1 consists of $n_{B-D1} = 19$ patients. The trial would proceed to Stage 2 if there are at least $C_{R1} = 2$ responses *and* there are also $C_{T1} = 12$ or fewer patients with high toxicity. The Stage 2 trial size is a further 21 patients, to a total of $N_{B-D} = 40$ for the whole trial, and sufficient efficacy with acceptable toxicity would be concluded if there were $C_R = 6$ or more responses observed *and* $C_T = 27$ or fewer with high toxicity.

16.5 References

A'Hern RP (2001). Sample size tables for exact single stage Phase II designs. *Statistics in Medicine*, **20**, 859–866.

Altman DG, Machin D, Bryant TN and Gardner MJ (eds) (2000). *Statistics with Confidence*, 2nd edn. British Medical Journal, London.

Bryant J and Day R (1995). Incorporating toxicity considerations into the design of two-stage Phase II clinical trials. *Biometrics*, **51**, 1372–1383.

Case LD and Morgan TM (2003). Design of Phase II cancer trials evaluating survival probabilities. *BMC Medical Research Methodology*, **3**, 6.

Chao Y, Chan W-K, Birkhofer MJ, Hu OY-P, Wang S-S, Huang Y-S, Liu M, Whang-Peng J, Chi K-H, Lui W-Y and Lee S-D (1998). Phase II and pharmacokinetic study of paclitaxel therapy for unresectable hepatocellular carcinoma patients. *British Journal of Cancer*, **78**, 34–39.

Cheung YK and Thall PF (2002). Monitoring the rates of composite events with censored data in Phase II clinical trials. *Biometrics*, **58**, 89–97.

Fleming TR (1982). One-sample multiple testing procedure for Phase II clinical trial. *Biometrics*, **38**, 143–151.

Foo K-F, Tan E-H, Leong S-S, Wee JTS, Tan T, Fong K-W, Koh L, Tai B-C, Lian L-G and Machin D (2002). Gemcitabine in metastatic nasopharyngeal carcinoma of the undifferentiated type. *Annals of Oncology*, **13**, 150–156.

Gajewski BJ and Mayo MS (2006). Bayesian sample size calculations in Phase II clinical trials using a mixture of informative priors. *Statistics in Medicine*, **25**, 2554–2566.

Gehan EA (1961). The determination of the number of patients required in a preliminary and follow-up trial of a new chemotherapeutic agent. *Journal of Chronic Diseases*, **13**, 346–353.

González-Martín A, Crespo C, García-López JL, Pedraza M, Garrido P, Lastra E and Moyano A (2002). Ifosfamide and vinorelbine in advanced platinum-resistant ovarian cancer: excessive toxicity with a potentially active regimen. *Gynecologic Oncology*, **84**, 368–373.

Iaffaioli RV, Formato R, Tortoriello A, Del Prete S, Caraglia M, Pappagallo G, Pisano A, Fanelli F, Ianniello G, Cigolari S, Pizza C, Marano O, Pezzella G, Pedicini T, Febbraro A, Incoronato P, Manzione L, Ferrari E, Marzano N, Quattrin S, Pisconti S, Nasti G, Giotta G, Colucci G and other Goim authors (2005). Phase II study of sequential hormonal therapy with anastrozole/exemestane in advanced and metastatic breast cancer. *British Journal of Cancer*, **92**, 1621–1625.

Itoh K, Ohtsu T, Fukuda H, Sasaki Y, Ogura M, Morishima Y, Chou T, Aikawa K, Uike N, Mizorogi F, Ohno T, Ikeda S, Sai T, Taniwaki M, Kawano F, Niimi M, Hotta T, Shimoyama M and Tobinai K (2002). Randomized phase II study of biweekly CHOP and dose-escalated CHOP with prophylactic use of lenograstim (glycosylated G-CSF) in aggressive non-Hodgkin's lymphoma: Japan Clinical Oncology Group Study 9505. *Annals of Oncology*, **13**, 1347–1355.

Lehnert M, Mross K, Schueller J, Thuerlimann B, Kroeger N and Kupper H (1998). Phase II trial of dexverapamil and epirubicin in patients with non-responsive metastatic breast cancer. *British Journal of Cancer*, **77**, 1155–1163.

Leong SS, Tay MH, Toh CK, Tan SB, Thng CH, Foo KF, Wee JTS, Lim D, See HT, Tan T, Fong KW and Tan EH (2005). Paclitaxel, carboplatin and gemcitabine in metastatic nasopharyngeal carcinoma: A Phase II trial using a triplet combination. *Cancer*, **103**, 569–575.

Leong SS, Toh CK, Lim WT, Lin X, Tan SB, Poon D, Tay MH, Foo KF, Ho J and Tan EH (2007). A randomized phase II trial of single agent gemcitabine, vinorelbine or docetaxel in patients with advanced non-small cell lung cancer who have poor performance status and/or are elderly. *Journal of Thoracic Oncology*, **2**, 230–236.

Liu PY (2001). Phase II selection designs. In: Crowley J (ed) *Handbook of Statistics in Clinical Oncology*, Marcel Dekker, New York, pp. 119–127.

Machin D and Campbell MJ (2005). *Design of Studies for Medical Research*. John Wiley & Sons, Chichester.

Mayo MS and Gajewski BJ (2004). Bayesian sample size calculations in Phase II clinical trials using informative conjugate priors. *Controlled Clinical Trials*, **25**, 157–167.

Mick R, Crowley JJ and Carroll RJ (2000). Phase II clinical trial design for noncytotoxic anticancer agents for which time to disease progression is the primary endpoint. *Controlled Clinical Trials*, **21**, 343–359.

Simon R (1989). Optimal two-stage designs for Phase II clinical trials. *Controlled Clinical Trials*, **10**, 1–14.

Simon R, Wittes RE and Ellenberg SS (1985). Randomized Phase II clinical trials. *Cancer Treatment Reports*, **69**, 1375–1381.

Tan SB and Machin D (2002). Bayesian two-stage designs for Phase II clinical trials. *Statistics in Medicine*, **21**, 1991–2012.

Tan SB, Machin D, Tai BC, Foo KF and Tan EH (2002). A Bayesian re-assessment of two Phase II trials of gemcitabine in metastatic nasopharyngeal cancer. *British Journal of Cancer* **86**, 843–850.

Tan SB, Wong EH and Machin D (2004). Bayesian two-stage design for Phase II clinical trials. In *Encyclopedia of Biopharmaceutical Statistics*, 2nd edn (online) (Chow SC, ed.), http://www.dekker.com/servlet/product/DOI/101081EEBS120023507. Marcel Dekker, New York.

Wang YG, Leung DHY, Li M and Tan SB (2005). Bayesian designs for frequentist and Bayesian error rate considerations. *Statistical Methods in Medical Research*, **14**, 445–456.

Table 16.1 Fleming–A'Hern single-stage Phase II design. Sample size and minimum number of successes required to conclude that the drug is effective.

π_0	π_{New}	α			
		0.05		**0.01**	
		$1 - \beta$		$1 - \beta$	
		0.8	**0.9**	**0.8**	**0.9**
0.10	0.25	8 / 40	10 / 55	13 / 62	15 / 78
	0.30	6 / 25	7 / 33	9 / 37	11 / 49
	0.35	5 / 18	6 / 25	7 / 25	9 / 35
	0.40	4 / 13	5 / 18	6 / 19	7 / 24
	0.45	4 / 11	4 / 13	5 / 14	6 / 19
	0.50	3 / 8	4 / 12	5 / 12	5 / 14
	0.55	3 / 7	3 / 8	4 / 9	5 / 13
	0.60	3 / 6	3 / 7	4 / 8	4 / 9
0.20	0.35	17 / 56	22 / 77	27 / 87	34 / 115
	0.40	12 / 35	15 / 47	18 / 52	22 / 67
	0.45	8 / 21	10 / 29	14 / 36	16 / 44
	0.50	7 / 17	8 / 21	11 / 26	13 / 33
	0.55	6 / 13	7 / 17	9 / 19	10 / 23
	0.60	5 / 10	6 / 13	8 / 16	9 / 19
	0.65	4 / 7	5 / 10	7 / 13	8 / 16
	0.70	4 / 7	5 / 9	6 / 10	7 / 13
0.30	0.45	27 / 67	36 / 93	43 / 104	53 / 133
	0.50	17 / 39	22 / 53	27 / 60	34 / 79
	0.55	12 / 25	16 / 36	20 / 41	25 / 53
	0.60	9 / 17	12 / 25	14 / 26	18 / 36
	0.65	8 / 14	9 / 17	12 / 21	14 / 26
	0.70	6 / 10	8 / 14	10 / 16	12 / 21
0.40	0.55	36 / 71	46 / 94	58 / 113	72 / 144
	0.60	23 / 42	29 / 56	35 / 63	45 / 84
	0.65	16 / 28	19 / 34	25 / 42	31 / 54
	0.70	12 / 19	15 / 25	18 / 28	22 / 36
	0.75	10 / 15	12 / 19	15 / 22	17 / 26
	0.80	8 / 11	9 / 13	11 / 15	14 / 20
0.50	0.65	42 / 69	55 / 93	69 / 112	86 / 143
	0.70	24 / 37	33 / 53	42 / 64	51 / 80
	0.75	16 / 23	22 / 33	28 / 40	34 / 50
	0.80	13 / 18	16 / 23	20 / 27	25 / 35
	0.85	10 / 13	12 / 16	15 / 19	17 / 22
	0.90	7 / 8	9 / 11	12 / 14	14 / 17
0.60	0.75	44 / 62	59 / 85	74 / 103	92 / 131
	0.80	27 / 36	33 / 45	42 / 55	52 / 70
	0.85	17 / 21	21 / 27	26 / 32	33 / 42
	0.90	12 / 14	14 / 17	19 / 22	21 / 25
0.70	0.85	40 / 49	55 / 69	65 / 79	84 / 104
	0.90	24 / 28	31 / 37	38 / 44	45 / 53

Table 16.2 Gehan two-stage Phase II design—Stage 1. The initial sample size n_{G1} required for anticipated therapeutic effectiveness π_{New} for Stage 1 rejection error, η.

	η	
π_{New}	0.10	0.05
0.05	45	59
0.06	38	49
0.07	32	42
0.08	28	36
0.09	25	32
0.10	22	29
0.11	20	26
0.12	19	24
0.13	17	22
0.14	16	20
0.15	15	19
0.16	14	18
0.17	13	17
0.18	12	16
0.19	11	15
0.20	11	14
0.25	9	11
0.30	7	9
0.35	6	7
0.40	5	6
0.45	4	6
0.50	4	5
0.60	3	4
0.70	2	3
0.80	2	2
0.90	2	2

Table 16.3 Gehan two-stage Phase II design—Stage 2. The number of additional patients n_{G2} required in Stage 2, for anticipated therapeutic effectiveness π_{New}, for required standard error γ, Stage I rejection error η, and the number of responses in Stage 1 ranging from 1 to 6.

Therapeutic efficacy	Number of patients Stage 1	Number of responses in Stage 1, r_{G1}					
π_{New}	n_{G1}	1	2	3	4	5	6
$\gamma = 0.1$, $1 - \eta = 0.90$							
0.10	22	0	0	0	0	0	2
0.12	19	0	0	0	3	5	6
0.14	16	0	2	5	8	9	9
0.16	14	1	6	9	11	11	11
0.18	12	5	10	12	13	13	12
0.20	11	7	11	14	14	14	11
0.30	7	16	18	17	12	5	–
0.40	5	20	19	11	1	–	–
0.50	4	21	15	3	–	–	–
0.60	3	19	6	–	–	–	–
0.70	2	10	–	–	–	–	–
0.80	2	10	–	–	–	–	–
$\gamma = 0.1$, $1 - \eta = 0.95$							
0.10	29	0	0	0	0	0	0
0.12	24	0	0	0	0	0	0
0.14	20	0	0	0	1	3	4
0.16	18	0	0	2	4	6	7
0.18	16	0	2	5	8	9	9
0.20	14	1	6	9	11	11	11
0.30	9	11	15	16	15	12	7
0.40	6	18	19	15	8	–	–
0.50	5	20	19	11	1	–	–
0.60	4	21	15	3	–	–	–
0.70	3	19	6	–	–	–	–
0.80	2	10	–	–	–	–	–

Table 16.4 Simon Optimal and Minimax designs. The denominators in the table give the size of Stage 1, n_{S1}, and the total sample size, N_{Simon}, for circumstances when Stage 2 is necessary. The numerators give the minimum number of successes required, R_{S1}, to move to Stage 2 and to conclude that the drug is effective, R.

$\alpha = 0.05$			Optimal		Minimax	
π_0	π_{New}	$1 - \beta$	Stage 1	Overall	Stage 1	Overall
$\pi_{New} - \pi_0 = 0.15$			R_{S1}/n_{S1}	R/N_{Simon}	R_{S1}/n_{S1}	R/N_{Simon}
0.05	0.20	0.8	1 / 10	4 / 29	1 / 13	4 / 27
		0.9	2 / 21	5 / 41	2 / 29	5 / 38
0.10	0.25	0.8	3 / 18	8 / 43	3 / 22	8 / 40
		0.9	3 / 21	11 / 66	4 / 31	10 / 55
0.20	0.35	0.8	6 / 22	20 / 72	7 / 31	16 / 53
		0.9	9 / 37	23 / 83	9 / 42	22 / 77
0.30	0.45	0.8	10 / 27	31 / 81	17 / 46	26 / 65
		0.9	14 / 40	41 / 110	28 / 77	34 / 88
0.40	0.55	0.8	12 / 26	41 / 84	29 / 59	35 / 70
		0.9	20 / 45	50 / 104	25 / 62	46 / 94
0.50	0.65	0.8	16 / 28	49 / 83	40 / 66	41 / 68
		0.9	23 / 42	61 / 105	29 / 57	55 / 93
0.60	0.75	0.8	18 / 27	47 / 67	19 / 30	44 / 62
		0.9	22 / 34	65 / 95	49 / 72	58 / 84
0.70	0.85	0.8	15 / 19	47 / 59	17 / 23	40 / 49
		0.9	19 / 25	62 / 79	34 / 44	54 / 68
0.80	0.95	0.8	8 / 9	27 / 29	8 / 9	27 / 29
		0.9	17 / 19	38 / 42	32 / 35	36 / 40
$\pi_{New} - \pi_0 = 0.20$						
0.05	0.25	0.8	1 / 9	3 / 17	1 / 12	3 / 16
		0.9	1 / 9	4 / 30	1 / 15	4 / 25
0.10	0.30	0.8	2 / 10	6 / 29	2 / 15	6 / 25
		0.9	3 / 18	7 / 35	3 / 22	7 / 33
0.20	0.40	0.8	4 / 13	13 / 43	5 / 18	11 / 33
		0.9	5 / 19	16 / 54	6 / 24	14 / 45
0.30	0.50	0.8	6 / 15	19 / 46	7 / 19	17 / 39
		0.9	9 / 24	25 / 63	8 / 24	22 / 53
0.40	0.60	0.8	8 / 16	24 / 46	18 / 34	21 / 39
		0.9	12 / /25	33 / 66	13 / 29	28 / 54
0.50	0.70	0.8	9 / 15	27 / 43	13 / 23	24 / 37
		0.9	14 / 24	37 / 61	15 / 27	33 / 53
0.60	0.80	0.8	8 / 11	31 / 43	9 / 13	26 / 35
		0.9	13 / 19	38 / 53	16 / 26	33 / 45
0.70	0.90	0.8	5 / 6	23 / 27	20 / 23	22 / 26
		0.9	12 / 15	30 / 36	14 / 18	27 / 32

Table 16.5 Bayesian single threshold design (STD). Sample sizes and cut-off values for Stage 1 and overall trial size for π_{Prior} and π_{New}. The two rows correspond to designs for the pairs (λ_1, λ_2) of (0.6, 0.7) and (0.6, 0.8) respectively. A implies designs for which $N_{T\text{-}M} < 2$; and B those with $N_{T\text{-}M} \geq 2$ but $n_{T\text{-}M1} < 1$, and C those with $N_{T\text{-}M} > 90$ or $n_{T\text{-}M1} > 89$. The denominators in the table give the size of Stage 1, $n_{T\text{-}M1}$, and the total sample size, $N_{T\text{-}M}$, for circumstances when Stage 2 is necessary. The numerators give the minimum number of successes required to move to Stage 2, $R_{T\text{-}M1}$, and to conclude that the drug is effective, $R_{T\text{-}M}$.

π_{Prior}	0.1		0.3		0.5		0.7		0.9	
π_{New}	Stage 1	Overall	Stage 1	Overall	Stage 1	Overall	Stage 1	Overall	Stage 1	Overall
0.30	2/5	9/24	B		A		A		A	
	2/5	22/61	B		B		A		A	
0.35	4/10	12/30	1/2	9/22	B		A		A	
	4/10	28/70	1/2	25/62	B		B		A	
0.40	7/14	16/35	4/7	13/28	B		A		A	
	7/14	36/78	4/7	32/70	B		B		B	
0.45	9/17	20/40	6/11	17/33	2/4	13/25	B		A	
	9/17	42/84	6/11	38/76	2/4	34/68	B		B	
0.50	11/20	25/44	9/15	21/37	5/9	17/30	B		B	
	11/20	49/88	9/15	45/81	5/9	41/73	B		B	
0.55	14/23	29/47	11/18	25/41	8/12	21/34	4/6	16/26	B	
	C		11/18	51/84	8/12	47/77	4/6	42/69	B	
0.60	17/26	33/50	14/21	29/44	10/15	25/37	6/9	20/30	2/2	15/22
	C		14/21	56/86	10/15	51/78	6/9	47/71	2/2	41/63
0.65	21/29	37/52	17/24	33/46	13/18	28/39	10/13	23/32	5/6	18/25
	C		17/24	61/86	13/18	56/79	10/13	50/71	5/6	45/64
0.70	24/31	40/53	20/26	36/47	16/21	31/41	12/15	26/34	8/10	21/27
	C		20/26	63/84	16/21	58/77	12/15	53/70	8/10	48/63
0.75	27/33	43/53	23/28	39/48	19/23	34/42	15/18	28/35	10/12	24/29
	27/33	71/88	23/28	65/81	19/23	60/75	15/18	55/68	10/12	48/60
0.80	30/35	46/53	26/30	40/47	22/25	35/41	17/20	31/36	13/15	25/29
	30/35	71/83	26/30	66/77	22/25	60/70	17/20	54/63	13/15	48/56
0.85	33/36	46/51	28/31	42/46	24/26	36/40	19/21	32/35	15/16	27/29
	33/36	69/76	28/31	63/70	24/26	58/64	19/21	52/57	15/16	45/50
0.90	35/36	47/49	31/32	42/44	26/27	37/38	22/23	32/33	18/18	26/27
	35/36	64/67	31/32	58/61	26/27	53/55	22/23	47/49	18/18	41/43
0.95	36/36	44/44	32/32	39/39	27/27	34/34	23/23	30/30	19/19	25/25
	36/36	55/55	32/32	49/49	27/27	44/44	23/23	38/38	19/19	33/33

Table 16.6 Bayesian dual threshold design (DTD). Sample sizes and cut-off values for Stage 1 and overall trial size for π_{Prior} and π_0. The two rows correspond to designs for the pairs (λ_1, λ_2) of (0.6, 0.7) and (0.6, 0.8) respectively. A implies designs for which $N_{T-M} < 2$; B those with $N_{T-M} \geq 2$ but $n_{T-M1} < 1$; and C those with $N_{T-M} > 90$ or $n_{T-M1} > 89$. The denominators in the table give the size of Stage 1, n_{T-M1}, and the total sample size, N_{T-M}, for circumstances when Stage 2 is necessary. The numerators give the minimum number of successes required to move to Stage 2, R_{T-M1}, and to conclude that the drug is effective, R_{T-M}.

π_0	π_{New}	π_{Prior} 0.1 Stage 1 n_{T-M1}	Overall N_{T-M}	0.3 Stage 1 n_{T-M1}	Overall N_{T-M}	0.5 Stage 1 n_{T-M1}	Overall N_{T-M}	0.7 Stage 1 n_{T-M1}	Overall N_{T-M}	0.9 Stage 1 n_{T-M1}	Overall N_{T-M}
0.1	0.2	4/18	5/19	5/23	6/24	6/27	7/28	6/32	7/33	7/36	8/37
		1/18	10/38	2/23	8/29	6/27	7/28	7/32	8/33	8/36	9/37
0.2	0.3	3/15	9/24	7/20	9/21	8/25	9/26	10/30	11/31	11/35	12/36
		3/15	22/61	4/20	19/53	4/25	16/44	8/30	12/34	12/35	13/36
0.3	0.4	3/10	16/35	4/15	13/28	9/21	10/22	11/26	12/27	13/31	14/32
		3/10	36/78	4/15	32/70	6/21	28/62	7/26	24/53	8/31	20/44
0.4	0.5	1/2	25/44	4/9	21/37	6/15	17/30	12/21	13/22	14/26	15/27
		1/2	49/88	4/9	45/81	6/15	41/73	8/21	36/65	10/26	32/57
0.5	0.6	B		B		5/9	25/37	7/15	20/30	13/20	15/22
		C		B		5/9	51/78	7/15	47/71	10/20	41/63
0.6	0.7	B		B		B		4/7	26/34	8/14	21/27
		C		B		B		4/7	53/70	8/14	48/63
0.7	0.8	B		B		B		B		4/5	25/29
		B		B		B		B		4/5	48/56
0.1	0.25	5/18	6/19	6/23	7/24	7/27	8/28	8/32	9/33	9/36	10/37
		1/18	16/51	2/23	13/42	5/27	10/32	9/32	10/33	10/36	11/37
0.2	0.35	3/15	12/30	7/20	9/22	10/25	11/26	11/30	12/31	13/35	14/36
		3/15	28/70	4/20	25/62	4/25	22/54	5/30	18/45	14/35	15/36
0.3	0.45	3/10	20/40	4/15	17/33	9/21	13/25	13/26	14/27	15/31	16/32
		3/10	42/84	4/15	38/76	6/21	34/68	7/26	30/60	8/31	26/51
0.4	0.55	1/2	29/47	4/9	25/41	6/15	21/34	11/21	16/26	15/26	16/27
		C		4/9	51/84	6/15	47/77	8/21	42/69	10/26	37/61
0.5	0.65	B		B		5/9	28/39	7/15	23/32	13/20	18/25
		C		B		5/9	56/79	7/15	50/71	10/20	45/64
0.6	0.75	B		B		B		4/7	28/35	9/14	24/29
		B		B		B		4/7	55/68	8/14	48/60
0.7	0.85	B		B		B		B		4/5	27/29
		B		B		B		B		4/5	45/50
0.1	0.3	3/18	9/24	8/23	9/24	9/27	10/28	10/32	11/33	11/36	12/37
		1/18	22/61	2/23	19/53	2/27	16/44	10/32	12/34	12/36	13/37
0.2	0.4	3/15	16/35	5/20	13/28	11/25	12/26	13/30	14/31	15/35	16/36
		3/15	36/78	4/20	32/70	4/25	28/62	5/30	24/53	11/35	20/44
0.3	0.5	3/10	25/44	4/15	21/37	8/21	17/30	14/26	15/27	17/31	18/32
		3/10	49/88	4/15	45/81	6/21	41/73	7/26	36/65	8/31	32/57
0.4	0.6	1/2	35/50	4/9	29/44	6/15	25/37	11/21	20/30	17/26	18/27
		C		4/9	56/86	6/15	51/78	8/21	47/71	10/26	41/63
0.5	0.7	B		B		5/9	31/41	7/15	26/34	14/20	21/27
		C		B		5/9	58/77	7/15	53/70	10/20	48/63
0.6	0.8	B		B		B		4/7	31/36	10/14	25/29
		B		B		B		4/7	54/63	8/14	48/56
0.7	0.9	B		B		B		B		4/5	26/27
		B		B		B		B		4/5	41/43

Table 16.7 Case and Morgan EDA design with $\alpha = 0.05$. n_{C-M1} gives the size of Stage 1, C_1 the threshold to move to Stage 2, N_{C-M} the total sample size and C_2 the threshold for efficacy, if Stage 2 is initiated.

$S_0(T)$	$S_A(T)$	R	Power $1 - \beta = 0.8$				Power $1 - \beta = 0.9$			
			C_1	C_2	n_{C-M1}	N_{C-M}	C_1	C_2	n_{C-M1}	N_{C-M}
0.30	0.45	2	0.166	1.567	46	75	0.082	1.590	65	102
		2.5	0.264	1.554	42	77	0.188	1.581	60	103
		3	0.322	1.544	39	78	0.252	1.574	57	105
	0.50	2	0.177	1.565	27	44	0.082	1.590	37	58
		2.5	0.270	1.552	24	45	0.193	1.579	34	59
		3	0.315	1.545	23	45	0.250	1.573	33	60
0.35	0.50	2	0.177	1.567	46	76	0.088	1.591	67	105
		2.5	0.270	1.553	42	78	0.192	1.580	62	107
		3	0.328	1.544	40	79	0.249	1.574	58	108
	0.55	2	0.188	1.564	28	46	0.097	1.590	37	58
		2.5	0.274	1.552	26	47	0.208	1.578	34	59
		3	0.330	1.543	24	48	0.252	1.574	33	60
0.40	0.55	2	0.180	1.567	48	80	0.094	1.591	66	103
		2.5	0.268	1.554	44	81	0.202	1.580	61	105
		3	0.318	1.547	41	82	0.249	1.574	57	106
	0.60	2	0.188	1.565	29	47	0.091	1.590	39	61
		2.5	0.286	1.550	26	48	0.217	1.577	36	63
		3	0.331	1.542	24	49	0.262	1.573	34	63
0.45	0.60	2	0.195	1.565	47	79	0.097	1.591	68	107
		2.5	0.280	1.553	43	80	0.211	1.579	63	110
		3	0.322	1.545	40	81	0.256	1.574	59	110
	0.65	2	0.185	1.567	29	47	0.108	1.590	38	59
		2.5	0.280	1.552	26	48	0.211	1.579	35	60
		3	0.331	1.544	24	49	0.262	1.573	33	61
0.50	0.65	2	0.192	1.567	47	77	0.105	1.590	65	102
		2.5	0.278	1.553	42	79	0.211	1.579	60	104
		3	0.322	1.546	40	80	0.256	1.574	56	105
	0.70	2	0.208	1.562	25	42	0.123	1.588	37	58
		2.5	0.289	1.550	23	43	0.209	1.579	34	59
		3	0.325	1.545	21	43	0.264	1.572	32	60
0.55	0.70	2	0.204	1.565	47	79	0.108	1.591	64	101
		2.5	0.292	1.552	43	80	0.224	1.578	59	103
		3	0.331	1.546	40	81	0.268	1.573	56	104
	0.75	2	0.205	1.564	25	42	0.117	1.589	35	55
		2.5	0.287	1.551	23	43	0.212	1.578	32	56
		3	0.346	1.541	22	43	0.256	1.574	30	57
0.60	0.75	2	0.201	1.567	42	70	0.126	1.589	59	94
		2.5	0.297	1.551	38	71	0.209	1.581	54	95
		3	0.331	1.546	36	72	0.265	1.574	51	96
	0.80	2	0.208	1.564	24	41	0.129	1.588	32	50
		2.5	0.293	1.552	22	42	0.220	1.579	29	50
		3	0.340	1.543	21	42	0.272	1.572	27	51
0.65	0.80	2	0.209	1.565	37	62	0.126	1.589	52	82
		2.5	0.296	1.552	34	63	0.218	1.579	48	84
		3	0.335	1.544	32	64	0.277	1.572	45	85
	0.85	2	0.211	1.565	21	35	0.126	1.589	29	46
		2.5	0.284	1.553	19	36	0.205	1.580	27	47
		3	0.346	1.542	18	36	0.271	1.573	26	48

Table 16.8 Case and Morgan ETSL design with $\alpha = 0.05$. n_{C-M1} gives the size of Stage 1, C_1 the threshold to move to Stage 2, N_{C-M} the total sample size and C_2 the threshold for efficacy, if Stage 2 is initiated.

$S_0(T)$	$S_A(T)$	R	Power $1 - \beta = 0.8$				Power $1 - \beta = 0.9$			
			C_1	C_2	n_{C-M1}	N_{C-M}	C_1	C_2	n_{C-M1}	N_{C-M}
0.3	0.45	2	0.662	1.485	53	83	0.639	1.520	77	111
		2.5	0.634	1.490	48	83	0.611	1.525	70	111
		3	0.606	1.494	44	83	0.577	1.532	65	110
	0.50	2	0.667	1.482	31	48	0.634	1.521	44	63
		2.5	0.631	1.490	28	48	0.614	1.522	40	64
		3	0.617	1.492	26	48	0.583	1.528	37	63
0.35	0.5	2	0.664	1.486	54	84	0.637	1.522	79	115
		2.5	0.634	1.490	48	84	0.608	1.525	72	115
		3	0.609	1.497	45	84	0.591	1.529	67	114
	0.55	2	0.667	1.482	33	51	0.643	1.520	44	63
		2.5	0.634	1.490	29	51	0.605	1.526	40	63
		3	0.611	1.493	27	51	0.592	1.527	37	63
0.40	0.55	2	0.669	1.484	56	88	0.645	1.520	78	113
		2.5	0.639	1.491	50	88	0.604	1.528	70	112
		3	0.614	1.495	47	88	0.584	1.531	65	112
	0.60	2	0.671	1.484	33	52	0.646	1.520	46	67
		2.5	0.639	1.489	30	52	0.602	1.528	42	67
		3	0.621	1.492	28	52	0.584	1.531	39	67
0.45	0.60	2	0.669	1.484	55	87	0.649	1.522	81	117
		2.5	0.642	1.491	50	87	0.609	1.527	73	117
		3	0.615	1.494	46	87	0.589	1.530	68	117
	0.65	2	0.674	1.484	33	52	0.642	1.521	45	65
		2.5	0.644	1.487	30	52	0.611	1.526	40	65
		3	0.618	1.494	28	52	0.587	1.529	37	65
0.50	0.65	2	0.673	1.485	54	86	0.650	1.522	77	111
		2.5	0.639	1.491	49	85	0.618	1.525	69	111
		3	0.617	1.495	45	85	0.592	1.530	64	111
	0.70	2	0.675	1.483	29	46	0.653	1.520	44	63
		2.5	0.646	1.488	26	46	0.611	1.527	39	63
		3	0.628	1.491	24	46	0.589	1.530	37	63
0.55	0.70	2	0.672	1.487	55	87	0.650	1.522	75	110
		2.5	0.640	1.491	49	87	0.615	1.527	68	110
		3	0.616	1.495	46	86	0.596	1.529	64	110
	0.75	2	0.679	1.483	29	46	0.656	1.519	41	60
		2.5	0.639	1.491	26	46	0.620	1.524	37	60
		3	0.625	1.492	24	46	0.589	1.530	35	60
0.60	0.75	2	0.677	1.485	48	77	0.652	1.521	70	102
		2.5	0.645	1.490	44	77	0.618	1.528	63	101
		3	0.621	1.494	40	77	0.592	1.531	59	101
	0.80	2	0.683	1.482	28	45	0.650	1.522	37	54
		2.5	0.642	1.490	25	45	0.617	1.526	34	54
		3	0.623	1.494	24	45	0.593	1.530	31	54
0.65	0.80	2	0.680	1.484	43	68	0.656	1.521	61	90
		2.5	0.645	1.492	39	68	0.618	1.526	55	90
		3	0.625	1.493	36	68	0.592	1.530	52	90
	0.85	2	0.687	1.481	24	39	0.655	1.521	35	50
		2.5	0.644	1.490	22	39	0.620	1.526	31	50
		3	0.625	1.493	20	39	0.594	1.530	29	50

Table 16.9 Simon, Wittes and Ellenberg design. For the probability of correctly selecting the best treatment $P_{CS} = 0.9$, the table gives the number of patients m in each group required to identify the best drug under investigation for the number of treatments g, the worst response rate π_{Worst} and difference in the superior response rate δ.

Smallest response rate, π_{Worst}	$\delta = 0.1$, $P_{CS} = 0.9$				
	Number of treatments, g				
	2	3	4	5	6
0.10	42	62	74	83	90
0.15	53	79	95	106	115
0.20	62	93	111	125	136
0.25	69	104	125	141	153
0.30	75	113	136	153	166
0.35	79	119	144	162	175
0.40	82	123	149	167	181
0.45	82	124	150	169	183
0.50	82	123	149	167	182
0.55	79	120	145	162	177
0.60	75	113	137	154	168
0.65	69	105	127	142	155
0.70	62	94	113	127	138
0.75	53	80	97	109	118
0.80	42	63	77	86	94
0.85	29	44	53	60	65

	$\delta = 0.15$, $P_{CS} = 0.9$				
0.10	21	31	37	41	45
0.15	26	38	45	51	55
0.20	29	44	52	59	64
0.25	32	48	58	65	71
0.30	35	52	62	70	76
0.35	36	54	65	73	79
0.40	37	55	67	75	81
0.45	37	55	67	75	81
0.50	36	54	65	73	80
0.55	35	52	63	71	77
0.60	32	49	59	66	72
0.65	29	44	53	60	65
0.70	26	39	47	53	57
0.75	21	32	38	43	47
0.80	16	24	29	32	35

Table 16.9 (*continued*): Simon, Wittes and Ellenberg design. For the probability of correctly selecting the best treatment $P_{CS} = 0.9$, the table gives the number of patients m in each group required to identify the best drug under investigation for the number of treatments g, the worst response rate π_{Worst} and the superior difference in response rate δ.

$\delta = 0.2, P_{CS} = 0.9$

Smallest response rate, π_{Worst}	Number of treatments, g				
	2	3	4	5	6
0.10	13	19	23	25	27
0.15	16	23	27	31	33
0.20	18	26	31	35	38
0.25	19	28	34	38	41
0.30	20	30	36	40	44
0.35	21	31	37	42	45
0.40	21	31	38	42	46
0.45	21	31	37	42	45
0.50	20	30	36	41	44
0.55	19	28	34	39	42
0.60	18	26	32	36	39
0.65	16	23	28	32	34
0.70	13	20	24	27	29
0.75	11	16	19	21	23

$\delta = 0.25, P_{CS} = 0.9$

	2	3	4	5	6
0.10	9	13	16	18	19
0.15	11	16	19	21	22
0.20	12	17	21	23	25
0.25	13	19	22	25	27
0.30	13	19	23	26	28
0.35	13	20	24	27	29
0.40	13	20	24	27	29
0.45	13	20	24	26	29
0.50	13	19	23	25	28
0.55	12	18	21	24	26
0.60	11	16	19	22	23
0.65	9	14	17	19	20
0.70	8	11	13	15	16

Table 16.10 Bryant and Day design. Sample sizes and rejection criteria for π_{R0}, π_{RNew}, π_{T0}, π_{TNew} with odds ratio, $\phi = 1$. $n_{B\text{-}D1}$ is the number of Stage 1 patients and $N_{B\text{-}D}$ is the total to be accrued to both stages. At the end of Stage 1, the treatment will be rejected if the number of positive responses is $< C_{R1}$ or when the number who do not experience toxicity is C_{T1}. At the end of Stage 2, the treatment will be rejected if the number of responses is $< C_R$ or the number who do not experience toxicity is C_T.

π_{R0}	π_{RNew}	π_{T0}	π_{TNew}	$n_{B\text{-}D1}$	C_{R1}	C_{T1}	$N_{B\text{-}D}$	C_R	C_T
				$\alpha_R = 0.10$; $\alpha_T = 0.10$; $\beta = 0.15$					
0.1	0.3	0.60	0.80	19	3	13	40	7	28
0.2	0.4	0.60	0.80	20	5	13	41	12	29
0.3	0.5	0.60	0.80	20	7	13	43	17	30
0.4	0.6	0.60	0.80	20	9	13	46	23	32
0.5	0.7	0.60	0.80	17	9	11	43	26	30
0.6	0.8	0.60	0.80	18	12	12	43	30	30
0.1	0.3	0.75	0.95	9	1	7	25	5	22
0.2	0.4	0.75	0.95	18	5	15	34	10	29
0.3	0.5	0.75	0.95	19	7	16	37	15	31
0.4	0.6	0.75	0.95	14	6	11	37	19	32
0.5	0.7	0.75	0.95	16	9	13	39	24	34
0.6	0.8	0.75	0.95	13	9	11	37	26	31
				$\alpha_R = 0.10$; $\alpha_T = 0.10$; $\beta = 0.10$					
0.1	0.3	0.60	0.80	21	3	14	46	8	32
0.2	0.4	0.60	0.80	24	6	16	54	15	37
0.3	0.5	0.60	0.80	23	8	15	57	22	39
0.4	0.6	0.60	0.80	25	11	16	53	26	37
0.5	0.7	0.60	0.80	22	12	14	52	31	36
0.6	0.8	0.60	0.80	20	13	13	49	34	34
0.1	0.3	0.75	0.95	14	2	12	34	6	29
0.2	0.4	0.75	0.95	18	4	14	37	11	32
0.3	0.5	0.75	0.95	22	8	18	46	18	39
0.4	0.6	0.75	0.95	22	10	18	46	23	39
0.5	0.7	0.75	0.95	20	11	16	43	26	37
0.6	0.8	0.75	0.95	19	13	16	43	30	36

Table 16.10 (*continued*): Bryant and Day design. Sample sizes and rejection criteria for π_{R0}, π_{RNew}, π_{T0}, π_{TNew} with odds ratio, $\phi = 1$. $n_{B\text{-}D1}$ is the number of Stage 1 patients and $N_{B\text{-}D}$ is the total to be accrued to both stages. At the end of Stage 1, the treatment will be rejected if the number of positive responses is $< C_{R1}$ or when the number who do not experience toxicity is $< C_{T1}$. At the end of Stage 2, the treatment will be rejected if the number of responses is $< C_R$ or the number who do not experience toxicity is C_T.

π_{R0}	π_{RNew}	π_{T0}	π_{TNew}	$n_{B\text{-}D1}$	C_{R1}	C_{T1}	$N_{B\text{-}D}$	C_R	C_T
				$\alpha_R = 0.15$; $\alpha_T = 0.15$; $\beta = 0.15$					
0.1	0.3	0.60	0.80	15	2	10	30	5	21
0.2	0.4	0.60	0.80	17	4	11	36	10	25
0.3	0.5	0.60	0.80	19	6	12	33	13	23
0.4	0.6	0.60	0.80	20	9	13	37	18	26
0.5	0.7	0.60	0.80	17	9	14	37	22	27
0.6	0.8	0.60	0.80	14	9	9	33	23	23
0.1	0.3	0.75	0.95	12	2	10	22	4	19
0.2	0.4	0.75	0.95	12	3	10	28	8	24
0.3	0.5	0.75	0.95	13	4	10	27	11	23
0.4	0.6	0.75	0.95	17	8	14	30	15	25
0.5	0.7	0.75	0.95	17	10	14	30	18	25
0.6	0.8	0.75	0.95	14	9	12	25	18	21
				$\alpha_R = 0.15$; $\alpha_T = 0.15$; $\beta = 0.10$					
0.1	0.3	0.60	0.80	16	2	10	36	6	25
0.2	0.4	0.60	0.80	24	6	16	41	11	28
0.3	0.5	0.60	0.80	22	7	14	42	16	29
0.4	0.6	0.60	0.80	26	11	17	41	20	28
0.5	0.7	0.60	0.80	24	13	15	39	23	27
0.6	0.8	0.60	0.80	18	11	11	36	25	25
0.1	0.3	0.75	0.95	13	2	11	31	5	26
0.2	0.4	0.75	0.95	16	4	13	36	10	30
0.3	0.5	0.75	0.95	20	7	16	36	14	30
0.4	0.6	0.75	0.95	17	7	13	36	18	30
0.5	0.7	0.75	0.95	15	8	12	37	22	31
0.6	0.8	0.75	0.95	15	10	12	33	23	28

17 Sample size software ^SS_S

SUMMARY

The sample size software, ^SS_S, implements the sample-size computation methods and dose-finding study designs discussed in this book.

17.1 Introduction

There are three ways in which ^SS_S may be used:

Sample-size calculator

The first is as a sample-size calculator, which can be accessed under **Sample Size Calculator** in the main menu, to compute sample sizes corresponding to various choices of input values. The calculator can be used for all methods described except those of Chapter 15 on dose finding studies.

Sample-size table printer

The second use of ^SS_S is as a sample-size table printer, which can be accessed under **Tabulation** in the main menu, for computing sample sizes for a range of input values, with the ability to print out the corresponding sample-size tables. This will facilitate discussions amongst the Study Team during the design of a trial as to the appropriate sample size to be used. This use of ^SS_S is available for all sample size methods discussed except those of Chapter 15 on dose finding studies and Chapter 16 on Phase II trials.

Database for early phase trials

For the implementation of dose finding studies, ^SS_S provides a database to allow for the capture of key data relevant to the trial design. This feature is also available for use with Phase II trials (Chapter 16). However, it should be noted that the included database is not meant to take the place of a full trial database, which would still need to be set up so as to capture all relevant information from the trial.

17.2 System requirements

It is essential to make sure that your computer meets the minimum system requirements of the program in order for it to run smoothly. If you are experiencing poor performance, kindly

Sample Size Tables for Clinical Studies, 3rd edition. By David Machin, Michael J. Campbell, Say Beng Tan, and Sze Huey Tan. Published 2009 by Blackwell Publishing, ISBN: 978-1-4051-4650-0

check to make sure that your system hardware supports the requirements. The minimum system requirements are:

Operating System: Windows XP, 2000;
CPU: 500 MHz;
RAM: 128 MB;
Disc drive: 16x CD drive;
Hard drive: 10 MB of free space

17.3 Installation instructions

To install the software, insert the ^SS_S CD into the CD-ROM/DVD drive, and follow the instructions that appear on the screen. If autorun has been disabled, the program can be run manually by clicking the setup icon in the appropriate drive.

There may be situations during the installation of the software whereby the system will prompt the user that his/her system files are older than the version required by the software. Should this happen, the user should run the Windows Update that comes with the Operating System so as to update the system files from the Microsoft website, prior to re-installing ^SS_S.

17.4 Help guide

For more details on using ^SS_S, users should refer to the Help file available under **Help** in the main menu of the software.

Cumulative references

Abernethy AP, Currow DC, Frith P, Fazekas BS, McHugh A and Bui C (2003). Randomised, double blind, placebo controlled crossover trial of sustained release morphine for the management of refractory dyspnoea. *British Medical Journal*, **327**, 523–528. [7]

A'Hern RP (2001). Sample size tables for exact single stage Phase II designs. *Statistics in Medicine*, **20**, 859–866. [1, 16]

Ahnn S and Anderson SJ (1995). Sample size determination for comparing more than two survival distributions. *Statistics in Medicine*, **14**, 2273–2282. [8]

Altman DG (1991). *Practical Statistics for Medical Research*. Chapman & Hall/CRC, Boca Raton. [13]

Altman DG and Gardner MJ (2000). Means and their differences. In Altman DG, Machin D, Bryant TN and Gardner MJ (eds). *Statistics with Confidence*, 2nd edn. British Medical Journal Books, London, 31–32. [10]

Altman DG, Machin D, Bryant TN and Gardner MJ (eds) (2000). *Statistics with Confidence*, 2nd edn. British Medical Journal, London. [2, 16]

Anderson LJ, Holden S, Davis B, Prescott E, Charrier CC, Bunce NH, Firmin DN, Wonke B, Porter J, Walker JM and Pennell DJ (2001). Cardiovascular T2-star (T2*) magnetic resonance for the early diagnosis of myocardial iron overload. *European Heart Journal*, **22**, 2171–2179. [13]

Ang ES-W, Lee S-T, Gan CS-G, See PG-J, Chan Y-H, Ng L-H and Machin D (2001). Evaluating the role of alternative therapy in burn wound management: randomized trial comparing moist exposed burn ointment with conventional methods in the management of patients with second-degree burns. *Medscape General Medicine*, 6 March 2001, **3**, 3. [3]

Armitage P, Berry G and Matthews JNS (2002). *Statistical Methods in Medical Research*, 4th edn. Blackwell Science, Oxford. [5]

Baker SG, Freedman LS and Parmar MKB (1991). Using replicate observations in observer agreement studies with binary assessments. *Biometrics*, **47**, 1327–1338. Erratum (1996) *Biometrics*, **52**, 1530. [14]

Barthel FM-S, Babiker A, Royston P and Parmar MKB (2006). Evaluation of sample size and power for multi-arm survival trials allowing for non-uniform accrual, non-proportional hazards, loss to follow-up and cross-over. *Statistics in Medicine*, **25**, 2521–2542. [8]

Bennett JE, Dismukes WE, Duma RJ, Medoff G, Sande MA, Gallis H, Leonard J, Fields BT, Bradshaw M, Haywood H, McGee Z, Cate TR, Cobbs CG, Warner JF and Alling DW (1979). A comparison of amphotericin B alone and combined with flucytosine in the treatment of cryptococcal meningitis. *New England Journal of Medicine*, **301**, 126–131. [9]

Bidwell G, Sahu A, Edwards R, Harrison RA, Thornton J and Kelly SP (2005). Perceptions of blindness related to smoking: a hospital-based cross-sectional study. *Eye*, **19**, 945–948. [10]

Biostat (2001). *Power & Precision: Release 2.1*. Englewood, NJ. [1]

Blackwelder WC (1982). 'Proving the null hypothesis' in clinical trials. *Controlled Clinical Trials*, **3**, 345–353. [9]

Bonett DG (2002). Sample size requirements for estimating intraclass correlations with desired precision. *Statistics in Medicine*, **21**, 1331–1335. [14]

Bristol DR (1989). Sample sizes for constructing confidence intervals and testing hypotheses. *Statistics in Medicine*, **8**, 803–811. [10]

Browne RH (1995). On the use of a pilot study for sample size determination. *Statistics in Medicine*, **14**, 1933–1940. [1]

Bryant J and Day R (1995). Incorporating toxicity considerations into the design of two-stage Phase II clinical trials. *Biometrics*, **51**, 1372–1383. [16]

Campbell MJ (1982). The choice of relative group sizes for the comparison of independent proportions. *Biometrics*, **38**, 1093–1094. [3]

Campbell MJ (2000). Cluster randomized trials in general (family) practice research. *Statistical Methods in Medical Research*, **9**, 81–94. [6]

Campbell MJ, Donner A and Klar N (2007). Developments in cluster randomized trials and *Statistics in Medicine*. *Statistics in Medicine*, **26**, 2–19. [6]

Campbell MJ and Gardner MJ (2000). Medians and their differences. In Altman DG, Machin D, Bryant TN and Gardner MJ (eds) *Statistics with Confidence*, 2nd edn. British Medical Journal, London, 171–190. [13]

Campbell MJ, Julious SA and Altman DG (1995). Sample sizes for binary, ordered categorical, and continuous outcomes in two group comparisons. *British Medical Journal*, **311**, 1145–1148. [3, 4]

Campbell MJ, Machin D and Walters SJ (2007). *Medical Statistics: A Textbook for the Health Sciences*, 4th edn. John Wiley & Sons, Chichester. [2, 3, 12]

Cantor AB (1996). Sample size calculations for Cohen's kappa. *Psychological Methods*, **2**, 150–153. [14]

Casagrande JT, Pike MC and Smith PG (1978). An improved approximate formula for comparing two binomial distributions. *Biometrics*, **34**, 483–486. [3]

Case LD and Morgan TM (2003). Design of Phase II cancer trials evaluating survival probabilities. *BMC Medical Research Methodology*, **3**, 6. [16]

Chant ADB, Turner DTL and Machin D (1983). Metronidazole v. Ampicillin: differing effects on the post-operative recovery. *Annals of the Royal College of Surgeons of England*, **66**, 96–97. [8]

Chao Y, Chan W-K, Birkhofer MJ, Hu OY-P, Wang S-S, Huang Y-S, Liu M, Whang-Peng J, Chi K-H, Lui W-Y and Lee S-D (1998). Phase II and pharmacokinetic study of paclitaxel therapy for unresectable hepatocellular carcinoma patients. *British Journal of Cancer*, **78**, 34–39. [16]

Cheung YK and Thall PF (2002). Monitoring the rates of composite events with censored data in Phase II clinical trials. *Biometrics*, **58**, 89–97. [16]

Chevret S (1993). The continual reassessment method for Phase I clinical trials: A simulation study. *Statistics in Medicine*, **12**, 1093–1108. [15]

CHMP (2005). Guideline on the choice of the non-inferiority margin. Doc EMEA/CPMP/EWP/2158/99. Available at URL: http://www.emea.europa.eu/pdfs/human/ewp/215899en.pdf. [9]

CHMP (2006). Guideline on the choice of the non-inferiority margin. *Statistics in Medicine*, **25**, 1628–1638. [9]

Chow PK-H, Tai B-C, Tan C-K, Machin D, Johnson PJ, Khin M-W and Soo K-C (2002). No role for high-dose tamoxifen in the treatment of inoperable hepatocellular carcinoma: An Asia-Pacific double-blind randomised controlled trial. *Hepatology*, **36**, 1221–1226. [1]

Chow S-C, Shao J and Wang H (2008). *Sample Size Calculations in Clinical Research*, 2nd edn. Marcel Dekker, New York. [1]

Chow S-C and Liu J-P (1992). *Design and Analysis of Bioavailability and Bioequivalence Studies*, Chapter 5. Marcel Dekker, New York. [9]

Cicchetti DV (2001). The precision of reliability and validity estimates re-visited: distinguishing between clinical and statistical significance of sample size requirements. *Journal of Clinical and Experimental Neuropsychology*, **23**, 695–700. [14]

Cohen J (1988). *Statistical Power Analysis for the Behavioral Sciences*, 2nd edn. Lawrence Earlbaum, New Jersey. [1, 7, 12]

Connett JE, Smith JA and McHugh RB (1987). Sample size and power for pair-matched case-control studies. *Statistics in Medicine*, **6**, 53–59. [7]

Coviello V and Boggess M (2004). Cumulative incidence estimation in the presence of competing risks. *The Stata Journal*, **4**, 103–112. [8]

CPMP Working Party on Efficacy of Medicinal Products (1995). Biostatistical methodology in clinical trials in applications for marketing authorizations for medical products. *Statistics in Medicine*, **14**, 1659–1682. [1]

CPMP (1998). Notes for guidance on the investigation of bioavailability and bioequivalence. Doc. CPMP/EWP/QWP1401/98. Available at URL: http://www.emea.eu.int/pdfs/human/ewp/140198en.pdf. [9]

CPMP (2000). Points to consider on switching between superiority and non-inferiority. Doc. CPMP/EWP/482/99. Available at URL: http://www.emea.eu.int/pdfs/human/ewp/048299en.pdf. [9]

CPMP (2004). Notes for guidance on the evaluation of medicinal products indicated for the treatment of bacterial infections. Doc. CPMP/EWP/558/95. Available at URL: http://www.emea.eu.int/pdfs/human/ewp/055895en.pdf. [9]

Crisp A and Curtis P (2007). Sample size estimation for non-inferiority trials of time-to-event data. *Pharmaceutical Statistics*, in press. [9]

Cruciani RA, Dvorkin E, Homel P, Malamud S, Culliney B, Lapin J, Portenoy RK and Esteban-Cruciani N (2006). Safety, tolerability and symptom outcomes associated with L-carnitine supplementation in patients with cancer, fatigue, and carnitine deficiency: a Phase I/II study. *Journal of Pain and Symptom Management*, **32**, 551–559. [7]

Cuschieri A, Weeden S, Fielding J, Bancewicz J, Craven J, Joypaul V, Sydes M and Fayers P (1999). Patient survival after D_1 and D_2 resections for gastric cancer: long-term results of the MRC randomized surgical trial. *British Journal of Cancer*, **79**, 1522–1530. [1, 8]

Day SJ (1988). Clinical trial numbers and confidence intervals of a pre-specified size. *Lancet*, **ii**, 1427. [10]

Demidenko E (2007). Sample size determination for logistic regression revisited. *Statistics in Medicine*, **26**, 3385–3397. [3]

Diletti E, Hauschke D and Steinijans VW (1991). Sample size determination for bioequivalence assessment by means of confidence intervals. *International Journal of Clinical Pharmacology, Therapy and Toxicology*, **29**, 1–8. [9]

Donner A and Eliasziw M (1992). A goodness-of-fit approach to inference procedures for the kappa statistic: confidence interval construction, significance-testing and sample size estimation. *Statistics in Medicine*, **11**, 1511–1519. [14]

Donner A and Klar N (2000). *Design and Analysis of Cluster Randomised Trials*. Edward Arnold, London [6]

Drummond M and O'Brien B (1993). Clinical importance, statistical significance and the assessment of economic and quality-of-life outcomes. *Health Economics*, **2**, 205–212. [1]

Dupont WD (1988). Power calculations for matched case-control studies. *Biometrics*, **44**, 1157–1168. [11]

Edwardes MD (2001). Sample size requirements for case-control study designs. *BMC Medical Research Methodology*, **1**, 11. [11]

Estlin EJ, Pinkerton CR, Lewis IJ, Lashford L, McDowell H, Morland B, Kohler J, Newell DR, Boddy AV, Taylor GA, Price L, Ablett S, Hobson R, Pitsiladis M, Brampton M, Cledeninn N, Johnston A and Pearson AD (2001). A Phase I study of nolatrexed dihydrochloride in children with advanced cancer. A United Kingdom Children's Cancer Study Group Investigation. *British Journal of Cancer*, **84**, 11–18. [15]

Eypasch E, Lefering R, Kum CK and Troidl H (1995). Probability of adverse events that have not yet occurred: a statistical reminder. *British Medical Journal*, **311**, 619–620.

Family Heart Study Group (1994). Randomized controlled trial evaluating cardiovascular screening and intervention in general practice: general results of British family heart study. *British Medical Journal*, **308**, 313–320. [6]

Farrington CP and Manning G (1990). Test statistics and sample size formulae for comparative binomial trials with null hypothesis of non-zero risk difference or non-unity relative risk. *Statistics in Medicine*, **9**, 1447–1454. [9]

Feng Z and Grizzle JE (1992). Correlated binomial variates: Properties of estimator of intraclass correlation and its effect on sample size calculation. *Statistics in Medicine*, **11**, 1607–1614. [6]

FDA (1988). *Guidelines for the Format and Content of the Clinical and Statistics Section of New Drug Applications*. US Department of Health and Human Services, Public Health Service, Food and Drug Administration, Washington D.C. [1]

FDA (1992a). Statistical procedures for bioequivalence studies using a standard two-treatment crossover design. US Department of Health and Human Services, Public Health Service, Food and Drug Administration, Washington D.C. [9]

FDA (1992b). Points to consider. Clinical evaluation of anti-infective drug products. Available at URL: http://www.fda.gov/cder/guidance/old043fn.pdf. [9]

FDA (2000). Guidance for industry. Bioavailability and bioequivalence studies for orally administered drug products—general considerations. Available at URL: http://www.fda.gov/cder/guidance/3615fnl.pdf. [9]

FDA (2001). Statistical approaches to establishing bioequivalence. Available at URL: http://www.fda.gov/cder/guidance/3616fnl.pdf. [9]

Fleiss JL (1986). *The Design and Analysis of Clinical Experiments*. John Wiley & Sons, New York. [6]

Fleiss JL, Levin B and Paik MC (2003). *Statistical Methods for Rates and Proportions.* John Wiley & Sons, Chichester. [3]

Fleming TR (1982). One-sample multiple testing procedure for Phase II clinical trial. *Biometrics,* **38,** 143–151. [1, 16]

Flinn IW, Goodman SN, Post L, Jamison J, Miller CB, Gore S, Diehl L, Willis C, Ambinder RF and Byrd JC (2000). A dose-finding study of liposomal daunorubicin with CVP (COP-X) in advanced NHL. *Annals of Oncology,* **11,** 691–695. [15]

Foo K-F, Tan E-H, Leong S-S, Wee JTS, Tan T, Fong K-W, Koh L, Tai B-C, Lian L-G and Machin D (2002). Gemcitabine in metastatic nasopharyngeal carcinoma of the undifferentiated type. *Annals of Oncology,* **13,** 150–156. [16]

Freedman LS (1982). Tables of the number of patients required in clinical trials using the logrank test. *Statistics in Medicine,* **1,** 121–129. [8]

Freedman LS, Parmar MKB and Baker SG (1993). The design of observer agreement studies with binary assessments. *Statistics in Medicine,* **12,** 165–179. [14]

Frison L and Pocock SJ (1992). Repeated measures in clinical trials: analysis using mean summary statistics and its implications for design. *Statistics in Medicine,* **11,** 1685–1704. [6]

Gajewski BJ and Mayo MS (2006). Bayesian sample size calculations in Phase II clinical trials using a mixture of informative priors. *Statistics in Medicine,* **25,** 2554–2566. [16]

Gehan EA (1961). The determination of the number of patients required in a preliminary and follow-up trial of a new chemotherapeutic agent. *Journal of Chronic Diseases,* **13,** 346–353. [2, 16]

George SL and Desu MM (1974). Planning the size and duration of a clinical trial studying the time to some critical event. *Journal of Chronic Diseases,* **27,** 15–24. [8]

González-Martín A, Crespo C, García-López JL, Pedraza M, Garrido P, Lastra E and Moyano A (2002). Ifosfamide and vinorelbine in advanced platinum-resistant ovarian cancer: excessive toxicity with a potentially active regimen. *Gynecologic Oncology,* **84,** 368–373. [16]

Goodman SN, Zahurak ML and Piantadosi S (1995). Some practical improvements in the continual reassessment method for Phase I studies. *Statistics in Medicine,* **14,** 1149–1161. [15]

Guenther WC (1981). Sample size formulas for normal theory *t*-tests. *The American Statistician,* **35,** 243–244. [5]

Hanley JA and Lippman-Hand A (1983). If nothing goes wrong, is everything alright? *Journal of the American Medical Association,* **259,** 1743–1745. [11]

Harris EK and Boyd JC (1995). *Statistical Bases of Reference Values in Laboratory Medicine.* Marcel Dekker, New York. [13]

Heyd JM and Carlin BP (1999). Adaptive design improvements in the continual reassessment method for Phase I studies. *Statistics in Medicine,* **18,** 1307–1321. [15]

Hosmer DW and Lemeshow S (2000). *Applied Logistic Regression,* 2nd edn. John Wiley & Sons, Chichester. [3]

Hosselet J-J, Ayappa I, Norman RG, Krieger AC and Rapoport DM (2001). Classification of sleep-disordered breathing. *American Journal of Respiratory Critical Care Medicine,* **163,** 398–405. [13]

Iaffaioli RV, Formato R, Tortoriello A, Del Prete S, Caraglia M, Pappagallo G, Pisano A, Fanelli F, Ianniello G, Cigolari S, Pizza C, Marano O, Pezzella G, Pedicini T, Febbraro A,

Incoronato P, Manzione L, Ferrari E, Marzano N, Quattrin S, Pisconti S, Nasti G, Giotta G, Colucci G and other Goim authors (2005). Phase II study of sequential hormonal therapy with anastrozole/exemestane in advanced and metastatic breast cancer. *British Journal of Cancer*, **92**, 1621–1625. [1, 16]

International Conference on Harmonisation of Technical Requirements for Registration of Pharmaceuticals for Human Use (1998). *Statistical Principles for Clinical Trials E9.* Available at www.ich.org [1]

ICH E10 (2000). Choice of control group in clinical trials. Available at URL: http://www.ifpma.org/ich5e.html. [9]

Itoh K, Ohtsu T, Fukuda H, Sasaki Y, Ogura M, Morishima Y, Chou T, Aikawa K, Uike N, Mizorogi F, Ohno T, Ikeda S, Sai T, Taniwaki M, Kawano F, Niimi M, Hotta T, Shimoyama M and Tobinai K (2002). Randomized Phase II study of biweekly CHOP and dose-escalated CHOP with prophylactic use of lenograstim (glycosylated G-CSF) in aggressive non-Hodgkin's lymphoma: Japan Clinical Oncology Group Study 9505. *Annals of Oncology*, **13**, 1347–1355. [16]

Jones B, Jarvis P, Lewis JA and Ebbutt AF (1996). Trials to assess equivalence: the importance of rigorous methods. *British Medical Journal*, **313**, 36–39. [9]

Julious SA (2004). Sample sizes for clinical trials with Normal data. *Statistics in Medicine*, **23**, 1921–1986. [5, 7, 9]

Julious SA (2005). Two-sided confidence intervals for the single proportion: comparison of seven methods. *Statistics in Medicine*, **24**, 3383–3384. [2]

Julious SA and Campbell MJ (1996). Sample size calculations for ordered categorical data (letter). *Statistics in Medicine*, **15**, 1065–1066. [3, 4]

Julious SA and Campbell MJ (1998). Sample sizes for paired or matched ordinal data. *Statistics in Medicine*, **17**, 1635–1642. [7]

Julious SA, Campbell MJ and Altman DG (1999). Estimating sample sizes for continuous, binary and ordinal outcomes in paired comparisons: practical hints. *Journal of Biopharmaceutical Statistics*, **9**, 241–251. [7]

Jung K, Perganda M, Schimke E, Ratzmann KP and Ilius A (1988). Urinary enzymes and low-molecular-mass proteins as indicators of diabetic nephropathy. *Clinical Chemistry*, **34**, 544–547. [10]

Kinmonth A-L, Fulton Y and Campbell MJ (1992). Management of feverish children at home. *British Medical Journal*, **305**, 1134–1136. [4]

Korn EL, Midthune D, Chen TT, Rubinstein LV, Christian MC and Simon RM (1994). A comparison of two Phase I trial designs. *Statistics in Medicine*, **13**, 1799–1806. [15]

Kupper LL and Hafner KB (1989). How appropriate are popular sample size formulas? *American Statistician*, **43**, 101–105. [9]

Lehnert M, Mross K, Schueller J, Thuerlimann B, Kroeger N and Kupper H (1998). Phase II trial of dexverapamil and epirubicin in patients with non-responsive metastatic breast cancer. *British Journal of Cancer*, **77**, 1155–1163. [2, 16]

Lehr R (1992). Sixteen s-squared over d-squared: a relation for crude sample size estimates. *Statistics in Medicine*, **11**, 1099–1102. [5]

Lemeshow S, Hosmer DW and Klar J (1988). Sample size requirements for studies estimating odds ratios or relative risks. *Statistics in Medicine*, **7**, 759–764. [10]

Lemeshow S, Hosmar DW, Klar J and Lwanga SK (1990). *Adequacy of Sample Size in Health Studies*. John Wiley & Sons, Chichester. [1]

Lenth RV (2006). *Java Applets for Power and Sample Size*. Available at URL: http://www.stat.uiowa.edu/~rlenth/Power. [1]

Leong SS, Tay MH, Toh CK, Tan SB, Thng CH, Foo KF, Wee JTS, Lim D, See HT, Tan T, Fong KW and Tan EH (2005). Paclitaxel, carboplatin and gemcitabine in metastatic naso-pharyngeal carcinoma: A Phase II trial using a triplet combination. *Cancer*, **103**, 569–575. [16]

Leong SS, Toh CK, Lim WT, Lin X, Tan SB, Poon D, Tay MH, Foo KF, Ho J and Tan EH (2007). A randomized Phase II trial of single agent gemcitabine, vinorelbine or docetaxel in patients with advanced non-small cell lung cancer who have poor performance status and/or are elderly. *Journal of Thoracic Oncology*, **2**, 230–236. [16]

Lesaffre E, Scheys I, Fröhlich J and Bluhmki E (1993). Calculation of power and sample size with bounded outcome scores. *Statistics in Medicine*, **12**, 1063–1078. [4]

Lewis JA (1981). Post-marketing surveillance: how many patients? *Trends in Pharmacological Sciences*, **2**, 93–94. [11]

Lewis JA (1983). Clinical trials: statistical developments of practical benefit to the pharmaceut-ical industry. *Journal of the Royal Statistical Society (A)*, **146**, 362–393. [11]

Li J and Fine J (2004). On sample size for sensitivity and specificity in prospective diagnostic accuracy studies. *Statistics in Medicine*, **23**, 2537–2550. [13]

Lin SC (1995). Sample size for therapeutic equivalence based on confidence intervals. *Drug Information Journal*, **29**, 45–50. [9]

Lindholm LH, Ekbom T, Dash C, Eriksson M, Tibblin G and Schersten B (1995). The impact of health care advice given in primary care on cardiovascular risk. *British Medical Journal*, **310**, 1105–1109. [6]

Linnet K (1987). Two-stage transformation systems for normalization of reference distribu-tions evaluated. *Clinical Chemistry*, **33**, 381–386. [13]

Lipsey MW (1990). *Design sensitivity. Statistical Power for Experimental Research*. Sage Publications, London. [1]

Liu PY (2001). Phase II selection designs. In Crowley J (ed) *Handbook of Statistics in Clinical Oncology*, Marcel Dekker Inc, New York, pp. 119–127. [16]

Loke YC, Tan SB, Cai Y and Machin D (2006). A Bayesian dose finding design for dual end-point Phase I trials. *Statistics in Medicine*, **25**, 3–22. [15]

Machin D and Campbell MJ (1987) *Statistical Tables for the Design of Clinical Trials*. Blackwell Scientific Publications, Oxford. [9]

Machin D and Campbell MJ (2005). *Design of Studies for Medical Research*. John Wiley & Sons, Chichester. [1, 9, 16]

Machin D, Campbell MJ, Fayers PM and Pinol A (1997). *Statistical Tables for the Design of Clinical Studies*, 2nd edn. Blackwell Scientific Publications, Oxford. [1]

Machin D, Cheung Y-B and Parmar MKB (2006). *Survival Analysis: A Practical Approach*, 2nd edn. John Wiley & Sons, Chichester. [2, 8]

Makuch R and Simon R (1978). Sample size requirements for evaluating a conservative therapy. *Cancer Treatment Reports*, **62**, 1037–1040. [9]

Mayo MS and Gajewski BJ (2004). Bayesian sample size calculations in Phase II clinical trials using informative conjugate priors. *Controlled Clinical Trials*, **25**, 157–167. [16]

Metzler CM (1991). Sample sizes for bioequivalence studies (with discussion). *Statistics in Medicine*, **10**, 961–970. [9]

Mick R, Crowley JJ and Carroll RJ (2000). Phase II clinical trial design for noncytotoxic anticancer agents for which time to disease progression is the primary endpoint. *Controlled Clinical Trials*, **21**, 343–359. [16]

Morrison JM, Gilmour H and Sullivan F (1991). Children seen frequently out of hours in one general practice. *British Medical Journal*, **303**, 1111–1114. [7]

Multicenter Study Group (1980). Long-term oral acetycysteine in chronic bronchitis. A double-blind controlled study. *European Journal of Respiratory Diseases*, **61** (Suppl.111), 93–108. [8]

National Council for Social Studies (2005). *Power Analysis and Sample Size Software (PASS): Version 2005*. NCSS Statistical Software, Kaysville, UT. [1]

Naylor CD and Llewellyn-Thomas HA (1994). Can there be a more patients-centred approach to determining clinically important effect size for randomized treatments? *Journal of Clinical Epidemiology*, **47**, 787–795. [1]

Newcombe RG and Altman DG (2000). Proportions and their differences. In Altman DG, Machin D, Bryant TN and Gardner MJ (eds). *Statistics with Confidence*, 2nd edn. British Medical Journal Books, London, pp. 45–56. [2, 10]

Nomura Y, Tamaki Y, Tanaka T, Arakawa H, Tsurumoto A, Kirimura K, Sato T, Hanada N and Kamoi K (2006). Screening of periodontitis with salivary enzyme tests. *Journal of Oral Science*, **48**, 177–183. [13]

Obuchowski NA and McClish DN (1997). Sample size determination for diagnostic accuracy studies involving binormal ROC curve indices. *Statistics in Medicine*, **16**, 1529–1542. [13]

O'Quigley J (2001). Dose-finding designs using continual reassessment method. In Crowley J (ed) *Handbook of Statistics in Clinical Oncology*, Marcel Dekker Inc, New York, pp. 35–72. [15]

O'Quigley J, Hughes MD and Fenton T (2001). Dose finding designs for HIV studies. *Biometrics*, **57**, 1018–1029. [15]

O'Quigley J, Pepe M and Fisher L (1990). Continual reassessment method: a practical design for Phase I clinical trials in cancer. *Biometrics*, **46**, 33–48. [15]

Peduzzi P, Concato J, Kemper E, Holford TR and Feinstein AR (1996). A simulation study of the number of events per variable in logistic regression analysis. *Journal of Clinical Epidemiology*, **49**, 1372–1379. [3]

Piaggio G, Elbourne DR, Altman DG, Pocock SJ and Evans SJW (2006). Reporting of non-inferiority and equivalence randomized trials: An extension of the CONSORT statement. *Journal of the American Medical Association*, **295**, 1152–1172. [9]

Philips KE (1990). Power of the two one-sided tests procedure in bioequivalence. *Journal of Pharmacokinetics and Biopharmaceutics*, **18**, 137–143. [9]

Piantadosi S and Liu G (1996). Improved designs for dose escalation studies using pharma-cokinetic measurements. *Statistics in Medicine*, **15**, 1605–1618. [15]

Pintilie M (2002). Dealing with competing risks: testing covariates and calculating sample size. *Statistics in Medicine*, **21**, 3317–3324. [8]

Poon CY, Goh BT, Kim M-J, Rajaseharan A, Ahmed S, Thongsprasom K, Chaimusik M, Suresh S, Machin D, Wong-HB and Seldrup J (2006). A randomised controlled trial to compare steroid with cyclosporine for the topical treatment of oral lichen planus. *Oral Surgery, Oral Medicine, Oral Pathology, Oral Radiolology and Endodontics*, **102**, 47–55. [1]

Richards B, Parmar MK, Anderson CK, Ansell ID, Grigor K, Hall RR, Morley AR, Mostofi FK, Risdon RA and Uscinska BM (1991). The interpretation of biopsies of 'normal' urothelium in patients with superficial bladder cancer. *British Journal of Urology*, **67**, 369–375. [14]

Roebruck P and Kühn A (1995). Comparison of tests and sample size formulae for proving therapeutic equivalence based on the difference of binomial probabilities. *Statistics in Medicine*, **14**, 1583–1594. [9]

Royston P (1993). Exact conditional and unconditional sample size for pair-matched studies with binary outcome: a practical guide. *Statistics in Medicine*, **12**, 699–712. [7]

Sahai H and Khurshid A (1996). Formulae and tables for the determination of sample sizes and power in clinical trials for testing differences in proportions for the two-sample design: A review. *Statistics in Medicine*, **15**, 1–21. [3]

SAS Institute (2004). *Getting Started with the SAS Power and Sample Size Application: Version 9.1*, SAS Institute, Cary, NC. [1]

Saville DJ (1990). Multiple comparison procedures: The practical solution. *The American Statistician*, **44**, 174–180. [1]

Schlesseman JJ (1982). *Case-control Studies*. Oxford University Press, Oxford. [7]

Schouten HJA (1999). Sample size formula with a continuous outcome for unequal group sizes and unequal variances. *Statistics in Medicine*, **18**, 87–91. [5]

Schuster JJ (1993). *Practical Handbook of Sample Size Guidelines for Clinical Trials*. CRC Press, Florida. [1]

Senn S (2002). *Cross-over Trials in Clinical Research*, 2nd edn. John Wiley & Sons, Chichester. [7, 9]

Silverstein FE, Faich G, Goldstein JL *et al.* (2000). Gastrointestinal toxicity with celecoxib vs nonsteroidal anti-inflammatory drugs for osteoarthritis and rheumatoid arthritis. *Journal of the American Medical Association*, **284**, 1247–1255. [11]

Simon R (1989). Optimal two-stage designs for Phase II clinical trials. *Controlled Clinical Trials*, **10**, 1–14. [16]

Simon R, Wittes RE and Ellenberg SS (1985). Randomized Phase II clinical trials. *Cancer Treatment Reports*, **69**, 1375–1381. [16]

Simpson AG (2004). A comparison of the ability of cranial ultrasound, neonatal neurological assessment and observation of spontaneous general movements to predict outcome in preterm infants. PhD Thesis, University of Sheffield. [2]

Skegg DCG and Doll R (1977). The case for recording events in clinical trials. *British Medical Journal*, **2**, 1523–1524. [11]

Smith LFP (1992). Roles, risks and responsibilities in maternal care: trainees' beliefs and the effects of practice obstetric training. *British Medical Journal*, **304**, 1613–1615. [7]

Speigelhalter DJ, Freedman LS and Parmar MKB (1994). Bayesian approaches to randomized trials (with discussion). *Journal of the Royal Statistical Society (A)*, **157**, 357–416. [1]

StataCorp (2007). *Stata Statistical Software: Release 10*. College Station, TX. [1, 8]

Statistical Solutions (2006). *nQuery Adviser: Version 6.0*. Saugus, MA. [1]

Storer BE (2001). Choosing a Phase I design. In Crowley J (ed) *Handbook of Statistics in Clinical Oncology*, Marcel Dekker, New York, pp. 73–91. [15]

Strom BL (2005). Sample size considerations for pharmacoepidemiology studies. In Strom BL (ed) *Pharmacoepidemiology*, 4th edn. John Wiley & Sons, Chichester, pp. 29–56. [11]

Swinscow TDV and Campbell MJ (2002). *Statistics at Square One*, 10th edn. British Medical Journal Books, London. [4]

Tan SB and Machin D (2002). Bayesian two-stage designs for Phase II clinical trials. *Statistics in Medicine*, **21**, 1991–2012. [16]

Tan SB, Machin D, Tai BC, Foo KF and Tan EH (2002). A Bayesian re-assessment of two Phase II trials of gemcitabine in metastatic nasopharyngeal cancer. *British Journal of Cancer*, **86**, 843–850. [16]

Tan SB, Wong EH and Machin D (2004). Bayesian two-stage design for Phase II clinical trials. In *Encyclopedia of Biopharmaceutical Statistics*, 2nd edn (online) (Ed. Chow SC). URL: http://www.dekker.com/servlet/product/DOI/101081EEBS120023507. Marcel Dekker, New York. [16]

Thall PF and Russel KE (1998). A strategy for dose-finding and safety monitoring based on efficacy and adverse outcomes in Phase I/II clinical trials. *Biometrics*, **54**, 251–264. [15]

Tubert-Bitter P, Begaud B, Moride Y and Abenhaim L (1994). Sample size calculations for single group post-marketing cohort studies. *Journal of Clinical Epidemiology*, **47**, 435–439. [11]

Valerius NH, Koch C and Hoiby N (1991). Prevention of chronic *Pseudomonas aeruginosa* colonisation in cystic fibrosis by early treatment. *Lancet*, **338**, 725–726. [8]

Van Belle G (2002). *Statistical Rules of Thumb*. John Wiley & Sons, Chichester. [1]

Van Breukelen GJP, Candel MJJM and Berger MPF (2007). Relative efficiency of unequal *versus* equal cluster sizes in cluster randomized and multicentre trials. *Statistics in Medicine*, **26**, 2589–2603. [6]

Wallentin L, Wilcox RG, Weaver WD, Emanuelsson H, Goodvin A, Nyström P and Bylock A (2003). Oral ximelagatran for secondary prophylaxis after myocardial infarction: the ESTEEM randomised controlled trial. *Lancet*, **362**, 789–797. [6]

Walter SD, Eliasziw M and Donner A (1998). Sample size and optimal designs for reliability studies. *Statistics in Medicine*, **17**, 101–110. [14]

Wang YG, Leung DHY, Li M and Tan SB (2005). Bayesian designs for frequentist and Bayesian error rate considerations. *Statistical Methods in Medical Research*, **14**, 445–456. [16]

Whitehead J and Williamson D (1998). An evaluation of Bayesian decision procedures for dose-finding studies. *Journal of Biopharmaceutical Medicine*, **8**, 445–467. [15]

Whiteley W, Al-Shahi R, Warlow CP, Zeideler M and Lueck CJ (2006). CSF opening pressure: Reference interval and the effect of body mass index. *Neurology*, **67**, 1690–1691. [13]

Wight J, Jakubovic M, Walters S, Maheswaran R, White P and Lennon V (2004). Variation in cadaveric organ donor rates in the UK. *Nephrology Dialysis Transplantation*, **19**, 963–968. [2]

Wilson AB (1977). Post-marketing surveillance of adverse reactions to new medicines. *British Medical Journal*, **2**, 1001–1003. [11]

Wooding WM (1994). *Planning Pharmaceutical Clinical Trials*. John Wiley & Sons, New York. [9]

Zhou Y, Whitehead J, Bonvini E and Stevens JW (2006). Bayesian decision procedures for binary and continuous bivariate dose-escalation studies. *Pharmaceutical Statistics*, **5**, 125–133. [15]

Author index

Subject index

Note. Page references in *italic* refer to tables.